NON-CODING RNA TRANSCRIPTS IN CANCER THERAPY

Pre-clinical and Clinical Implications

Editors

Gautam Sethi

National University of Singapore, Singapore

Milad Ashrafizadeh

Sabanci University, Turkey

World Scientific

NEW JERSEY • LONDON • SINGAPORE • BEIJING • SHANGHAI • HONG KONG • TAIPEI • CHENNAI • TOKYO

Published by

World Scientific Publishing Co. Pte. Ltd.
5 Toh Tuck Link, Singapore 596224
USA office: 27 Warren Street, Suite 401-402, Hackensack, NJ 07601
UK office: 57 Shelton Street, Covent Garden, London WC2H 9HE

British Library Cataloguing-in-Publication Data
A catalogue record for this book is available from the British Library.

NON-CODING RNA TRANSCRIPTS IN CANCER THERAPY
Pre-clinical and Clinical Implications

ISBN 978-981-126-738-3 (hardcover)
ISBN 978-981-126-739-0 (ebook for institutions)
ISBN 978-981-126-740-6 (ebook for individuals)

For any available supplementary material, please visit
https://www.worldscientific.com/worldscibooks/10.1142/13172#t=suppl

Typeset by Stallion Press
Email: enquiries@stallionpress.com

https://doi.org/10.1142/9789811267390_fmatter

Preface

Genome has been always an interesting subject for researchers and biologists around the world, and with advances in the field of biology and next-generation sequencing technology, new aspects of the genome are revealed that can be beneficial for the development of new therapeutics in the near future and treatment of genetic-based diseases. In the human genome, there are introns and exons and during the process of transcription, messenger RNAs (mRNAs) are produced that can finally be translated into proteins for vital functions in cells. However, one of the important aspects of the genome is that all the RNA molecules are not transcribed into proteins and there are a high number of RNAs that do not translate proteins, called noncoding RNAs (ncRNAs). Although the discovery of ncRNAs was not significant due to the lack of attention to these molecules and they were considered as "junks" in cells, advances in high-throughput sequencing led to the identification of their roles in cells and their importance in biological events. In a certain cell during physiological conditions, various functions are performed such as autophagy at the basic level for preserving homeostasis. Furthermore, there are other important biological functions, such as apoptosis, migration, and differentiation that need to be coordinated and controlled in an optimal manner to prevent any disturbance in cell homeostasis. Notably, ncRNAs have been shown to be the master regulators of these biological functions in cells and they can coordinate a wide variety of signaling networks to regulate apoptosis, autophagy, differentiation, migration, and other important mechanisms in cells to maintain their homeostasis. After recognizing the function of ncRNAs as important regulators in cells, researchers focused on evaluating their functions in disease pathogenesis. Since ncRNAs are important effectors in cells, changes in their expression level can lead to the development of diseases. Accumulating data now displays that ncRNAs undergo dysregulation during disease pathogenesis and aberrant expression of ncRNAs has been demonstrated in neurological disorders, cardiovascular diseases, diabetes mellitus, and inflammatory diseases, among others. However, one of the most important aspects of ncRNAs is their function in cancer, since cancer is the second leading cause of death worldwide, and based on the studies, researchers have shown that dysregulation of ncRNAs can result in the development of cancer and can improve tumor progression. Therefore, targeting ncRNAs has been of importance in cancer therapy, and based on these, both anti-cancer compounds and genetic tools such as small interfering RNA, short hairpin RNA, and CRISPR/Cas9 system have been utilized in regulating the expression level of ncRNAs in cancer therapy. More importantly, the function of ncRNAs in clinical trials for prognosis and diagnosis of cancer in patients has been highlighted in recent years.

Editors

Associate Professor Gautam Sethi (PhD), Department of Pharmacology, NUS Centre for Cancer Research (N2CR), Yong Loo Lin School of Medicine, National University of Singapore, 117600, Singapore, Email: phcgs@nus.edu.sg

Dr. Milad Ashrafizadeh (DVM), Faculty of Engineering and Natural Sciences, Sabanci University, Orta Mahalle, Üniversite Caddesi No. 27, Orhanlı, Tuzla, 34956 Istanbul, Turkey, Email: milad.ashrafizadeh@sabanciuniv.edu; dvm.milad1994@gmail.com

Contents

https://doi.org/10.1142/9789811267390_0001

Chapter 1

MicroRNAs (miRNAs) in cancer proliferation: Molecular interactions and possible therapeutic targets

Shokooh Salimimoghadam[1], Mahshid Deldar Abad Paskeh[2,3], Sepideh Mirzaei[4], Mehrdad Hashemi[2,3]*, Azuma Kalu[5,6] and Noushin Nabavi[7]

[1]*Department of Biochemistry and Molecular Biology, Faculty of Veterinary Medicine, Shahid Chamran University of Ahvaz, Ahvaz, Iran*
[2]*Farhikhtegan Medical Convergence Sciences Research Center, Farhikhtegan Hospital Tehran Medical Sciences, Islamic Azad University, Tehran, Iran*
[3]*Department of Genetics, Faculty of Advanced Science and Technology, Tehran Medical Sciences, Islamic Azad University, Tehran, Iran*
[4]*Department of Biology, Faculty of Science, Islamic Azad University, Science and Research Branch, Tehran, Iran*
[5]*School of Life, Health & Chemical Sciences, The Open University, Milton Keynes, United Kingdom*
[6]*Laboratory Medicine Directorate, Sheffield Teaching Hospital, Sheffield, United Kingdom*
[7]*Department of Urologic Sciences and Vancouver Prostate Centre, University of British Columbia, Vancouver, BC, Canada*

*Corresponding author: Mehrdad Hashemi, Farhikhtegan Medical Convergence Sciences Research Center, Farhikhtegan Hospital Tehran Medical Sciences, Islamic Azad University, Tehran, Iran, Email: mhashemi@iautmu.ac.ir

Abstract

Cancer is one of the most life-threatening diseases worldwide and is characterized by uncontrolled cell division, suppressed cell death, promoted metastasis, and angiogenesis. MicroRNAs (miRNAs) are single-stranded RNA molecules at ~22 nucleotides in length belonging to the family of small non-coding RNAs. They exert critical regulatory roles in cells and shape various cellular activities. Tumor suppressor miRNAs work in a way to suppress oncogenic pathways, while tumor-promoting miRNAs mediate genes responsible for oncogenesis and suppress tumor inhibitory genes. However, there are miRNAs with dual roles in suppressing or promoting tumor growth in different cancer types. miRNAs regulate gene expression and protein function in cells by targeting mainly the 3′ untranslated region of a gene. Studies on the role of miRNAs in cancer illuminate the complex interaction between miRNAs and pathways involved in cancer. This chapter reviews the current knowledge regarding the importance and role of miRNAs in cancer focusing on proliferation, apoptosis, autophagy, and cell cycle arrest.

1. Introduction

Cancer is one of the most common causes of death in the world, and the number of new cases and cancer deaths are estimated to be 1,918,030 and 609,360 by 2022, respectively [1]. Cancer is characterized by certain hallmarks of functional capabilities developed by cells during their transition from normalcy to neoplasm. In contrast to normal cells, tumor cells and cancer stem cells (CSCs) are capable of retaining their entrance to the cell cycle to proliferate. Douglas Hanahan and Bob Weinberg raised eight acquired characteristics as cancer hallmarks: preservation of proliferative signaling, escape from growth suppressors, resistance against cell death mechanisms, empowering replicative immortality, induction of vasculature, inducing invasion and metastasis, reprogramming cellular metabolism, and immune evasion. By reprogramming cellular metabolism, cancer cells increase nutrient uptake and catabolism to sustain anabolic cell growth through the rewiring of their metabolic mechanisms. These alterations significantly affect cellular characteristics. In addition to the cancer hallmarks, tumor microenvironment (TME) also plays a critical role in tumorigenesis and tumor malignancy. TME comprised a population of interactive heterogeneous cancer and CSCs along with a high number of stromal cell types [2, 3].

Cancer is a life-threatening disease that has led to the development of various therapies, including surgery, radiation therapy, chemotherapy, and targeted therapy, among others. Although these methods do not completely eliminate cancer, they significantly decrease the incidence and morbidity [4]. Because of the malignancy of cancer, its heterogenic nature, chemo-resistance, radio-resistance, and immune evasion, it remains a difficult-to-treat disease. Therefore, different therapeutic methods are developed besides the conventional therapies, such as agents targeting CSCs [5], immune checkpoint immunotherapy [6], agents directly targeting apoptotic pathways [7], targeting host–microbiome [8], and non-coding RNA (ncRNA)-based therapeutics [9].

ncRNAs comprise a large proportion of the genome and although they are not coding protein, they have been linked to a myriad of vital cellular mechanisms and therefore play critical roles in the regulation of protein functions, genes expression, coding, decoding, and regulation [9–16]. It has been found that genetic alteration enacted by ncRNAs can lead to cancer development. ncRNAs are divided into two classes based on their length: small ncRNAs (sncRNAs) which have less than 200 nucleotides and long ncRNAs (lncRNAs) which are greater than 200 nucleotides in length. sncRNAs with proven roles in cancer comprise microRNAs (miRNAs), Piwi-interacting RNA, and transfer RNA-derived small RNAs [10]. The purpose of this chapter is to discuss the critical role of miRNAs in cancer by focusing on cancer hallmark of apoptosis and related processes including autophagy and cell cycle arrest.

2. miRNA: Biogenesis and function

The first miRNAs, *Lineage defective-4 (lin-4)* and *lethal-7 (let-7)*, were detected during the studies on the developmental timing of

Caenorhabditis elegans in the 1990s [17, 18]. Approximately, 2300 human mature miRNAs were annotated by March 2019 [19]. miRNAs are ~22 nucleotides in length and are transcribed from DNA by RNA polymerase II/III (Pol II/III) into primary miRNA (pri-miRNA) with at least one hairpin substrate, which is a part of miRNA folds. pri-miRNAs have 5′ cap, but they do not have a polyadenylated 3′ tail which could result from transcriptional processing by microprocessors. Hairpin structures are substrates for microprocessors, heterotrimeric complexes containing double-stranded RNA-specific proteins including two molecules of DiGeorge Syndrome Critical Region 8 (DGCR8) and one molecule of Drosha. Drosha has two domains of RNase III in its structure. In the next step, the microprocessor cleaves pri-miRNA to release a stem-loop structure named precursor miRNA (pre-miRNA), approximately 60 nucleotides long. For this purpose, DGCR8 which is the non-catalytic subunit of microprocessor identifies a region of N6-methyl adenylated CGAC in the pri-miRNA sequence and each one of RNase III domains of Drosha cut one strand of pri-miRNA stem to produce a 2-base pair offset at 3′ end. Once formed, pre-miRNA is exported by Exportin 5 and Ras-related nuclear protein (RAN)–GTP complex to the cytoplasm for further processing. Pre-miRNAs are then processed by another RNase III endonuclease called Dicer which cut the pre-miRNA stem near its loop. Dicer has five domains consisting of a helicase-like domain for recognizing the pre-miRNA molecule through interacting with its terminal loop; a Piwi–Argonaute–Zwille domain for recognizing and binding to the 3′ overhang end of pre-miRNA; two RNase III (types A and B) for cutting the miRNA; and a double-stranded RNA-binding domain. Dicer action results in the production of a miRNA–miRNA* duplex and its passenger strands. The function of Drosha and Dicer ultimately produces a double-stranded miRNA with each strand having ~2 nucleotides overhang at its 3′ end. miRNAs derived from 5′ and 3′ ends are called 5p and 3p miRNAs, respectively. miRNA duplex is then loaded onto an Argonaute (AGO) protein in association with chaperone proteins in an ATP-dependent manner. AGO then returns to its base-state conformation and leads to exiting the passenger strand to generate a single strand of mature miRNA. Subsequently, AGO mediates the assembly of RNA-induced silencing complex (RISC) to be used in the detection of miRNA targets to suppress translation or degrade target mRNAs (Figure 1) [9, 10, 20–24].

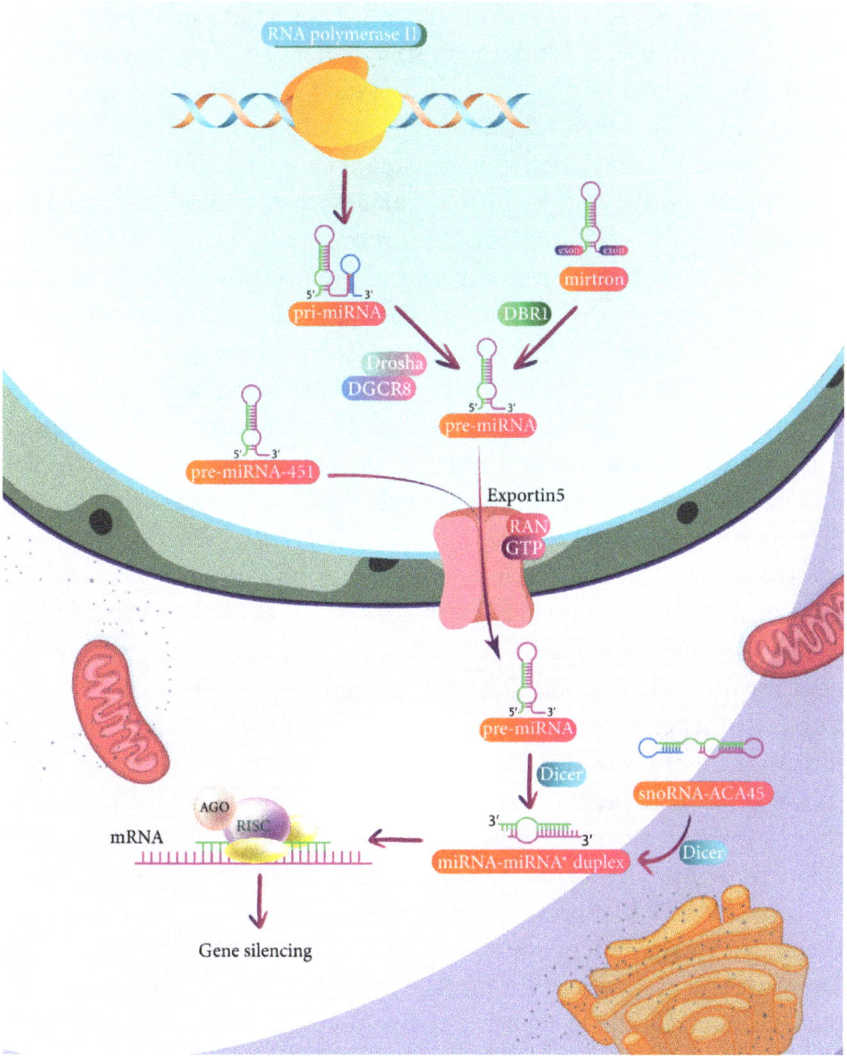

Figure 1. The biogenesis of miRNA and its origins.

In addition to the canonical path, miRNAs could also be generated from alternative precursors through non-canonical pathways by bypassing canonical pathway steps. An example of miRNAs produced in this way is mirtrons whose biogenesis is independent of the Drosha function and use splicing instead of Drosha activity. Mirtrons are short hairpin RNAs inside introns and have splice site-match ends. After identifying and binding to splice sites, splicing factors cleave short hairpin introns from exons to generate mirtron lariat. Then, DBR1 which is a lariat-debranching enzyme processes the lariat to make pre-miRNAs. Thus, mirtrons can be called pre-miRNA after transcription as they undergo cleavage by Dicer without the need for Drosha and DGCR8 activities. Moreover, a subclass of mirtrons, called tailed mirtrons, have only one of the pre-miRNA ends that are generated through the splicing process [24, 25]. Furthermore, miRNAs can be generated from small nucleolar RNAs (snoRNAs). For instance, ACA45 is a snoRNA processed by Dicer to a short RNA with functions similar to miRNAs in a Drosha-independent manner [26]. In another pathway of miRNA biogenesis, these molecules are derived from short hairpin RNAs (shRNAs). As they are structurally like miRNAs, shRNAs bypass Drosha/DGCR8 function and are transported to the cytoplasm to be further processed by Dicer. Like mirtrons, shRNAs could also be included in a tail that is removed by a nuclease but is not identified yet [27]. Same as the miRNAs generated through non-canonical pathways, miRNA-320 is produced in a Drosha-independent, Dicer-dependent manner. miRNA-320 is directly transcribed from endogenous shRNA by Pol II. In contrast to the previously mentioned miRNAs, miRNA-320 is transported to the cytoplasm through the function of another member of the Exportin family, Exportin 1, which is dependent on phosphorylated adaptor for RNA export (PHAX) [28]. In addition to biogenesis through Drosha-independent manner, there is Dicer-independent, Drosha-dependent non-canonical pathways. miRNA-451 is an example generated by this method. For this purpose, the pre-miRNA-451 produced by Drosha is translocated into cytoplasm and loaded into AGO2 to undergo further processing toward maturity (Figure 1) [29–31].

After the production of a mature miRNA–RISC complex, miRNA is ready to exert its function by either regulating translation or mRNA degradation. This depends on the quality of miRNA–target mRNA binding to its seed region (nucleotides 2–8), required for identifying their target. miRNAs bind to the 3′ untranslated region (3′UTR) of their target. Indeed, perfect or partial complementarity of miRNA to its target results in mRNA degradation and suppression of translation process, respectively [24]. In addition to 3′UTR region, miRNAs have other binding sites as their targets. For instance, miRNA-532-5p binds to the 5′UTR site of its target to apply its inhibitory activity [32]. Moreover, it has been shown that miRNA-324-3p could mediate promoter-based transcriptional activation [33]. Furthermore, the site of miRNA activity is not only in the cytoplasm but also in the nucleus where post-transcriptional gene regulation occurs [22].

An overwhelming number of studies now suggest that such naturally occurring miRNAs have critical roles in cellular mechanisms and the biology of disease as a whole. Dysregulation of miRNAs has been well-documented in cancers [16, 34–37]. It is estimated that approximately 17% of miRNAs are predominantly expressed in specific tissues [38]. Similarly, there are cancer-specific miRNAs whose alteration in expression is variable in specific cancers. For example, the expression of miRNA-155 is high in pediatric Burkitt lymphoma and the expression level of miRNA-143 is found to be low in colorectal neoplasia. miRNA signatures could be a reflection of the developmental history of cancer and a biomarker [20]. As mentioned before, one of the cancer cell characteristics is the uninhibited proliferation and inactivated apoptotic pathways. To gain and maintain this feature, cancer cells undergo metabolic reprogramming. Cancer cells need to provide energy as ATP molecules to support mechanisms involved in uncontrolled proliferation. In addition to ATP, other molecules such as nicotinamide adenine dinucleotide phosphate (NADPH), required for ATP generation, are necessary. It is well known for a century that alteration in glucose metabolism through different mechanisms such as glycolysis is an indispensable factor in the viability of cancer cells. As well, other metabolic alterations observed in cancer cells for maintaining cell growth include elevation of glutaminolysis for NADPH rebuilding; increased macromolecule generation by alteration flux via tricarboxylic acid cycle and pentose phosphate pathway; improvement of lipid uptake by cells and lipogenesis; upturn of one-carbon metabolism to increase the generation of nucleotides, ATP, NADPH, and glutathione; modified amino acid metabolism; increased usage of metabolic substrates like acetate and lactate; and suppression of apoptosis by metabolic reprogramming [39].

Growing evidence from numerous studies suggests the critical role of miRNAs in cancer hallmarks including apoptosis, proliferation, invasion, and metastasis. In the case of cell growth, proliferation, and apoptosis, miRNAs affect various cellular mechanisms which affect these hallmarks (Table 1).

3. miRNAs and apoptosis regulation

Apoptosis and autophagy are programmed cell death (PCD) mechanisms in living organisms. Apoptosis, a hallmark of cancer, has been extensively studied. The primary mode of PCD is in cell homeostasis, development, and deregulation. Apoptotic cells are identified by characteristics that include round shape, condensed chromatin, shrunk cytoplasm, cell membrane protrusions, and fragmented DNA [48, 50]. Apoptosis is initiated by damaging stress signals and has two overlapping pathways, namely intrinsic (known as mitochondrial pathway) and extrinsic (known as death receptor pathway).

In the intrinsic pathway, pro-apoptotic proteins [BH3-only "activators" of apoptosis such as p53-upregulated modulator of apoptosis (PUMA), truncated form of BH3-interacting domain death agonist (tBID), and BCL-2-interacting mediator of cell death (BIM)] are released at first. Pro-apoptotic proteins interact with pro-survival factors such as BCL-2, myeloid cell leukemia 1 (MCL1), B cell lymphoma W (BCL-W), B cell lymphoma extra-large (BCL-X_L), and BCL-2-related isolated from fetal liver (BFL1) to inhibit them. In the absence of pro-survival proteins, the pro-apoptotic factors could activate BCL-2 antagonist/killer (BAK) and BCL-2-associated X protein (BAX). BAK and BAX form pores in the mitochondrial outer membrane that leads to unleashing apoptotic proteins, such as cytochrome

Table 1. A summary of miRNAs regulating the proliferation of cancer cells.

miRNA	Cancer Type	Function	Signaling Network	Remark(s)	Ref
miRNA-199a-5p	Esophageal cancer	Tumor suppressor	JUN-B	Downregulation of JUN-B by miRNA-199a-5p. Impairing cancer cell proliferation.	[40]
miRNA-543	Triple-negative breast cancer	Tumor suppressor	ACTL6A	ACTL6A is involved in the modification of DNA–histone interaction and regulating transcription process. ACTL6A downregulation by miRNA-543 to reduce proliferation, tumor growth, and impairing invasion and metastasis.	[41]
miRNA-16-5p	Colorectal cancer	Tumor suppressor	PI3K/Akt/mTOR	Downregulation of FOXK1 by miRNA-16-5p results in proliferation and angiogenesis inhibition via suppression of PI3K/Akt/mTOR signaling.	[42]
miRNA-190b	Pancreatic cancer	Tumor suppressor	MEF2C TCF4	miRNA-190b hampers cancer cell proliferation, invasion, and metastasis by the inhibition of MEF2C and TCF4. miRNA-190b is a predictor of good prognosis.	[43]
miRNA-338-3p	Glioma	Tumor suppressor	MYT1L	miRNA-338-3p reduces tumor cell proliferation, invasion, and metastasis and induces apoptosis via inhibition of MYT1L.	[44]
miRNA-671-5p	Ovarian cancer	Tumor suppressor	HDAC5 HIF-1α	Downregulation of HDAC5 and HIF-1α by miRNA-671-5p to decrease tumor cells' proliferation, invasion, and migration.	[42]

(*Continued*)

Table 1. (*Continued*)

miRNA	Cancer Type	Function	Signaling Network	Remark(s)	Ref
miRNA-146a-5p	Hepatocellular carcinoma	Oncogene	FLAP	FLAP is involved in the metabolic pathway of arachidonic acid. miRNA-146a-5p promotes proliferation and cell growth and induces invasion and metastasis via inhibiting FLAP.	[44]
miRNA-19a-3p	Gastric cancer	Oncogene	SMOC2	miRNA-19a-3p promotes proliferation, invasion, and migration via suppression of SMOC2.	[45]
miRNA-21	Head and neck squamous cell carcinoma	Oncogene	PTEN	Inhibition of PTEN by miRNA-21 results in increased cell proliferation and apoptosis inhibition. Cisplatin resistance mediated by miRNA-21 via targeting PTEN pathway.	[46]
miRNA-181a	Papillary thyroid carcinoma	Oncogene	KDM5C	KDM5C is a tumor suppressor factor that inhibits S100A2 via histone demethylation to inhibit cell proliferation and migration. miRNA-181a diminish KDM5C to increase S100A2 and enhance proliferation.	[47]
miRNA-486-3p	Cutaneous squamous cell carcinoma	Oncogene	FLOT2	Downregulation of FLOT2 by miRNA-486-3p increases proliferation and tumorigenicity in vivo and in vitro.	[48]
miRNA-196-5p	Cholangiocarcinoma	Oncogene	HAND1/Wnt/β-catenin	miRNA-196-5p upregulation is positively related to metastasis situation, TNM stage, and tumor size. Upregulation of N-cadherin and downregulation of E-cadherin by miRNA-196-5p to increase EMT level. miRNA-196-5p exerts its function by upturning HAND1/Wnt/β-catenin axis function.	[49]

c, second mitochondrial-derived activator of caspase (SMAC), and serine protease OMI from the mitochondrial space of intermembrane into the cytoplasm. Next, cytochrome *c* binds to a factor named apoptotic protease-activating factor 1 (APAF1) resulting in the formation of apoptosome, required for the activation of caspase 9, and subsequent activation of its effectors — caspase 3 and 7. Subsequently, cells are dismantled and ready for phagocytosis. X-linked inhibitor of apoptosis protein (XIAP) can inactivate caspase proteins. In turn, OMI and SMAC proteins have inhibitory functions on XIAP. Apoptosis activator signals can also induce BH3-only "sensitizer" proteins [such as BCL-2-associated agonist of cell death (BAD), activator of apoptosis hara-kiri (Hrk)] that directly inactivate the pro-survival BCL-2 family.

During the extrinsic pathway that is elaborated by caspase proteins, an interaction between the death receptor ligand and other receptors is established. Fas-ligand (FAS-L) and FAS receptor interactions are known examples that result in the activation of apoptosis. Then, caspase 8 is activated to mediate the cleavage and activation of caspase 3/7 and subsequent apoptosis [51, 52].

During the process of transition from normal to cancer, excessive cell growth signals are generated and this creates a microenvironmental stress, which increases the risk of DNA damage. Besides, most of the genes involved in cell metabolism, proliferation, and growth are under the control of Myc oncoproteins, proteins that belong to the family of pleiotropic transcription factors [51, 53]. Interestingly, the mechanisms for escaping from apoptosis are very different between cancers, which resulted in a heterogeneous expression of BCL-2 family proteins. Typically, the mechanisms for inhibiting apoptosis include the upturning of pro-survival proteins; downregulation or suppression of pro-apoptotic proteins through phosphorylation, mutation, transcriptional and post-transcriptional regulation; and down turning of pore-forming proteins of BAK and BAX [51].

miRNAs regulate apoptosis in cancer by targeting different factors involved in this process. An example of such miRNA, miRNA-29-3p, with tumor suppressor activities is observed in prostate cancer. miRNA-29-3p exerts its function by upregulation of BIM and subsequent apoptotic induction [54]. In contrast, miRNA-148a exerts oncogenic activities in glioblastoma. It has been demonstrated that miRNA-148a downregulates BIM protein to inhibit apoptosis and increase cell survival, growth, invasion, and metastasis [55].

Forkhead box protein O3a (FOXO3a) is a tumor suppressor in different cancers. As an upstream regulator, FOXO3a induces apoptosis by targeting PUMA and increasing its expression [56–58]. A study by Adlakha and Saini shows that miRNA-128 expression is downregulated in cancer. They suggest that miRNA-128 induces apoptosis by inducing PUMA activation by FOXO3a. They also stated that FOXO3a could bind to the promoter region of PUMA regardless of p53. Thus, FOXO3a affects PUMA in a p53-dependent and p53-independent manner to induce apoptosis [59]. Like PUMA, limited studies evaluate the effect of miRNAs on apoptosis. The oncogenic miRNA-500a is a tumor-promoting molecule with increased expression in hepatocellular carcinoma. miRNA-500a post-transcriptionally regulates BID by binding to its 3′UTR site to mediate BID suppression and subsequently inhibit apoptosis initiation [60]. Furthermore, miRNA-20a is another oncogene highly expressed in colorectal cancer. miRNA-20a inhibits apoptosis by targeting 3′UTR of BID and suppresses its function. Moreover, the anti-apoptotic activity of miRNA-20a results in tumor necrosis factor–related apoptosis-inducing ligand (TRAIL) resistance in these cancer cells. For exerting its apoptotic function in cells, TRAIL activates caspase-8 to bind its substrate, BID. Caspase-8 cleaves BID to generate tBID, and then translocation of tBID from the cytoplasm to mitochondria leads to the activation of apoptosis [61].

In contrast to the pro-apoptotic factors, pro-survival proteins are widely studied and the role of miRNAs in their regulation is shown. miRNA-3614-5p's regulatory effect on MCL-1 in prostate cancer has recently been studied for the first time. The downregulation of miRNA-3641-5p is accompanied by tumor progression in prostate cancer. In contrast, overexpression of miRNA-3641-5p induces apoptosis through suppression of MCL-1 expression [62]. Pro-survival

Bcl-2 protein could be affected by miRNAs directly or indirectly. For example, miRNA-331-3p is a tumor suppressor with decreased levels in osteosarcoma. miRNA-331-3p binds to the 3′UTR site of *N*-acetylglucosaminyltransferase I (MGAT1) and mediates its suppression. Downregulation of MGAT1 results in the inhibition of its downstream target, BCL-2. Therefore, miRNA-331-3p induces apoptosis by indirect targeting of BCL-2. Moreover, miRNA-331-3p inhibits proliferation by targeting Wnt/b-catenin pathway [63]. On the contrary, miRNA-34a-5p directly targets BCL-2 to regulate its downregulation and induce apoptosis in cervical cancer cells [64]. Similarly, tumor suppressor miRNA-342-3p induces apoptosis in lung cancer cells by inhibiting BCL-2 directly [65]. Another member of pro-survival protein is BCL-W that has been found to play a role in carcinogenesis. It has been shown that decreased expression levels of BCL-W by tumor suppressor miRNA-519-3p lead to the induction of apoptosis in lung cancer cells [66]. Moreover, miRNA-148b exerts tumor inhibitory functions in lymphoma. To exert its function, miRNA-148b directly targets BCL-W to inhibit its activity and subsequently induce apoptosis and decrease cell viability and colony formation. Furthermore, targeting BCL-W by miRNA-148b leads to mitochondrial membrane dysfunction, cytochrome *c* unleashing, and increased levels of activated form of caspase 3 and 9 [67]. As mentioned previously, XIAP is an apoptosis suppressor that negatively affects caspase 9 and 3. miRNA-CHA1 is a novel tumor inhibitor molecule and its expression is decreased in lung cancer cells. miRNA-CHA1 induces apoptosis and regulates cell proliferation and survival by inhibiting XIAP in vivo and in vitro [68]. In the same way, miRNA-3607-3p and miRNA-3607-5p induce apoptosis in hepatocellular carcinoma by inhibiting XIAP as their common target [69]. miRNA-644a is a tumor suppressor factor with low expression level in hepatocellular carcinoma. For exerting its inhibitory function in tumor cells, miRNA-644a adversely affects heat shock factor 1 (HSF1) to induce apoptosis via increasing the expression of BIM, BID, SMAC, BAD, and APAF1 and upregulating activated form of caspase 3 and 9 (Figure 2) [70].

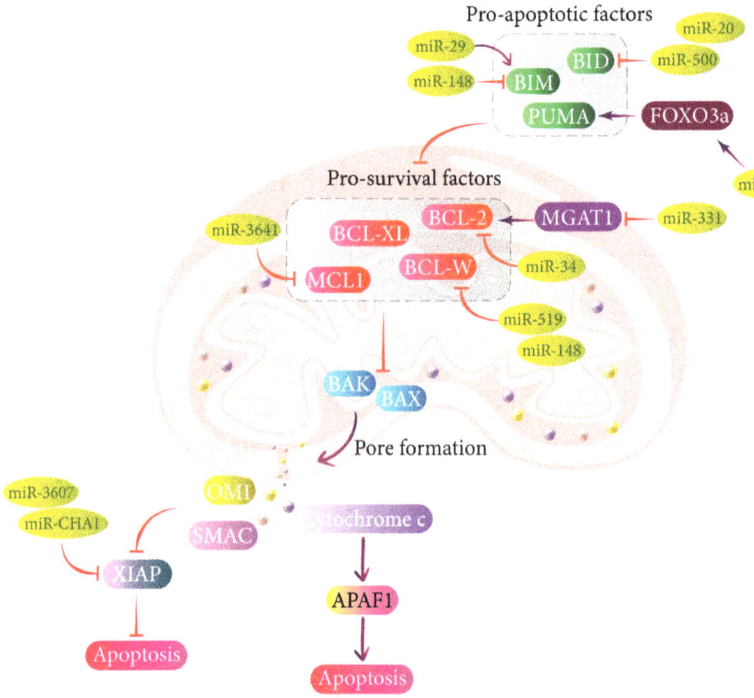

Figure 2. The intrinsic signaling pathway of apoptosis and its regulation by miRNAs.

4. miRNAs and autophagy regulation

As another type of PCD, autophagy eliminates misfolded, mutant, and long-lived proteins and dysfunctional organelles through the lysosomal system. Three types of autophagy include microautophagy, macroautophagy, and chaperone mediated. Autophagy starts with the engulfment of cargo molecules into the autophagosome which is a double-membrane vesicle. After the closure of the vesicle, lysosomes and endosomes are fused to it to form another structure named autolysosome. Then, lysosomal hydrolases function to degrade cargo molecules. Some stimuli and stress situations such as deprivation, hypoxia and chemicals are activators of autophagy [71]. It is noteworthy that the factors which induce organismal and cellular stress in cells lead to the dysregulation of miRNAs. Overexpression and downregulation or reduction of miRNA levels lead to the activation of mechanisms responsible for cellular response to stress, such as autophagy. Interestingly, as miRNAs and their machinery are degraded through autophagy, it could be suggested that the autophagy process may control its regulation. miRNAs target factors involved in different stages of autophagy [72]. Most of the autophagy-related signals are downstream targets of mTOR signaling pathway. To promote cell growth, mTORC1 suppresses autophagy regulators such as Unc-51-like autophagy activating kinase 1 (ULK1) that is involved in the formation of autophagosomes [73]. Several miRNAs were suggested as regulators of mTOR signaling in the context of autophagy, including miRNA-216b [74], miRNA-381 [75], miRNA-495-3p [76], miRNA-126 [77], miRNA-22 [78], and miRNA-100 [79]. miRNA-489 is reported to be a molecule with tumor suppressor activities in breast cancer. miRNA-489 directly targets ULK1 to suppress its function and subsequently inhibit autophagy. Furthermore, miRNA-489 induces the accumulation of autophagosomes in cancer cells [80]. miRNA-100 is a tumor suppressor agent with low levels of expression in hepatocellular carcinoma. It has been demonstrated that miRNA-100 induces autophagy by upregulation of LC3B-II and downregulation of mTOR [81]. Nearly all the autophagy signaling pathway elements are targeted by miRNAs. For example, in hepatocellular carcinoma, targeting ATG14 by miRNA-375 results in the suppression of autophagy and sensitization of cancer cells to sorafenib therapy [82]. Furthermore, direct targeting of BECN1 by miRNA-516A promotes the autophagy process in bladder cancer cells [83]. Besides, negative regulation of ATG5 and ATG16L1 by miRNA-142-3p results in autophagy inhibition in hepatocellular carcinoma and decreasing sorafenib resistance [84]. Furthermore, miRNA-20a targets ATG5/Fip200 to suppress autophagy induced by hypoxia in colorectal cancer cells [85]. Additionally, in colorectal cancer, overexpression of miRNA-183 results in the inhibition of rapamycin- and starvation-induced autophagy pathway via targeting UVRAG [86].

5. miRNAs and cell cycle regulation

Cell cycle is highly controlled and regulated by an extensive network of cellular mechanisms. Predominantly, it is assumed that cancer cells have an uncontrolled cell cycle accompanied by dysregulated cell cycle checkpoints. In fact, faults in any part of the cell cycle are enough for cancer cells to continue their division. In cancer cells, checkpoints of DNA damage are defective. In marked contrast, checkpoints for controlling the replication stress are highly conserved and rarely undergo mutations in their gene. Cyclin-dependent kinases (CDK) are master regulators of cell cycle progression [87]. miRNAs target CDK activity in addition to the cyclins involved in different stages of the cell cycle. For instance, Xie *et al.* demonstrated that miRNA-424 functions as a breast cancer inhibitor through its effect on CDK1 and mediating cell cycle arrest in the G2/M cell phase [88]. Another miRNA, miRNA-524-5p inhibits the expression of CDK6, drives cell cycle arrest at G1 phase, and suppresses proliferation in osteosarcoma [89]. On the other hand, Li *et al.* identified that miRNA-582-3p targeted cyclin B2 to induce cell cycle arrest at G2/M phase in leukemia [90]. Another study demonstrated the role of CDKs and cyclins in regulating miRNA-4779 in colon cancer. miRNA-4779 negatively regulates CDK2, CDK4, cyclin D3, and D2 and promotes CDK inhibitor p27Kip1, resulting in cell cycle arrest at G1 phase (Figure 3) [91].

6. Tumor suppressor miRNAs

miRNAs are frequently placed at fragile sites and breakpoint regions involved in cancer [92]. It is well accepted now that miRNAs with tumor suppressor activity have low expression levels in cancer. miRNAs expressions can be epigenetically regulated by DNA methylation and the activity of histone deacetylase inhibitors. In fact, DNA hypermethylation and generation of a closed chromatin structure around the promoter region of tumor suppressor miRNAs could mediate the suppression of these miRNAs, as observed in human cancer cells [93]. For instance, miRNA-127, a miRNA that is expressed in normal cells but not in cancer cells, directly targets BCL6 proto-oncogene

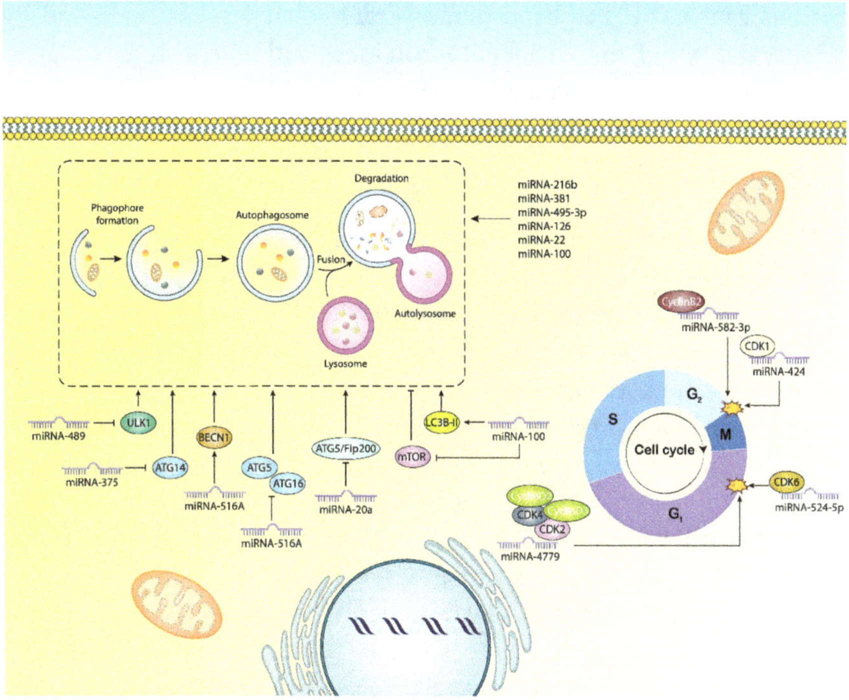

Figure 3. Role of miRNAs regulating autophagy and cell cycle progression in cancers.

protein. In this study, the treatment of cancer cells with chromatin-modifying drugs of 4-phenylbutyric acid and 5-aza-2′-deoxycytidine resulted in the overexpression of miRNA-127 [94]. In addition to chromatin modification, mutations also take part in the regulation of tumor suppressor miRNAs. As an example, miRNA-16-1 and miRNA-15a are tumor suppressor molecules with low expression levels in chronic lymphocytic leukemia which results from mutations in these genes [95]. Another example of genetic alterations is identified in miRNA-34a, which is a tumor suppressor molecule in lung and breast cancer, and miRNA-123 which functions as a tumor inhibitor in lung cancer cells [96]. Interestingly, miRNAs can be regulated by extracellular matrix elements. For instance, let-7 miRNA expression mostly involved in inhibiting cellular growth is downregulated in various cancers. It has been demonstrated that let-7 is regulated by membrane type I-matrix metalloproteinase and its substrate collagen type I in pancreatic ductal adenocarcinoma [97].

7. Tumor-promoting miRNAs

miRNAs that act in a way that promotes tumor cell growth, proliferation, and metastasis are considered oncogene miRNAs, also known as oncomiRs. Like tumor suppressor miRNAs, these molecules are regulated in cells. For instance, miRNA-17-92 cluster has oncogenic activities in human cancers. miRNA-17-92 cluster increases tumor proliferation and promotes angiogenesis by suppressing connective tissue growth factor and anti-angiogenic thrombospondin-1 and inhibits apoptosis by suppressing PTEN and p21. miRNA-17-92 family is controlled by c-Myc, which is an overexpressed transcriptional factor [98]. miRNA-31 is the first mammalian miRNA identified with roles in the oncogenesis of several cancers. It has been demonstrated that miRNA-31 targets genes, such as RhoA, SIRT3, VEGF, and ACOX1, and signaling pathways like Wnt, Akt, ERK, and hippo signaling pathways [99]. Furthermore, miRNA-31 has been demonstrated to be involved in radiosensitivity in colorectal cancer cells. In fact, miRNA-31 adversely controls STK40 expression to regulate radiosensitivity [100]. In another study, anti-apoptotic, proliferative, invasive, and metastasis-promoting roles were detected for miRNA-31. Specifically,miRNA-31 targets RhoA, ROCK2, and FOXO1 [101].

miRNAs can either act as tumor suppressor (inhibiting oncogenes or apoptosis-inducing genes) or tumor-promoting (inducing oncogenesis or suppression of anti-tumor genes) factors. However, several miRNAs exist that have dual roles in cancer; in another word, they are context-dependent miRNAs. For example, miRNA-125 and miRNA-155 have different roles of tumor suppressor or oncogene in different cancers [102]. In cancer, the upregulation of miRNAs is associated with tumor-promoting function and conversely, their downregulation is linked with tumor suppression [102]. Another example of miRNAs with dual roles is miRNA-338-3p which affects cell proliferation, metastasis, radiosensitivity, and chemosensitivity in different cancers. Besides, lncRNAs and circular RNAs could also regulate the expression level and function of miRNA-338-3p [103].

8. Conclusion and remarks

This chapter details the critical role of miRNAs in cancer proliferation by focusing on apoptosis, autophagy, and cell cycle arrest processes. Furthermore, we discuss miRNAs' role in cancer as tumor suppressors or promoter molecules. The heterogeneous nature of cancer makes it hard to find a precise treatment. Cancer is characterized by its hallmarks including uncontrolled proliferation, inhibited apoptosis, angiogenesis, and metastasis. Conventional therapies include surgery, radiation therapy, and chemotherapy. However, ncRNAs such as miRNAs and lncRNAs are a new group of therapeutic tools. Recent studies and clinical trials demonstrate the critical role of miRNAs in cancer and suggest their promising role in cancer therapy. However, it has become increasingly apparent that more studies are needed to overcome the challenges of cancer therapy.

Conflict of interest:

The authors declare no conflict of interest.

References

1. Siegel, R.L., et al., *Cancer statistics, 2022.* CA: A Cancer Journal for Clinicians, 2022. **72**(1): p. 7–33.
2. Hanahan, D., *Hallmarks of cancer: new dimensions.* Cancer Discovery, 2022. **12**(1): p. 31–46.
3. Intlekofer, A.M. and L.W. Finley, *Metabolic signatures of cancer cells and stem cells.* Nature Metabolism, 2019. **1**(2): p. 177–188.
4. Yang, L., et al., *Targeting cancer stem cell pathways for cancer therapy.* Signal Transduction and Targeted Therapy, 2020. **5**(1): p. 1–35.
5. Batlle, E. and H. Clevers, *Cancer stem cells revisited.* Nature Medicine, 2017. **23**(10): p. 1124–1134.

6. Robert, C., *A decade of immune-checkpoint inhibitors in cancer therapy.* Nature Communications, 2020. **11**(1): p. 1–3.
7. Carneiro, B.A. and W.S. El-Deiry, *Targeting apoptosis in cancer therapy.* Nature Reviews Clinical Oncology, 2020. **17**(7): p. 395–417.
8. Helmink, B.A., et al., *The microbiome, cancer, and cancer therapy.* Nature Medicine, 2019. **25**(3): p. 377–388.
9. Winkle, M., et al., *Noncoding RNA therapeutics — Challenges and potential solutions.* Nature Reviews Drug Discovery, 2021. **20**(8): p. 629–651.
10. Slack, F.J. and A.M. Chinnaiyan, *The role of non-coding RNAs in oncology.* Cell, 2019. **179**(5): p. 1033–1055.
11. Paskeh, M.D.A., et al., *Emerging role of exosomes in cancer progression and tumor microenvironment remodeling.* Journal of Hematology & Oncology, 2022. **15**(1): p. 1–39.
12. Hashemi, M., et al., *Long non-coding RNA (lncRNA) H19 in human cancer: From proliferation and metastasis to therapy.* Pharmacological Research, 2022. **184**: p. 106418.
13. Entezari, M., et al., *LncRNA-miRNA axis in tumor progression and therapy response: An emphasis on molecular interactions and therapeutic interventions.* Biomedicine & Pharmacotherapy, 2022. **154**: p. 113609.
14. Mirzaei, S., et al., *Molecular landscape of LncRNAs in prostate cancer: A focus on pathways and therapeutic targets for intervention.* Journal of Experimental & Clinical Cancer Research, 2022. **41**(1): p. 1–26.
15. Sadrkhanloo, M., et al., *Non-coding RNAs in EMT regulation: Association with tumor progression and therapy response.* European Journal of Pharmacology, 2022: p. 175212.
16. Mirzaei, S., et al., *The long and short non-coding RNAs modulating EZH2 signaling in cancer.* Journal of Hematology & Oncology, 2022. **15**(1): p. 18.
17. Lee, R.C., R.L. Feinbaum, and V. Ambros, *The C. elegans heterochronic gene lin-4 encodes small RNAs with antisense complementarity to lin-14.* Cell, 1993. **75**(5): p. 843–854.
18. Reinhart, B.J., et al., *The 21-nucleotide let-7 RNA regulates developmental timing in Caenorhabditis elegans.* Nature, 2000. **403**(6772): p. 901–906.

19. Alles, J., et al., *An estimate of the total number of true human miRNAs.* Nucleic Acids Research, 2019. **47**(7): p. 3353–3364.
20. Anastasiadou, E., et al., *The nefarious nexus of noncoding RNAs in cancer.* International Journal of Molecular Sciences, 2018. **19**(7): p. 2072.
21. Bartel, D.P., *Metazoan micrornas.* Cell, 2018. **173**(1): p. 20–51.
22. O'Brien, J., et al., *Overview of microRNA biogenesis, mechanisms of actions, and circulation.* Frontiers in Endocrinology, 2018. **9**: p. 402.
23. Saliminejad, K., et al., *An overview of microRNAs: biology, functions, therapeutics, and analysis methods.* Journal of Cellular Physiology, 2019. **234**(5): p. 5451–5465.
24. Salim, U., et al., *Biogenesis, characterization, and functions of mirtrons.* Wiley Interdisciplinary Reviews: RNA, 2022. **13**(1): p. e1680.
25. Castellano, L. and J. Stebbing, *Deep sequencing of small RNAs identifies canonical and non-canonical miRNA and endogenous siRNAs in mammalian somatic tissues.* Nucleic Acids Research, 2013. **41**(5): p. 3339–3351.
26. Ender, C., et al., *A human snoRNA with microRNA-like functions.* Molecular Cell, 2008. **32**(4): p. 519–528.
27. Babiarz, J.E., et al., *Mouse ES cells express endogenous shRNAs, siRNAs, and other Microprocessor-independent, Dicer-dependent small RNAs.* Genes & Development, 2008. **22**(20): p. 2773–2785.
28. Xie, M., et al., *Mammalian 5′-capped microRNA precursors that generate a single microRNA.* Cell, 2013. **155**(7): p. 1568–1580.
29. Cheloufi, S., et al., *A dicer-independent miRNA biogenesis pathway that requires Ago catalysis.* Nature, 2010. **465**(7298): p. 584–589.
30. Cifuentes, D., et al., *A novel miRNA processing pathway independent of Dicer requires Argonaute2 catalytic activity.* Science, 2010. **328**(5986): p. 1694–1698.
31. Yang, J.-S., et al., *Conserved vertebrate mir-451 provides a platform for Dicer-independent, Ago2-mediated microRNA biogenesis.* Proceedings of the National Academy of Sciences, 2010. **107**(34): p. 15163–15168.
32. Zhang, J., et al., *Oncogenic role of microRNA-532-5p in human colorectal cancer via targeting of the 5'UTR of RUNX3.* Oncology Letters, 2018. **15**(5): p. 7215–7220.
33. Dharap, A., et al., *MicroRNA miR-324-3p induces promoter-mediated expression of RelA gene.* PloS One, 2013. **8**(11): p. e79467.

34. Syllaios, A., et al., *The role of miR-101 in esophageal and gastric cancer.* Personalized Medicine, 2021. **18**(5): p. 491–499.
35. Guo, Y.X., et al., *The role of miR-23b in cancer and autoimmune disease.* Journal of Clinical Oncology, 2021. **2021**: p. 6473038.
36. Zou, Y., et al., *MiR-873-5p: A potential molecular marker for cancer diagnosis and prognosis.* Frontiers in Oncology, 2021. **11**: p. 743701.
37. Paskeh, M.D.A., et al., *Revealing the role of miRNA-489 as a new onco-suppressor factor in different cancers based on pre-clinical and clinical evidence.* International Journal of Biological Macromolecules, 2021. **191**: p. 727–737.
38. Ludwig, N., et al., *Distribution of miRNA expression across human tissues.* Nucleic Acids Research, 2016. **44**(8): p. 3865–3877.
39. Schiliro, C. and B.L. Firestein, *Mechanisms of metabolic reprogramming in cancer cells supporting enhanced growth and proliferation.* Cells, 2021. **10**(5): p. 1056.
40. Phatak, P., M.E. Tulapurkar, and J.M. Donahue, *MicroRNA (miR) 199a-5p targets JUN-B to decrease cell proliferation in esophageal cancer cells.* Cancer Research, 2022. **82**(12_Supplement): p. 1486–1486.
41. Li, Y., et al., *MicroRNA-190b expression predicts a good prognosis and attenuates the malignant progression of pancreatic cancer by targeting MEF2C and TCF4.* Oncology Reports, 2022. **47**(1): p. 1–13.
42. Peng, D., et al., *microRNA-671-5p reduces tumorigenicity of ovarian cancer via suppressing HDAC5 and HIF-1α expression.* Chemico-Biological Interactions, 2022. **355**: p. 109780.
43. Wang, H., et al., *MicroRNA-146a promotes proliferation, migration, and invasion of HepG2 via regulating FLAP.* Cancer Cell International, 2022. **22**(1): p. 1–12.
44. Yu, Z., et al., *miRNA-338-3p inhibits glioma cell proliferation and progression by targeting MYT1L.* Brain Research Bulletin, 2022. **179**: p. 1–12.
45. Xu, H., et al., *MicroRNA-19a-3p acts as an oncogene in gastric cancer and exerts the effect by targeting SMOC2.* Applied Biochemistry and Biotechnology, 2022. **194**: p. 3833–3842.
46. Li, X., et al., *MicroRNA-486–3p promotes the proliferation and metastasis of cutaneous squamous cell carcinoma by suppressing flotillin-2.* Journal of Dermatological Science, 2022. **105**(1): p. 18–26.

47. Wang, Y., et al., *microRNA-181a promotes the oncogene S100A2 and enhances papillary thyroid carcinoma growth by mediating the expression of histone demethylase KDM5C.* Journal of Endocrinological Investigation, 2022. **45**(1): p. 17–28.
48. Lopez, A., et al., *Co-targeting of BAX and BCL-XL proteins broadly overcomes resistance to apoptosis in cancer.* Nature Communications, 2022. **13**(1): p. 1–18.
49. Liu, C., et al., *MiRNA-196-5p promotes proliferation and migration in cholangiocarcinoma via HAND1/Wnt/β-catenin signaling pathway.* Journal of Oncology, 2022. **2022**: p. 4599676.
50. Wang, S., et al., *PEBP balances apoptosis and autophagy in whitefly upon arbovirus infection.* Nature Communications, 2022. **13**(1): p. 1–13.
51. Singh, R., A. Letai, and K. Sarosiek, *Regulation of apoptosis in health and disease: the balancing act of BCL-2 family proteins.* Nature reviews Molecular Cell Biology, 2019. **20**(3): p. 175–193.
52. Bock, F.J. and S.W. Tait, *Mitochondria as multifaceted regulators of cell death.* Nature Reviews Molecular Cell Biology, 2020. **21**(2): p. 85–100.
53. Whitfield, J.R., M.-E. Beaulieu, and L. Soucek, *Strategies to inhibit Myc and their clinical applicability.* Frontiers in Cell and Developmental Biology, 2017. **5**: p. 10.
54. Sur, S., et al., *miRNA-29b inhibits prostate tumor growth and induces apoptosis by increasing bim expression.* Cells, 2019. **8**(11): p. 1455.
55. Kim, J., et al., *microRNA-148a is a prognostic oncomiR that targets MIG6 and BIM to regulate EGFR and apoptosis in glioblastoma.* Cancer Research, 2014. **74**(5): p. 1541–1553.
56. Zhu, Y., et al., *WTIP upregulates FOXO3a and induces apoptosis through PUMA in acute myeloid leukemia.* Cell Death & Disease, 2021. **13**(1): p. 1–11.
57. Lou, J., et al., *OSI-027 Inhibits the tumorigenesis of colon cancer through mediation of c-Myc/FOXO3a/PUMA axis.* Cell Biology International, 2022. **46**: p. 1204–1214.
58. Li, X., et al., *Xanthohumol inhibits non-small cell lung cancer by activating PUMA-mediated apoptosis.* Toxicology, 2022. **470**: p. 153141.
59. Adlakha, Y. and N. Saini, *miR-128 exerts pro-apoptotic effect in a p53 transcription-dependent and-independent manner via PUMA-Bak axis.* Cell Death & Disease, 2013. **4**(3): p. e542–e542.

60. Bao, L., et al., *MicroRNA-500a promotes the progression of hepatocellular carcinoma by post-transcriptionally targeting BID.* Cellular Physiology and Biochemistry, 2018. **47**: p. 2046–2055.
61. Huang, G., et al., *miR-20a-directed regulation of BID is associated with the TRAIL sensitivity in colorectal cancer.* Oncology Reports, 2017. **37**(1): p. 571–578.
62. Hsieh, Y.-H., et al., *Targeting of Mcl-1 expression by MiRNA-3614-5p promotes cell apoptosis of human prostate cancer cells.* International Journal of Molecular Sciences, 2022. **23**(8): p. 4194.
63. Bi, W., et al., *MicroRNA miR-331-3p suppresses osteosarcoma progression via the Bcl-2/Bax and Wnt/β-Catenin signaling pathways and the epithelial-mesenchymal transition by targeting N-acetylglucosaminyltransferase I (MGAT1).* Bioengineered, 2022. **13**(6): p. 14159–14174.
64. Wang, X., Y. Xie, and J. Wang, *Overexpression of microRNA-34a-5p inhibits proliferation and promotes apoptosis of human cervical cancer cells by downregulation of Bcl-2.* Oncology Research, 2018. **26**(6): p. 977.
65. Chen, Z., et al., *miR-342-3p regulates the proliferation and apoptosis of NSCLC cells by targeting BCL-2.* Technology in Cancer Research & Treatment, 2021. **20**: p. 15330338211041193.
66. Choi, J.Y., et al., *miR-519d-3p suppresses tumorigenicity and metastasis by inhibiting Bcl-w and HIF-1α in NSCLC.* Molecular Therapy-Oncolytics, 2021. **22**: p. 368–379.
67. Liu, S.-h., et al., *MicroRNA-148b enhances the radiosensitivity of B-cell lymphoma cells by targeting Bcl-w to promote apoptosis.* International Journal of Biological Sciences, 2020. **16**(6): p. 935.
68. Yoo, J.K., et al., *The novel microRNA hsa-miR-CHA1 regulates cell proliferation and apoptosis in human lung cancer by targeting XIAP.* Lung Cancer, 2019. **132**: p. 99–106.
69. Lou, W., et al., *XIAP, commonly targeted by tumor suppressive miR-3607-5p and miR-3607-3p, promotes proliferation and inhibits apoptosis in hepatocellular carcinoma.* Genomics, 2021. **113**(3): p. 933–945.
70. Liang, W., et al., *MicroRNA-644a promotes apoptosis of hepatocellular carcinoma cells by downregulating the expression of heat shock factor 1.* Cell Communication and Signaling, 2018. **16**(1): p. 1–13.

71. Kocaturk, N.M. and D. Gozuacik, *Crosstalk between mammalian autophagy and the ubiquitin-proteasome system.* Frontiers in Cell and Developmental Biology, 2018: p. 128.
72. Akkoc, Y. and D. Gozuacik, *MicroRNAs as major regulators of the autophagy pathway.* Biochimica et Biophysica Acta (BBA)-Molecular Cell Research, 2020. **1867**(5): p. 118662.
73. Saxton, R.A. and D.M. Sabatini, *mTOR signaling in growth, metabolism, and disease.* Cell, 2017. **168**(6): p. 960–976.
74. Liu, T., et al., *MicroRNA-216b targets HK2 to potentiate autophagy and apoptosis of breast cancer cells via the mTOR signaling pathway.* International Journal of Biological Sciences, 2021. **17**(11): p. 2970.
75. Liao, W. and Y. Zhang, *MicroRNA-381 facilitates autophagy and apoptosis in prostate cancer cells via inhibiting the RELN-mediated PI3K/AKT/mTOR signaling pathway.* Life Sciences, 2020. **254**: p. 117672.
76. Chen, S., et al., *MicroRNA-495-3p inhibits multidrug resistance by modulating autophagy through GRP78/mTOR axis in gastric cancer.* Cell Death & Disease, 2018. **9**(11): p. 1–12.
77. Wei, L., et al., *MicroRNA-126 inhibit viability of colorectal cancer cell by repressing mTOR induced apoptosis and autophagy.* OncoTargets and Therapy, 2020. **13**: p. 2459.
78. Meng, C.Y., et al., *MicroRNA-22 mediates the cisplatin resistance of osteosarcoma cells by inhibiting autophagy via the PI3K/Akt/mTOR pathway.* Oncology Reports, 2020. **43**(4): p. 1169–1186.
79. Liu, X., et al., *MicroRNA-100 enhances autophagy and suppresses migration and invasion of renal cell carcinoma cells via disruption of NOX4-dependent mTOR pathway.* Clinical and Translational Science, 2022. **15**(2): p. 567–575.
80. Soni, M., et al., *Autophagy, cell viability, and chemoresistance are regulated by miR-489 in breast cancer.* Molecular Cancer Research, 2018. **16**(9): p. 1348–1360.
81. Ge, Y.-Y., et al., *MicroRNA-100 promotes the autophagy of hepatocellular carcinoma cells by inhibiting the expression of mTOR and IGF-1R.* Oncotarget, 2014. **5**(15): p. 6218.
82. Yang, S., et al., *MicroRNA-375 targets ATG14 to inhibit autophagy and sensitize hepatocellular carcinoma cells to sorafenib.* OncoTargets and Therapy, 2020. **13**: p. 3557.

83. Jin, H., et al., *Oncogenic role of MIR516A in human bladder cancer was mediated by its attenuating PHLPP2 expression and BECN1-dependent autophagy.* Autophagy, 2021. **17**(4): p. 840–854.
84. Zhang, K., et al., *PU. 1/microRNA-142-3p targets ATG5/ATG16L1 to inactivate autophagy and sensitize hepatocellular carcinoma cells to sorafenib.* Cell Death & Disease, 2018. **9**(3): p. 1–16.
85. Che, J., et al., *miR-20a inhibits hypoxia-induced autophagy by targeting ATG5/FIP200 in colorectal cancer.* Molecular Carcinogenesis, 2019. **58**(7): p. 1234–1247.
86. Huangfu, L., et al., *miR-183 regulates autophagy and apoptosis in colorectal cancer through targeting of UVRAG.* Oncotarget, 2016. 7(4): p. 4735.
87. Matthews, H.K., C. Bertoli, and R.A. de Bruin, *Cell cycle control in cancer.* Nature Reviews Molecular Cell Biology, 2022. **23**(1): p. 74–88.
88. Xie, D., et al., *MicroRNA-424 serves an anti-oncogenic role by targeting cyclin-dependent kinase 1 in breast cancer cells.* Oncology Reports, 2018. **40**(6): p. 3416–3426.
89. Chen, H., C. Cheng, and S. Gao, *microRNA-524-5p inhibits proliferation and induces cell cycle arrest of osteosarcoma cells via targeting CDK6.* Biochemical and Biophysical Research Communications, 2020. **530**(3): p. 566–573.
90. Li, H., et al., *MicroRNA-582–3p negatively regulates cell proliferation and cell cycle progression in acute myeloid leukemia by targeting cyclin B2.* Cellular & Molecular Biology Letters, 2019. **24**(1): p. 1–12.
91. Koo, K.H. and H. Kwon, *MicroRNA miR-4779 suppresses tumor growth by inducing apoptosis and cell cycle arrest through direct targeting of PAK2 and CCND3.* Cell Death & Disease, 2018. **9**(2): p. 1–14.
92. Calin, G.A., et al., *Human microRNA genes are frequently located at fragile sites and genomic regions involved in cancers.* Proceedings of the National Academy of Sciences, 2004. **101**(9): p. 2999–3004.
93. Saito, Y. and P.M. Jones, *Epigenetic activation of tumor suppressor microRNAs in human cancer cells.* Cell Cycle, 2006. **5**(19): p. 2220–2222.
94. Saito, Y., et al., *Specific activation of microRNA-127 with downregulation of the proto-oncogene BCL6 by chromatin-modifying drugs in human cancer cells.* Cancer Cell, 2006. **9**(6): p. 435–443.

95. Calin, G.A., et al., *A MicroRNA signature associated with prognosis and progression in chronic lymphocytic leukemia.* New England Journal of Medicine, 2005. **353**(17): p. 1793–1801.
96. Anfossi, S., et al., *MicroRNAs, regulatory messengers inside and outside cancer cells.* Exosomes, Stem Cells and MicroRNA, 2018: p. 87–108.
97. Dangi-Garimella, S., et al., *Collagen regulation of let-7 in pancreatic cancer involves TGF-β1-mediated membrane type 1-matrix metalloproteinase expression.* Oncogene, 2011. **30**(8): p. 1002–1008.
98. Lopez-Serra, P. and M. Esteller, *DNA methylation-associated silencing of tumor-suppressor microRNAs in cancer.* Oncogene, 2012. **31**(13): p. 1609–1622.
99. Lin, X., et al., *MicroRNA-31: a pivotal oncogenic factor in oral squamous cell carcinoma.* Cell Death Discovery, 2022. **8**(1): p. 1–9.
100. Zhang, W., et al., *miRNA-31 increases radiosensitivity through targeting STK40 in colorectal cancer cells.* Asia-Pacific Journal of Clinical Oncology, 2022. **18**(3): p. 267–278.
101. Zeng, X., et al., *MiroRNA-31-3p promotes the invasion and metastasis of non-small-cell lung cancer cells by targeting forkhead box 1 (FOXO1).* Computational and Mathematical Methods in Medicine, 2022. **2022**: p. 4597087.
102. Smolarz, B., et al., *miRNAs in cancer (review of literature).* International Journal of Molecular Sciences, 2022. **23**(5): p. 2805.
103. Mirzaei, S., et al., *The role of microRNA-338-3p in cancer: growth, invasion, chemoresistance, and mediators.* Life Sciences, 2021. **268**: p. 119005.

https://doi.org/10.1142/9789811267390_0002

Chapter 2

MicroRNAs (miRNAs) in cancer metastasis: Molecular interactions and possible therapeutic targets

Mahshid Deldar Abad Paskeh[1,2], Shokooh Salimimoghadam[3], Sepideh Mirzaei[4], Mehrdad Hashemi[1,2*], Azuma Kalu[5,6] and Noushin Nabavi[7]

[1]*Department of Genetics, Faculty of Advanced Science and Technology, Tehran Medical Sciences, Islamic Azad University, Tehran, Iran*
[2]*Farhikhtegan Medical Convergence Sciences Research Center, Farhikhtegan Hospital Tehran Medical Sciences, Islamic Azad University, Tehran, Iran*
[3]*Department of Biochemistry and Molecular Biology, Faculty of Veterinary Medicine, Shahid Chamran University of Ahvaz, Ahvaz, Iran*
[4]*Department of Biology, Faculty of Science, Islamic Azad University, Science and Research Branch, Tehran, Iran*
[5]*School of Life, Health & Chemical Sciences, The Open University, Milton Keynes, United Kingdom*
[6]*Laboratory Medicine Directorate, Sheffield Teaching Hospital, Sheffield, United Kingdom*
[7]*Department of Urologic Sciences and Vancouver Prostate Centre, University of British Columbia, Vancouver, BC, Canada*

*Corresponding author: Mehrdad Hashemi, Farhikhtegan Medical Convergence Sciences Research Center, Farhikhtegan Hospital Tehran Medical Sciences, Islamic Azad University, Tehran, Iran, Email: mhashemi@iautmu.ac.ir

Abstract

As a global disease with a high mortality rate, cancer remains a difficult-to-treat disorder, which is still challenging despite the numerous studies carried out in this field. Cancers have a heterogeneous nature which helps them to escape from the immune system and therapies. Conventional cancer therapies include surgery, radiation therapy, and chemotherapy. However, studies of targeted therapy and combinational therapies show promising results. Non-coding RNAs are molecules with critical regulatory functions in cells and can be divided into two main types: short non-coding RNAs including microRNAs (miRNAs) and long non-coding RNAs. miRNAs regulate gene expression at transcription and post-transcription levels and regulate protein function. They also play key regulatory roles in cancer and mediate various hallmarks of cancer including metastasis. For survival, cancer cells alter their microenvironment and neighboring cellular metabolism, with their increasing need for energy. Epithelial–mesenchymal transition is one of the mechanisms that enhance metastasis and invasion of tumor cells. This chapter discusses our current knowledge of miRNAs' regulatory role in cancer metastasis.

1. Introduction

MicroRNAs (miRNAs), molecules with ~22 nucleotides length, were first identified in *Caenorhabditis elegans* in the 1990s [1, 2]. miRNAs belong to non-coding RNAs (ncRNAs) and are synthesized through canonical or non-canonical pathways, and the difference is the use of Drosha or Dicer enzymes. The canonical pathway is initiated by the activity of RNA polymerase II to produce primary miRNA (pri-miRNA). Pri-miRNA is characterized by a hairpin structure and a 5′ cap and a 3′ polyadenylated tail which is not essential. Hairpin structure is a substrate for Drosha–DGCR8 complex, which generates precursor miRNA (pre-miRNA) with ~60 nucleotides. DGCR8's role is to find an N6-methyl adenylated GGAC in pri-miRNA for Drosha to function. Subsequently, pre-miRNA is transported into the cytoplasm by Exportin 5. Processed by Dicer, a miRNA–miRNA duplex is generated, which consists of a miRNA guide and passenger strands. The process is continued by loading the miRNA in RNA-induced silencing complex through Argonaute protein activity, which results in preparing miRNAs for doing their functions [3–5]. It has been shown that miRNA dysregulation is manifest in different disorders, particularly cancer [6]. Besides mutations or impairment in miRNA synthesis, machinery [7], rearrangement of chromosomes, genome amplification, and epigenetic alterations [8] also result in carcinogenesis. miRNA-15 and miRNA-16 are well-known examples of miRNAs with a decreased expression in B cell chronic lymphocytic leukemias [9]. miRNAs mainly interact with the 3′ untranslated region (3′ UTR) of their targets to exert their function. Besides, miRNAs could interact with the 5′ UTRs, gene promoters, and coding sequence of their targets. Binding to their target sites, miRNAs can suppress translation by decapping and deadenylation of mRNAs. In addition to their suppressor activity on transcription, miRNAs could also induce gene expression by interacting with the promoter region of genes. miRNAs are further involved in vital cellular processes including translation and gene regulation at transcriptional and post-transcriptional levels in the nucleus [10]. Because of the important role of miRNAs in cancer metastasis (Table 1), this chapter focuses on epithelial–mesenchymal transition (EMT) and matrix metalloproteinase (MMPs).

2. Role of miRNAs in regulating EMT

EMT was first described in embryo development as embryonic epithelial cells need to move to distant sites. However, EMT also takes part in physiological processes in adult tissues such as during wound healing, and pathological processes like cancer [19–21]. EMT is induced by paracrine signaling molecules such as transforming growth factor-β (TGF-β), Wnt and Notch signaling pathways, growth factors, hypoxia, cytokines, and integrins. These factors are leading to the activation of EMT master regulators including EMT-inducing transcription factors (EMT-TFs) consisting of TWIST family (TWIST1

Table 1. Summary of miRNAs involved in regulating cancer cell metastasis.

miRNA	Cancer Type	Function	Signaling Network	Remark	Ref
miR-328-3p	Breast cancer	Tumor suppressor	miR-328-3p/CPT1A/fatty acid β-oxidation	Downregulation of CPT1A by miR-328-3p. CPT1A increases invasion and metastasis by regulating fatty acid β-oxidation and influencing cell stemness.	[11]
miR-506-3p	Ovarian cancer	Tumor suppressor	miR-506-3p/EZH2	Downregulation of EZH2 by miR-506-3p resulted in decreasing invasion and metastasis.	[12]
miR-200b-3p	Gastric cancer	Tumor suppressor	miR-200b-3p/CXCL12/CXCR7	Downregulation of miR-200b-3p is associated with lymph node metastasis and a decrease in differentiation. Upregulation of miR-200b-3p suppresses tumor growth, invasion, and migration and induces cell cycle arrest via suppressing CXCL12. CXCR7 has inhibitory activity on tumor cells and is suppressed by CXCL12.	[13]
miR-29b-2/miR-338	Breast cancer	Tumor suppressor	FOXO3a-miRNA-VEGF-A/NRP1	FOXO3a enhances the expression of miR-29b-2 and miR-338. Overexpression of miR-29b-2/miR-338 inhibits EMT, invasion, and metastasis. miR-29b-2 targets VEGF-A and miR-338 targets NRP1.	[14]

(*Continued*)

Table 1. (*Continued*)

miR-27a-5p	Gastric cancer	Tumor suppressor	RAS/MEK/FOS PTEN/AKT/SMAD2	miR-27a-5p overexpression inhibits APEX1-induced cancer metastasis, proliferation, and doxorubicin resistance.	[15]
miR-335-5p	Colorectal cancer	Tumor promoting	miR-335-5p/RASA1	Exosome-transmitted miRNA-335-5p augments invasion and metastasis by facilitating EMT via targeting RASA1.	[16]
miR-4535	Melanoma cancer	Tumor promoting	miR-4535/autophagy	Exosomal miR-4535 of melanoma stem cells promotes metastasis by inhibiting the autophagy.	[17]
miR-23b-3p	Salivary adenoid cystic carcinoma	Tumor promoting	miR-23b-3p/PTEN	Exosomal miR-23b-3p increases the vascular permeability and decreases the expression of tight junction proteins. Exosomal miR-23b-3p overexpression promotes angiogenesis and migration. miR-23b-3p is a potential biomarker for distant metastasis.	[18]

and TWIST2), zinc-finger E-box-binding homeobox (ZEB1 and ZEB2) family, and factors encoded by SNAI1 (Snail) and SNAI2 (Slug). Additionally, forkhead box C2 (FOXC2), ovo-like transcriptional repressor (OVOL) family (OVOL1 and OVOL2), p53, grainyhead-like transcription factor 2 (GRHL2), paired-related homeobox 1 (PRRX1), and E74-like ETS transcription factor 5 (ELF5) are among the other transcription factors that regulate EMT induction [19, 22–24]. During EMT, cells acquire characteristics that help them to survive by increasing cancer progression pathways and gaining the ability to resist chemotherapy. For example, epithelial cells lose their E-cadherin, claudins, occludins, cytokeratins, apico-basal polarity, and cell–cell junctions while gaining mesenchymal characteristics including front–back polarity and increased N-cadherin, fibronectin, and vimentin to help them for metastasis and invasion [25–28].

Interestingly, miRNAs also play roles in mediating EMT. For instance, SNAIL-miRNA-34 and ZEB1-miRNA-200 participate in a feedback loop that controls EMT-TF function [19]. Extensive number of miRNAs are regulators of EMT in cancer cells by targeting EMT-TFs [29], such as miRNA-222-3p [30], miRNA-1246 [31], miRNA-490-5p [32], miRNA-543 [33], miRNA-375-3p [34], miRNA-1266-5p [35], and miRNA-16-5p [29]. Furthermore, direct targeting of eEF2k/MAPK/ERK signaling pathway by miRNA-193b-5p suppresses EMT in pancreatic cancer cells. Besides, miRNA-193b-5p promotes the expression of E-cadherin and claudin-1 but decreases Snail and TCF8/ZEB1 expression [36]. It is noteworthy that miRNAs can regulate downstream targets even if they are not the main members of EMT regulation. For example, miRNA-141-3p increases EMT by targeting nuclear factor kappa B (NF-κB) indirectly in prostate cancer. NF-κB has an oncogenic role and mediates the transcription of various genes involved in the regulation of EMT. miRNA-141-3p activates tumor necrosis factor receptor-associated factor 5 (TRAF5) and TRAF6 to mediate NF-κB and suppress EMT, invasion, and bone metastasis [37, 38]. As mentioned before, p53 affects tumor progression by regulating EMT. Zhang and colleagues reveal that miRNA-3622 family members including miRNA-3622a and miRNA-3622b have dual roles in prostate cancer. Indeed, miRNA-3622a exerts tumor suppression while miRNA-3622b is an oncomiR. They have shown that miRNA-3622b-3p regulates downstream targets of p53 such as AIFM2 to activate tumor cells. Besides, miRNA-3622b-3p mediates vimentin and induces EMT [39]. The regulatory effect of p53 on EMT has been the subject of studies in the past decade. p53 attenuates EMT-TFs by increasing the expression levels of EMT-inhibiting miRNAs. To increase EMT, EMT-TFs such as Snail suppress p53. For instance, p53 augments the expression levels of miRNA-340, miRNA-96, miRNA-183, miRNA-34, and miRNA-200 family to mediate EMT suppression via targeting ZEB1/2. In addition, p53 could suppress long non-coding RNAs (lncRNAs) via EMT-suppressing miRNAs. For instance, p53 suppresses lncRNA-H19 to reverse its function on tumor suppressor miRNA-200b and miRNA-200c [40]. Intriguingly, mutant p53, unlike its wild-type form, increases EMT by upregulating oncomiRs or downregulating tumor suppressor miRNAs.

miRNA-130b is a tumor inhibitor molecule with low expression levels in endometrial cancer cells. It has been demonstrated that miRNA-130b inhibits ZEB1 to attenuate EMT. Moreover, a mutant form of p53 downregulates the expression levels of miRNA-130b by binding to its promoter and hence increasing ZEB1 expression subsequently leading to EMT [41]. Conversely, miRNA-155 expression is positively regulated by mutant p53 to increase EMT in breast cancer. miRNA-155 suppresses a zinc-finger transcriptional repressor, ZNF652, by binding to its 3′UTR site. ZNF652 attenuates the key regulators of invasion and metastasis including TGFB1/2, epidermal growth factor receptor (EGFR), VIM, and SMAD2 [42]. On the other hand, miRNA-651-3p expression is downregulated in ovarian cancer cells. miRNA-651-3p targets zinc-finger protein 703 (ZNF703) and MEK/ERK signaling to inhibit EMT [17]. In other instances, miRNA-21-5p is highly expressed in laryngeal carcinoma by triggering EMT through the inhibition of Kruppel-like factor 6 (KLF6) [43].

miRNA-200 family is the key regulator of EMT by mainly targeting E-cadherin. There are five miRNAs in this family that forms two clusters including miRNA-200a/miRNA-141 and miRNA-200b/miRNA-200c/miRNA-429. They increase E-cadherin expression by targeting ZEB1 and ZEB2. As an example, the inhibitory effect of miRNA-200c/miRNA-141 on EMT through the targeting of ZEB1/2 in head and neck squamous cell carcinoma [44]. In another study, the results have demonstrated the regulation of EMT by two miRNA families in non-small cell lung cancer cells of which Foxf2 is their common target. Foxf2 expression is highly correlated with ZEB1 and is overexpressed in cancer cells to induce EMT, invasion, and metastasis. In one study, it was revealed that miRNA-200 family and miRNA-183/96/182 cluster target Foxf2 to inhibit EMT, metastasis, and invasion. Interestingly, Foxf2 adversely affects miRNA-200 and E-cadherin expression as a negative feedback loop [45].

miRNAs' regulatory effects on EMT can be controlled by other upstream ncRNAs and mediators. Circular RNA (CircRNA)-0087429 is downregulated in cervical cancer cells and has inhibitory roles on proliferation, invasion, metastasis, and angiogenesis. On the contrary, miRNA-5003-3p is upregulated and mediates EMT by decreasing osteoglycin. Osteoglycin is a member of the small leucine-rich proteoglycan family in the extracellular matrix (ECM) and is involved in various cellular processes, including cell adhesion, signal transduction, and DNA repair. To function, circRNA-0087429 binds to osteoglycin in competition with miRNA-5003-3p to reverse EMT [46]. Increased expression levels of miRNA-224-5p induce invasion, metastasis, and EMT in hepatocellular cancer cells. miRNA-224-5p is upregulated by E2F1 causing binding to its promoter site. miRNA-224-5p directly targets melanoregulin to increase its expression and subsequently induce EMT, invasion, and metastasis in cancer cells [47]. Furthermore, miRNA-92a is targeted by lncRNA-OIP5-AS1, as EMT inducer. lncRNA-OIP5-AS1 increases integrin alpha 6 by suppressing miRNA-92a to increase EMT, invasion, cell viability, and metastasis in ovarian cancer cells [48]. Furthermore, lncRNA1410 (LINC01410) is reported to act as a tumor promoter factor in bladder cancer with poor prognosis. Linc01410 sponges miRNA-4319 to suppress its function and promote Snail for increasing EMT, invasion, and metastasis [49]. Besides, lncRNA snoRNA host gene 6 (SNHG6) targets miRNA-125b to suppress its inhibitory function on Snail1/2 and thereby promoting EMT, metastasis, and invasion [50]. Interestingly, circRNA–miRNA–lncRNA pathway is suggested to be involved in mediating EMT in cancer. CircRTN4 suppresses miRNA-497-5p to increase lncRNA HOTTIP expression level and promote EMT. CircRNT4 function results in the elevation of Snail, Twist, ZEB1, Slug, and N-cadherin in pancreatic ductal adenocarcinoma [51]. Remarkably, EMT can interfere with autophagy pathway through the lncRNA/miRNA axis [52]. An example is a work done by Xiong *et al.* on the H19/let-7/Lin28 axis, which is involved in autophagic inhibition of EMT in breast cancer [53].

EMT pathway can also augment chemo- and radio-resistance in cancer cells by regulating miRNAs. For instance, miRNA-125b downregulates EVA1A to suppress EMT and autophagy to reverse oxaliplatin resistance in hepatocellular carcinoma [54]. On the other hand, miRNA-1275 inhibits EMT by increasing its radiosensitivity through direct suppression of Wnt/β-catenin signaling pathway [55]. Radiation therapy could also act as an EMT inducer in cancer cells. It has been demonstrated that ionizing radiation mediates smad2/3 phosphorylation resulting in TGF-β activation and subsequent activation of EMT [56]. In another study, PI3K/Akt/mTOR signaling pathways were studied in relation to radio-resistance in esophageal squamous cell carcinoma. In this study, tumor suppressor circVRK1 acts as an upstream mediator of miRNA-624-3p to regulate PTEN/PI3K/Akt signaling pathway and inhibit radio-resistance by reversing EMT [57]. In esophageal squamous cell carcinoma, miRNA-205 exerts radio-resistance function by activating DNA repair mechanisms, mediating apoptosis inhibition, and increasing EMT. Furthermore, Sp1 factor acts as an upstream mediator of miRNA-205 to promote radio-resistance through PTEN/PI3K/Akt axis [58]. In addition, miRNA-875-5p exerts its tumor-inhibitory role in prostate cancer to counteract radio-resistance. miRNA-875-5p downregulates EGFR–ZEB1 axis, which mediates CHK1-induced DNA repair and subsequently induces radiosensitivity (Figure 1) [59].

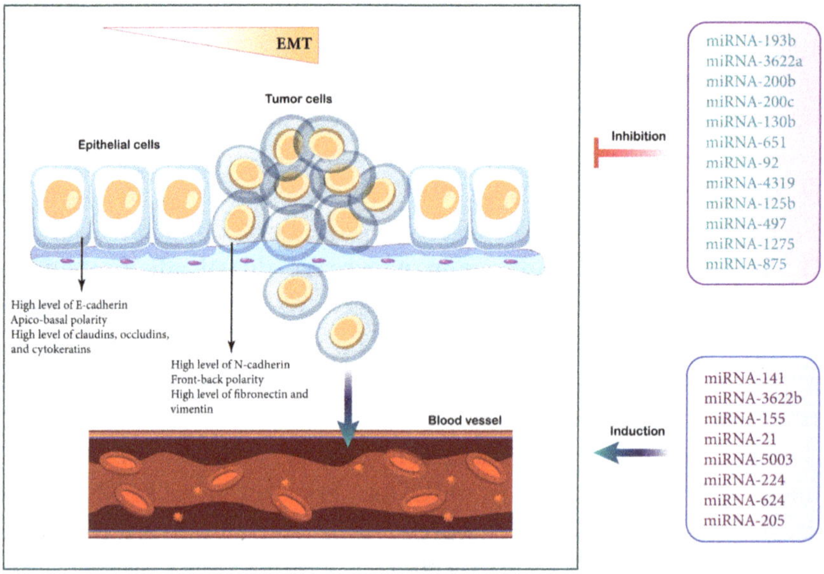

Figure 1. An illustration of the EMT pathway regulating metastasis through the inhibitory or inducing roles of miRNAs.

3. miRNAs regulating MMPs

Matrix metalloproteinases (MMPs) belong to a family of zinc-dependent endopeptidases that were initially identified as regulators of the ECM with functions in tissue remodeling accompanied by developmental processes and human diseases. At first, it was assumed that MMPs are only for matrix modulation, but we now know that their function is beyond the physiologic and pathologic regulation of the matrix. They are, in fact, the potent modulators of cellular response and the microenvironment. One of their important roles is to degrade the components of ECM for tissue modeling and remodeling during health and disease states. Importantly, MMPs increase the activity of growth factors and hormones in ECM. MMPs are classified based on their structure and substrate specificity into different groups, such as collagenases (MMP1, MMP8, MMP13), stromelysins (MMP3 and MMP10), and gelatinases (MMP2 and MMP9). Structurally, MMPs consist of (1) signal peptide, (2) *N*-terminal propeptide domain, (3) catalytic domain, (4) hinge region, and (5) *C*-terminal hemopexin-like domain. MMPs are overexpressed in many types of cancer and play a critical role in cancer cell invasion and migration [60–62]. MMPs' functions could facilitate tumor progression. In fact, they regulate cell growth, apoptosis, differentiation, metastasis, and angiogenesis [63]. MMPs also significantly affect the promotion of invasion and metastasis and specifically MMP1, MMP2, MMP3, MMP7, MMP9, MMP10, MMP11, MMP13, MMP14, MMP16, MMP26, and MMP28 are among them [64]. However, MMPs can also negatively affect tumor growth by regulating TNF-α and Fas [65] expression.

MMP2 and MMP9 increase invasion and metastasis through the degradation of collagen IV of the basement membrane [65]. Furthermore, the activation of MMP2 and MMP9 is positively related to tumor grade and poor prognosis. They can also be used as possible biomarkers for follow-up or assessing the response of diseases to therapy [66–68]. In a study on bladder cancer, miRNA-34a shows an antitumor activity. Indeed, miRNA-34a inhibits MMP-2 to suppress cancer cell motility, invasion, and metastasis. In addition, overexpression of miRNA-34a was reversely associated with lymph node metastasis, clinical disease stage, and overall survival [69]. On the other hand, miRNA-29b is shown to be a tumor suppressor in colorectal cancers. miRNA-29b attenuates the expression of E26 transformation-specific (ETS) variant 4 (ETV4) to decrease EGFR function. Subsequently, the function of extracellular signal-regulated kinase (ERK) signaling pathway is suppressed which results in the depletion of MMP2, MMP9, vimentin, and elevation of E-cadherin to decrease EMT and metastasis [70]. In contrast, miRNA-1297 silencing is accompanied by overexpression of PTEN, which results in the inhibition of metastasis in prostate cancer cells via MMP2, MMP9, and N-cadherin downturning [71]. Besides, a study on gastric cancers revealed that circRNA-101996 inhibits miRNA-143, a tumor suppressor agent. In fact, miRNA-143 mediates the downregulation of ten–eleven translocation (TET2) gene to suppress DNA methylation of MMP2 and MMP9, thereby suppressing malignancy of gastric cancer cells in vivo and in vitro [72]. In another example, tumor suppressor miRNA, miRNA-125b, is able to counteract the migration and invasion of hepatocellular carcinoma via downregulation of MMP2, MMP9, and MMP14 mRNA expression [73]. Moreover, inhibition of MMP13 is also shown to decrease tumor cell metastasis. miRNA-27b targets 3′UTR region of MMP13 to abolish its expression and suppresses the invasion and migration of cutaneous squamous cell carcinoma [74]. miRNAs, miRNA-377-3p also exerts tumor suppression activities in ovarian cancer. Targeted by miRNA-377-3p, MMP16 expression is decreased and is associated with reduced colony formation rate, growth, metastasis, and invasion [75].

MMP1 is another member of the MMPs family with metastasis-inducing roles. A recently published research reveals that miRNA-145-5p directly targets MMP1 to abolish its expression and thereby suppresses metastasis, stemness, and chemo-resistance induced by Imiquimod. As a confirmation, imiquimod inhibits miRNA-145 expression via DNA methylation and miRNA-145/MMP1 axis attenuation, restoring MMP1 activity [76]. Moreover, MMPs can act as upstream regulators of miRNAs thereby increasing metastasis. For example, MMP3 abrogates miRNA-421's negative effects on invasion, proliferation, and metastasis in hepatocellular carcinoma [77].

4. miRNAs decreasing cancer metastasis

The critical role of miRNAs in the regulation of gene expression and modulation of cancer hallmarks is already elucidated. However, the scope of miRNAs activity is not limited to these functions as they can also control metastasis by targeting vital metabolic processes and influencing malignancy characteristics. For survival, cancer cells need to increase their metabolism and energy production. Glucose-related pathways such as glycolysis, glycogenolysis, pentose phosphate pathway (PPP), and gluconeogenesis are the mechanisms for increasing energy required for cellular functions. Expression of glucose transporters (GLUTs) is increased in cancers and is associated with tumor malignancy, and they can be regulated by miRNAs. miRNA-199-5p inhibits glucose metabolism by targeting GLUT1 in non-small cell lung cancer to suppress metastasis and proliferation. Furthermore, miRNA-140 attenuates hexokinase 2, the key enzyme in the glycolysis pathway and the branching point of PPP, to suppress the migration of hepatocellular carcinoma. This affects miRNA-140 that can be reversely regulated by lncRNA-NR2F1-AS1.

Interestingly, focal adhesions are large molecular complexes that transmit cellular signaling from the inside to the outside, bi-directionally. They undergo various reorganizations in response to tumor microenvironment stimuli. Integrins are a group of focal adhesions, which form the adhesome with their associated complexes and are a potent target of miRNAs. miRNA-198 inhibits the actin filament branching and elongation, thereby suppressing migration and metastasis in head and neck squamous cell carcinoma [78–81].

miRNAs can also affect bone metastasis by targeting cells located in the bone microenvironment. For instance, conditioned medium of breast cancer cells that were transfected with miRNA-124 show an inhibitory effect on the expression of MMP13 by osteoblasts leading to the manifestation of breast cancer bone metastasis [82]. Suppressing the activity of miRNAs can affect metastasis through the regulation of upstream factors. The regulatory role of circRNAs and lncRNAs on miRNAs has been elucidated in previous studies. Based on the theory of competitive endogenous RNAs, there is a common site in lncRNAs and circRNAs for binding to miRNA. Furthermore, by regulating miRNAs, lncRNAs and circRNAs can also regulate the expression of miRNA targets. Regulation of miRNAs by circRNAs is evaluated in different cancer types [83]. Such examples suggest the association of metastasis with other ncRNAs such as circP4HB/miRNA-133a-5p/vimentin axis [84], circUBE2D2/miRNA-376a-3p/EIF4G2 axis [85] in lung cancer, circ-0008043/miRNA-326/RAB21 axis in hepatocellular carcinoma [86], and HNRNPC/circXRCC5/miRNA-655-3p/RREB1/UBA2 axis in gastric cancer [13]. In the case of LINC00205, an oncogenic lncRNA associated with a poor prognosis of gastric cancer cells is involved in their proliferation, tumor progression, invasion, and metastasis. miRNA-26a is a downstream target of

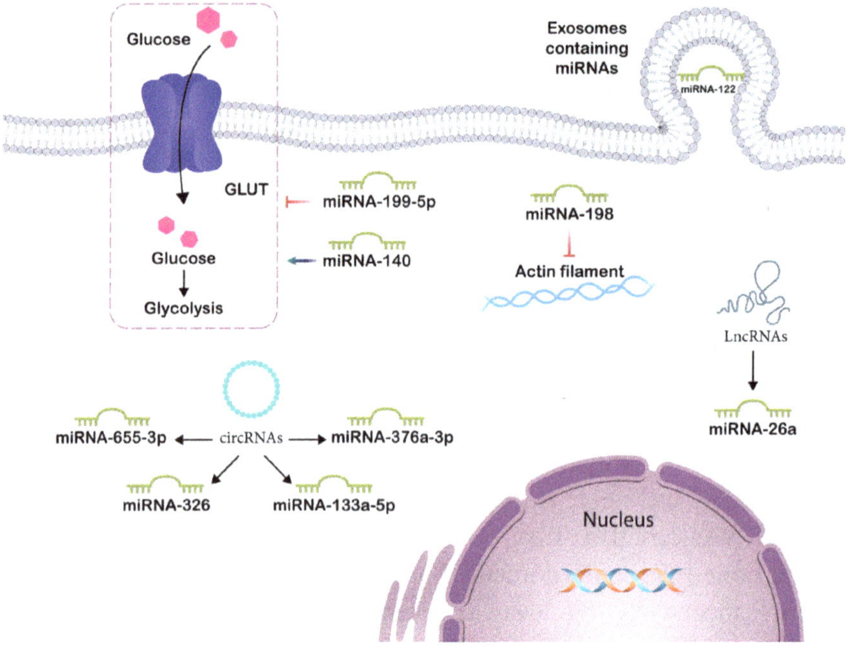

Figure 2. The mechanisms by which miRNAs regulate cancer metastasis. miRNAs can target cellular metabolism pathways such as glycolysis to suppress or increase metastasis. Besides, targeting elements involved in the metastasis process like actin are of importance for regulating metastasis. In addition, different upstream modulators such as circRNAs and lncRNAs can mediate the function of miRNA in metastasis.

LINC00205 and its inhibition by this lncRNA results in the activation of miRNA-26a which targets EZH2, HMGA2, and USP15, thereby promoting EMT and tumor progression [87] (Figure 2).

5. miRNAs enhancing cancer metastasis

In the case of oncogenic miRNAs, all the mechanisms regulated by tumor suppressor miRNAs could be affected by oncomiRs too. For instance, breast cancer cells secrete vesicles containing miRNA-122, which suppress glucose uptake. This is accomplished by the down-regulation of pyruvate kinase enzyme in non-tumor cells located in the pre-metastatic niche to then facilitate metastasis by increasing nutrients for tumor cells [88]. Interestingly, oncomiRs could augment metastasis by targeting the immune cell infiltration of the tumor microenvironment. miRNA-6852-3p involved in the metastasis of hepatocellular carcinoma cells regulates their susceptibility to natural killer cells via targeting ICAM-1. In fact, miRNA-6852-3p overexpression leads to less susceptibility of cancer cells to the natural killer cell-mediated cytotoxicity, thereby increasing metastasis [89].

In the tumor site, there is a small subgroup of cancer cells with properties like stem cells, named cancer stem cells. These cells are critical for cancer formation, metastasis, therapy resistance, and tumor recurrence. miRNA-210 expression is increased in hypoxic conditions and promotes the ability of breast cancer stem cells to metastasize and proliferate. Besides, miRNA-210 overexpression leads to the depletion of E-cadherin via targeting its suppressor, Snail [90]. In addition, EMT and cancer metastasis are key factors in developing drug resistance, regulated by numerous oncomiRs in various cancers [91, 92].

6. Conclusion and remarks

The recent two decades have seen exponential growth in the study of miRNAs' role and importance in cancer. This review touches on many of the facets of miRNA function in mediating cancer metastasis, including regulation of EMT and MMPs. The upstream regulators of miRNAs such as lncRNAs and circRNAs are also discussed in this chapter. It is noteworthy that a high number of studies elucidate miRNAs targets in the context of cancer metastasis. However, finding effective therapeutic targets among this extensive network of molecules is crucial for future studies to address.

Conflict of interest:

The authors declare no conflict of interest.

References

1. Lee, R.C., R.L. Feinbaum, and V. Ambros, *The C. elegans heterochronic gene lin-4 encodes small RNAs with antisense complementarity to lin-14.* Cell, 1993. **75**(5): p. 843–854.
2. Reinhart, B.J., et al., *The 21-nucleotide let-7 RNA regulates developmental timing in Caenorhabditis elegans.* Nature, 2000. **403**(6772): p. 901–906.
3. Bartel, D.P., *Metazoan micrornas.* Cell, 2018. **173**(1): p. 20–51.
4. Alarcón, C.R., et al., *N6-methyladenosine marks primary microRNAs for processing.* Nature, 2015. **519**(7544): p. 482–485.
5. Leitão, A.L. and F.J. Enguita, *A structural view of miRNA biogenesis and function.* Non-Coding RNA, 2022. **8**(1): p. 10.
6. Ha, M. and V.N. Kim, *Regulation of microRNA biogenesis.* Nature Reviews Molecular Cell Biology, 2014. **15**(8): p. 509–524.
7. Lin, S. and R.I. Gregory, *MicroRNA biogenesis pathways in cancer.* Nature Reviews Cancer, 2015. **15**(6): p. 321–333.
8. Annese, T., et al., *MicroRNAs biogenesis, functions and role in tumor angiogenesis.* Frontiers in Oncology, 2020. **10**: p. 581007.
9. Calin, G.A., et al., *Frequent deletions and down-regulation of micro-RNA genes miR15 and miR16 at 13q14 in chronic lymphocytic leukemia.* Proceedings of the National Academy of Sciences, 2002. **99**(24): p. 15524–15529.
10. O'Brien, J., et al., *Overview of microRNA biogenesis, mechanisms of actions, and circulation.* Frontiers in Endocrinology, 2018. **9**: p. 402.
11. Zeng, F., et al., *Fatty acid β-oxidation promotes breast cancer stemness and metastasis via the miRNA-328-3p-CPT1A pathway.* Cancer Gene Therapy, 2022. **29**(3): p. 383–395.
12. Sun, Y., C. Meng, and G. Liu, *MicroRNA-506-3p inhibits ovarian cancer metastasis by down-regulating the expression of EZH2.* Journal of Cancer, 2022. **13**(3): p. 943.
13. Liu, Z.-L., et al., *CircXRCC5 foster gastric cancer growth and metastasis by the HNRNPC/circXRCC5/miR-655-3p/RREB1/UBA2 positive feedback loop.* Cancer Gene Therapy, 2022: p. 1–14.
14. Song, Y., et al., *FOXO3a-driven miRNA signatures suppresses VEGF-A/NRP1 signaling and breast cancer metastasis.* Oncogene, 2021. **40**(4): p. 777–790.

15. He, H., et al., *The APEX1/miRNA-27a-5p axis plays key roles in progression, metastasis and targeted chemotherapy of gastric cancer.* International Journal of Pharmaceutics, 2021. **599**: p. 120446.
16. Sun, X., et al., *Exosome-transmitted miRNA-335-5p promotes colorectal cancer invasion and metastasis by facilitating EMT via targeting RASA1.* Molecular Therapy-Nucleic Acids, 2021. **24**: p. 164–174.
17. Liu, D., et al., *Exosomal microRNA-4535 of melanoma stem cells promotes metastasis by inhibiting autophagy pathway.* Stem Cell Reviews and Reports, 2022: p. 1–15.
18. Hou, C.-x., et al., *Exosomal microRNA-23b-3p promotes tumor angiogenesis and metastasis by targeting PTEN in salivary adenoid cystic carcinoma.* Carcinogenesis, 2022. **43**(7): p. 682–692.
19. Lambert, A.W. and R.A. Weinberg, *Linking EMT programmes to normal and neoplastic epithelial stem cells.* Nature Reviews Cancer, 2021. **21**(5): p. 325–338.
20. Dongre, A. and R.A. Weinberg, *New insights into the mechanisms of epithelial–mesenchymal transition and implications for cancer.* Nature Reviews Molecular Cell Biology, 2019. **20**(2): p. 69–84.
21. Ashrafizadeh, M., et al., *New insight towards development of paclitaxel and docetaxel resistance in cancer cells: EMT as a novel molecular mechanism and therapeutic possibilities.* Biomedicine & Pharmacotherapy, 2021. **141**: p. 111824.
22. Shibue, T. and R.A. Weinberg, *EMT, CSCs, and drug resistance: The mechanistic link and clinical implications.* Nature Reviews Clinical Oncology, 2017. **14**(10): p. 611–629.
23. Lamouille, S., J. Xu, and R. Derynck, *Molecular mechanisms of epithelial–mesenchymal transition.* Nature Reviews Molecular Cell Biology, 2014. **15**(3): p. 178–196.
24. Ashrafizadeh, M., et al., *MicroRNAs and their influence on the ZEB family: Mechanistic aspects and therapeutic applications in cancer therapy.* Biomolecules, 2020. **10**(7): p. 1040.
25. Nieto, M.A., et al., *EMT: 2016.* Cell, 2016. **166**(1): p. 21–45.
26. Sadrkhanloo, M., et al., *STAT3-EMT axis in tumors: Modulation of cancer metastasis, stemness and therapy response.* Pharmacological Research, 2022. **182**: p. 106311.

27. Ashrafizadeh, M., et al., *Role of microRNA/epithelial-to-mesenchymal transition axis in the metastasis of bladder cancer.* Biomolecules, 2020. **10**(8): p. 1159.
28. Ashrafizadeh, M., et al., *Association of the epithelial–mesenchymal transition (EMT) with cisplatin resistance.* International Journal of Molecular Sciences, 2020. **21**(11): p. 4002.
29. Feng, J., et al., *The role of microRNA in the regulation of tumor epithelial–mesenchymal transition.* Cells, 2022. **11**(13): p. 1981.
30. Gao, Y., et al., *BRAFV600E mutation-responsive miRNA-222-3p promotes metastasis of papillary thyroid cancer cells via snail-induced EMT.* Frontiers in Endocrinology, 2022. **13**: p. 843334.
31. Wang, Y., et al., *MicroRNA-543 inhibits the proliferation, migration, invasion, and epithelial-mesenchymal transition of triple-negative breast cancer cells via down-regulation of ACTL6A gene.* Clinical and Translational Oncology, 2022. **24**(1): p. 84–92.
32. Huang, X., et al., *MicroRNA-16-5p suppresses cell proliferation and angiogenesis in colorectal cancer by negatively regulating forkhead box K1 to block the PI3K/Akt/mTOR pathway.* European Journal of Histochemistry: EJH, 2022. **66**(2): p. 3333.
33. Li, Y., et al., *MicroRNA-190b expression predicts a good prognosis and attenuates the malignant progression of pancreatic cancer by targeting MEF2C and TCF4.* Oncology Reports, 2022. **47**(1): p. 1–13.
34. Jhan, J.-H., et al., *MicroRNA-375-3p suppresses upper tract urothelial carcinoma cell migration and invasion via targeting Derlin-1.* Cancers, 2022. **14**(4): p. 880.
35. Peng, D., et al., *MicroRNA-671-5p reduces tumorigenicity of ovarian cancer via suppressing HDAC5 and HIF-1α expression.* Chemico-Biological Interactions, 2022. **355**: p. 109780.
36. Gurbuz, N., et al., *miRNA-193b-5p suppresses pancreatic cancer cell proliferation, invasion, epithelial mesenchymal transition, and tumor growth by inhibiting eEF2K.* Anti-Cancer Agents in Medicinal Chemistry, 2022. **22**(14): p. 2607–2618.
37. Huang, S., et al., *Downregulation of miR-141-3p promotes bone metastasis via activating NF-κB signaling in prostate cancer.* Journal of Experimental & Clinical Cancer Research, 2017. **36**(1): p. 1–13.

38. Mirzaei, S., et al., *NF-κB as a regulator of cancer metastasis and therapy response: A focus on epithelial–mesenchymal transition*. Journal of Cellular Physiology, 2022. **237**(7): p. 2770–2795.
39. Zhang, Y., et al., *The microRNA-3622 family at the 8p21 locus exerts oncogenic effects by regulating the p53-downstream gene network in prostate cancer progression*. Oncogene, 2022: p. 1–11.
40. Parfenyev, S., et al., *Interplay between p53 and non-coding RNAs in the regulation of EMT in breast cancer*. Cell Death & Disease, 2021. **12**(1): p. 1–16.
41. Dong, P., et al., *Mutant p53 gain-of-function induces epithelial–mesenchymal transition through modulation of the miR-130b–ZEB1 axis*. Oncogene, 2013. **32**(27): p. 3286–3295.
42. Neilsen, P.M., et al., *Mutant p53 drives invasion in breast tumors through up-regulation of miR-155*. Oncogene, 2013. **32**(24): p. 2992–3000.
43. Xu, Y., *MiRNA-21-5p accelerates EMT and inhibits apoptosis of laryngeal carcinoma via inhibiting KLF6 expression*. Biochemical Genetics, 2022: p. 1–15.
44. Tamagawa, S., et al., *Role of miR-200c/miR-141 in the regulation of epithelial-mesenchymal transition and migration in head and neck squamous cell carcinoma*. International Journal of Molecular Medicine, 2014. **33**(4): p. 879–886.
45. Kundu, S.T., et al., *The miR-200 family and the miR-183~96~182 cluster target Foxf2 to inhibit invasion and metastasis in lung cancers*. Oncogene, 2016. **35**(2): p. 173–186.
46. Yang, M., et al., *EIF4A3-regulated circ_0087429 can reverse EMT and inhibit the progression of cervical cancer via miR-5003-3p-dependent upregulation of OGN expression*. Journal of Experimental & Clinical Cancer Research, 2022. **41**(1): p. 1–20.
47. Li, A., N. Wu, and J. Sun, *E2F1-induced microRNA-224-5p expression is associated with hepatocellular carcinoma cell migration, invasion and epithelial-mesenchymal transition via MREG*. Oncology Letters, 2022. **23**(3): p. 1–14.
48. Wang, Y., et al., *Long non-coding RNA OIP5-AS1 suppresses microRNA-92a to augment proliferation and metastasis of ovarian cancer cells through upregulating ITGA6*. Journal of Ovarian Research, 2022. **15**(1): p. 1–12.

49. Guo, W., et al., *LINC01410 leads the migration, invasion and EMT of bladder cancer cells by modulating miR-4319/Snail1.* Cancer Cell International, 2021. **21**(1): p. 1–12.
50. Wang, C., et al., *Upregulation of lncRNA snoRNA host gene 6 regulates NUAK family SnF1-like kinase-1 expression by competitively binding microRNA-125b and interacting with Snail1/2 in bladder cancer.* Journal of Cellular Biochemistry, 2019. **120**(1): p. 357–367.
51. Wong, C.H., et al., *CircRTN4 promotes pancreatic cancer progression through a novel CircRNA-miRNA-lncRNA pathway and stabilizing epithelial-mesenchymal transition protein.* Molecular Cancer, 2022. **21**(1): p. 1–15.
52. Si, L., et al., *Regulatory effects of incRNAs and miRNAs on the crosstalk between autophagy and EMT in cancer: A new era for cancer treatment.* Journal of Cancer Research and Clinical Oncology, 2022: p. 1–18.
53. Xiong, H., et al., *H19/let-7/Lin28 ceRNA network mediates autophagy inhibiting epithelial-mesenchymal transition in breast cancer.* International Journal of Oncology, 2020. **56**(3): p. 794–806.
54. Ren, W.-W., et al., *MicroRNA-125b reverses oxaliplatin resistance in hepatocellular carcinoma by negatively regulating EVA1A mediated autophagy.* Cell Death & Disease, 2018. **9**(5): p. 1–15.
55. Xie, C., et al., *MicroRNA-1275 induces radiosensitization in oesophageal cancer by regulating epithelial-to-mesenchymal transition via Wnt/β-catenin pathway.* Journal of Cellular and Molecular Medicine, 2020. **24**(1): p. 747–759.
56. Zhou, S., et al., *The role of epithelial-mesenchymal transition in regulating radioresistance.* Critical Reviews in Oncology/Hematology, 2020. **150**: p. 102961.
57. He, Y., et al., *CircVRK1 regulates tumor progression and radioresistance in esophageal squamous cell carcinoma by regulating miR-624-3p/PTEN/PI3K/AKT signaling pathway.* International Journal of Biological Macromolecules, 2019. **125**: p. 116–123.
58. Pan, F., et al., *Sp1-mediated transcriptional activation of miR-205 promotes radioresistance in esophageal squamous cell carcinoma.* Oncotarget, 2017. **8**(4): p. 5735.
59. El Bezawy, R., et al., *MiR-875-5p counteracts epithelial-to-mesenchymal transition and enhances radiation response in prostate cancer through repression of the EGFR-ZEB1 axis.* Cancer Letters, 2017. **395**: p. 53–62.

60. McCawley, L.J. and L.M. Matrisian, *Matrix metalloproteinases: They're not just for matrix anymore!* Current Opinion in Cell Biology, 2001. **13**(5): p. 534–540.
61. Liao, H.-Y., et al., *Roles of matrix metalloproteinase-7 (MMP-7) in cancer.* Clinical Biochemistry, 2021. **92**: p. 9–18.
62. Hofmann, U.B., et al., *Matrix metalloproteinases in human melanoma.* Journal of Investigative Dermatology, 2000. **115**(3): p. 337–344.
63. Welch, D.R. and D.R. Hurst, *Defining the hallmarks of metastasis.* Cancer Research, 2019. **79**(12): p. 3011–3027.
64. Niland, S., A.X. Riscanevo, and J.A. Eble, *Matrix metalloproteinases shape the tumor microenvironment in cancer progression.* International Journal of Molecular Sciences, 2021. **23**(1): p. 146.
65. Abdel-Hamid, N.M. and S.A. Abass, *Matrix metalloproteinase contribution in management of cancer proliferation, metastasis and drug targeting.* Molecular Biology Reports, 2021. **48**(9): p. 6525–6538.
66. Zhou, W., et al., *Increased expression of MMP-2 and MMP-9 indicates poor prognosis in glioma recurrence.* Biomedicine & Pharmacotherapy, 2019. **118**: p. 109369.
67. Fouad, H., et al., *MMP-2 and MMP-9 as prognostic markers for the early detection of urinary bladder cancer.* Journal of Biochemical and Molecular Toxicology, 2019. **33**(4): p. e22275.
68. Alrehaili, A.A., et al., *Clinical significance of plasma MMP-2 and MMP-9 levels as biomarkers for tumor expression in breast cancer patients in Egypt.* Molecular Biology Reports, 2020. **47**(2): p. 1153–1160.
69. Chou, K.Y., et al., *MicroRNA-34a-5p serves as a tumor suppressor by regulating the cell motility of bladder cancer cells through matrix metalloproteinase-2 silencing.* Oncology Reports, 2021. **45**(3): p. 911–920.
70. Leng, Y., et al., *Overexpression of microRNA-29b inhibits epithelial-mesenchymal transition and angiogenesis of colorectal cancer through the ETV4/ERK/EGFR axis.* Cancer Cell International, 2021. **21**(1): p. 1–19.
71. Wang, L., et al., *Silencing miRNA-1297 suppresses the invasion and migration of prostate cancer cells via targeting modulation of PTEN and blocking of the AKT/ERK pathway.* Experimental and Therapeutic Medicine, 2021. **22**(1): p. 1–9.
72. Huang, F., et al., *Circular RNA Hsa_circRNA_101996 promotes the development of gastric cancer via upregulating matrix*

metalloproteinases-2/matrixmetalloproteinases-9throughmicroRNA-143/ten-eleven translocation-2 pathway. Journal of Cancer, 2021. **12**(22): p. 6665.
73. Kim, H.S., et al., *Exosomal miR-125b exerts anti-metastatic properties and predicts early metastasis of hepatocellular carcinoma.* Frontiers in Oncology, 2021. **11**: p. 637247.
74. Liang, D. and Z. Zhang, *MicroRNA-27b-3p inhibits the proliferation and invasion of cutaneous squamous cell carcinoma by targeting EGFR and MMP-13.* Oncology Letters, 2021. **22**(4): p. 1–9.
75. Wang, H., C. Qi, and D. Wan, *MicroRNA-377-3p targeting MMP-16 inhibits ovarian cancer cell growth, invasion, and interstitial transition.* Annals of Translational Medicine, 2021. **9**(2): p. 124.
76. Zhu, S., et al., *The miR-145–MMP1 axis is a critical regulator for imiquimod-induced cancer stemness and chemoresistance.* Pharmacological Research, 2022. **179**: p. 106196.
77. Zhang, B. and J. Zhou, *CircSEC24A (hsa_circ_0003528) interference suppresses epithelial-mesenchymal transition of hepatocellular carcinoma cells via miR-421/MMP3 axis.* Bioengineered, 2022. **13**(4): p. 9050–9063.
78. Quirico, L., et al., *miRNA-guided reprogramming of glucose and glutamine metabolism and its impact on cell adhesion/migration during solid tumor progression.* Cellular and Molecular Life Sciences, 2022. **79**(4): p. 1–16.
79. Xu, Y., et al., *miRNA-199a-5p/SLC2A1 axis regulates glucose metabolism in non-small cell lung cancer.* Journal of Cancer, 2022. **13**(7): p. 2352.
80. Li, X., et al., *NR2F1-AS1/miR-140/HK2 axis regulates hypoxia-induced glycolysis and migration in hepatocellular carcinoma.* Cancer Management and Research, 2021. **13**: p. 427.
81. Sundaram, G.M., et al., *EGF hijacks miR-198/FSTL1 wound-healing switch and steers a two-pronged pathway toward metastasis.* Journal of Experimental Medicine, 2017. **214**(10): p. 2889–2900.
82. Haider, M.-T., D.J. Smit, and H. Taipaleenmäki, *MicroRNAs: Emerging regulators of metastatic bone disease in breast cancer.* Cancers, 2022. **14**(3): p. 729.

83. Guo, L., et al., *Critical roles of cCircular RNA in tumor metastasis via acting as a sponge of miRNA/isomiR*. International Journal of Molecular Sciences, 2022. **23**(13): p. 7024.
84. Wang, T., et al., *The circRNA circP4HB promotes NSCLC aggressiveness and metastasis by sponging miR-133a-5p*. Biochemical and Biophysical Research Communications, 2019. **513**(4): p. 904–911.
85. Tong, J., et al., *Circular RNA-UBE2D2 accelerates the proliferation and metastasis of non-small cell lung cancer cells via modulating microRNA-376a-3p/eukaryotic translation initiation factor 4γ2 axis*. Bioengineered, 2022. **13**(3): p. 5942–5953.
86. Zhang, K., et al., *Circular RNA Circ_0008043 promotes the proliferation and metastasis of hepatocellular carcinoma cells by regulating the microRNA (miR)-326/RAB21 axis*. Bioengineered, 2022. **13**(3): p. 6600–6614.
87. Huangfu, L., et al., *Novel prognostic marker LINC00205 promotes tumorigenesis and metastasis by competitively suppressing miRNA-26a in gastric cancer*. Cell Death Discovery, 2022. **8**(1): p. 1–10.
88. Fong, M.Y., et al., *Breast-cancer-secreted miR-122 reprograms glucose metabolism in premetastatic niche to promote metastasis*. Nature Cell Biology, 2015. **17**(2): p. 183–194.
89. Shi, M., et al., *Hsa_circ_0007456 regulates the natural killer cell-mediated cytotoxicity toward hepatocellular carcinoma via the miR-6852-3p/ICAM-1 axis*. Cell Death & Disease, 2021. **12**(1): p. 1–13.
90. Tang, T., et al., *Up-regulation of miR-210 induced by a hypoxic microenvironment promotes breast cancer stem cell metastasis, proliferation, and self-renewal by targeting E-cadherin*. The FASEB Journal, 2018. **32**(12): p. 6965–6981.
91. Pan, G., et al., *EMT-associated microRNAs and their roles in cancer stemness and drug resistance*. Cancer Communications, 2021. **41**(3): p. 199–217.
92. Dong, B., et al., *MiRNA-mediated EMT and CSCs in cancer chemoresistance*. Experimental Hematology & Oncology, 2021. **10**(1): p. 1–12.

https://doi.org/10.1142/9789811267390_0003

Chapter 3

MicroRNAs (miRNAs) in therapy response of human cancers: Biological aspects

Mahshid Deldar Abad Paskeh[1,2], Sepideh Mirzaei[3], Shokooh Salimimoghadam[4], Mehrdad Hashemi[1,2]* and Amir Reza Aref[5,6]

[1]*Department of Genetics, Faculty of Advanced Science and Technology, Tehran Medical Sciences, Islamic Azad University, Tehran, Iran*
[2]*Farhikhtegan Medical Convergence Sciences Research Center, Farhikhtegan Hospital Tehran Medical Sciences, Islamic Azad University, Tehran, Iran*
[3]*Department of Biology, Faculty of Science, Islamic Azad University, Science and Research Branch, Tehran, Iran*
[4]*Department of Biochemistry and Molecular Biology, Faculty of Veterinary Medicine, Shahid Chamran University of Ahvaz, Ahvaz, Iran*
[5]*Belfer Center for Applied Cancer Science, Dana-Farber Cancer Institute, Harvard Medical School, Boston, MA, USA*
[6]*Translational Sciences, Xsphera Biosciences Inc., Boston, MA 02210, USA*

*Corresponding author: Mehrdad Hashemi, Department of Genetics, Faculty of Advanced Science and Technology, Tehran Medical Sciences, Islamic Azad University, Tehran, Iran, Email: mhashemi@iautmu.ac.ir

Abstract

After the vast number of studies on the field of cancer, cancer therapy is still remaining as a major challenge in science. Conventional cancer therapeutic methods are chemotherapy, radiotherapy, and surgery, and their main aim is to suppress mechanisms related to cancer progression. However, in some conditions such as prolonged therapy resulted in chemo- and radio-resistance. DNA damage is one of the events that happened during cancer therapy, and resistant cells to therapy have been revealed to have a high level of factors responsible for DNA damage repair. MicroRNAs (miRNAs), molecules with ~22 nucleotides at length, belong to non-coding RNAs with critical roles in cellular functions and regulation of cancer cells hallmarks. miRNAs' role in cancer cells' response to therapy is the subject of many studies. miRNAs could act in a tumor suppressor and tumor-promoting way. Thus, miRNAs are mediating chemoresistance/radio-resistance or chemo-sensitivity/radio-sensitivity based on their initial function in cancer cells. To enhance the therapeutic efficacy, considering miRNA is of great importance. This chapter discussed the role of miRNAs in the regulation of mechanisms involved in sensitizing or resistance of cancer cells to chemotherapy/radiotherapy.

1. Introduction

Cancer is one of the most causes of death in developed countries. In 2020, the number of cancer cases was over 19 million, and almost 10 million deaths were counted for cancer deaths globally. Moreover, 2,370,000 new cancer cases and 640,000 cancer deaths in the USA have been estimated for 2022. Breast cancer and lung cancer are the most common type of cancer and the most leading cause of death in the USA, respectively [1]. During cancer, cell division mechanisms which are tightly regulated by cell cycle control mechanisms are disrupted, leading to continuous and excessive rounds of cell division [2]. Cancer cells have capabilities that help them in long-term survival including high rate of proliferation, suppressing apoptotic mechanisms, inducing, invasion, metastasis, immune evasion, and reprogramming the critical cellular metabolic pathways [3].

MicroRNAs (miRNAs) are ~22 nucleotides in length and belong to the family of non-coding RNAs and do not encode proteins [4–7]. miRNAs are responsible for gene expression and regulation of protein function in cells. miRNAs are estimate to regulate the expression of almost one-third of human genes. Besides, as they are highly tissue and cell specific and because of the significant difference between the expression levels of miRNAs in cancer and normal tissues, they are considered as valuable diagnostic and therapeutic biomarkers [8, 9]. miRNA expression is highly controlled by the tumor suppressor and promoting genes during mutations or deletions, thereby miRNAs are widely involved in cancer initiation and progression mechanisms such as tumor cell growth, proliferation, apoptosis, angiogenesis, invasion, metastasis, DNA repair mechanisms, metabolic regulation, and drug resistance [10]. Moreover, miRNAs are considered as the critical cytoplasmic regulators of gene expression. miRNA responsible gene is transcribed by RNA polymerase II to form a primary miRNA (pri-miRNA). Then, pri-miRNA is processed by two different endonuclease enzymes, the first time at the nucleus and the second time at the cytoplasm. miRNAs target the 3′-untranslated region (3′UTR) of their targets mostly, but they have also other interaction sites in their targets [11]. Regarding the critical role of miRNAs in the regulation of cancer progression mechanisms, this chapter is written to address the current cancer chemo- and radio-therapies.

2. Therapies for cancer

Current cancer therapeutic methods are chemotherapy, radiotherapy, immunotherapy, surgery, and hormonal therapy. Chemotherapy and radiation therapy are the first cancer therapeutic methods that radically changes after the emergence of targeted therapies. It bears noting that chemotherapeutics, which targets the endogenous dysregulated mechanisms of cancer cells, was the first introduced pharmacological approach for cancer therapy. In addition, other therapeutic methods are developed which include hormone therapy, cancer vaccines, combination therapies, stem cell–based therapies, and nanotechnology-based therapies [12]. Chemotherapies and radiotherapies are discussed in detail below.

2.1 *Chemotherapy*

The idea of chemotherapy was initially proposed after the findings indicated that mustard gas is able to kill lymphatic tissues. This theory was examined later in an animal model of mice using a derivative of gas, nitrogen mustard, and demonstrated an effective lymphoma tissue regression [13]. Chemotherapy primarily works as cytostatic (inhibiting proliferation) or cytotoxic (mediating tumor cell death). Chemotherapeutic agents can be administered before treatment (as neoadjuvants), after treatment (as adjuvants), or as palliative chemotherapy to ease the survival rate of patients [14]. Regarding their accelerated growth and division, cancer cells have high stress conditions than normal cells. Thus, they are destroyed by drugs rapidly compared to the surrounding cells [13]. It bears noting that systemic chemotherapy is often associated with severe side effects of toxicity, immediately or chronically, graded from mil to disabling [15].

Various chemotherapeutics exist which have performed different methods to induce cancer cell death. For instance, alkylating agents (such as nitrogen mustard–based drugs) act as anti-cancerous by adding alkyl groups onto bases in the DNA of cancer cells, and antimetabolites (such as fluorouracil and gemcitabine) stop the process of DNA replication. Despite these therapeutic agents, more effective drugs and therapies are still needed. [12]. Alkylating agents, which were discovered in 1942, are the frontline chemotherapeutic drugs that produce cytotoxic and mutagenic adducts onto DNA and are classified as mono-functional and bi-functional compounds. In fact, these agents act through intra- or inter-strand cross-linking DNA and RNA to suppress vital cellular processes such as transcription, translation, and DNA replication. Moreover, these molecules could induce cell death through mechanisms such as lipid peroxidation, increasing reactive oxygen and nitrogen species, inducing oxidative stress, and decreasing the level of NAD^+ required for DNA repair enzymes. However, different DNA damage–repair mechanisms such as base excision repair, direct DNA damage reversal, and mismatch repair are involved in repairing DNA, leading to unfavorable responses to these chemotherapies. Thus, considering these mechanisms and developing factors to modulate them is crucial for enhancing the efficacy of chemotherapeutic alkylating agents. Besides, as the response to these agents is varying from person to person, investigation of DNA repair capacity by patients helps to choose the best options. Alkylating agents are divided into six groups, including nitrogen mustards, ethyleneimines and methylmelamines (altretamine), piperazines, nitrosoureas, triazenes (dacarbazine), and alkyl sulfonates (busulfan) (Figure 1) [16–18]. Antimetabolites are another class of chemotherapeutics that could interfere with cellular metabolic processes by competing, replacing, or suppressing metabolites of cells. These agents are structurally similar to an enzyme substrate or cellular metabolites.

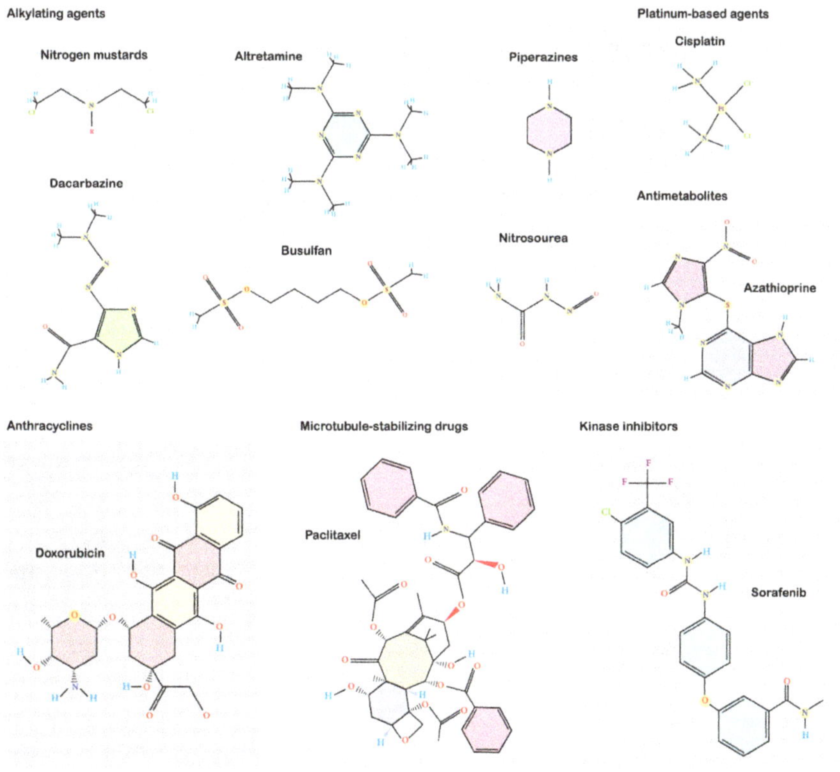

Figure 1. Various types of chemotherapeutics used in cancer therapy.

Examples of antimetabolites are azathioprine, gemcitabine, and mercaptopurine. A subgroup of antimetabolites is pyrimidine antagonists (pyrimidine-derived antimetabolites) which disturb the DNA synthesis process. 5-Fluorouracil (5-FU) and decitabine are the members of this subgroup [13]. Another class of chemotherapeutics is microtubule-stabilizing drugs, which induce mitotic arrest, mediating cell death during mitosis or by multi-nucleation, and target spindle apparatus. The most known example of this group is paclitaxel [19, 20]. Moreover, histone deacetylase inhibitors (HDACis) possess anti-cancer activities, such as mediation of cell cycle arrest, induction of apoptosis and autophagy, and angiogenesis suppression [21]. Topoisomerase I and II are proteins with critical functions in relaxing DNA supercoiling form produced after replication, transcription, and chromatin remodeling. Topoisomerases are highly susceptible to topoisomerase inhibitors, especially during the cleavage reaction. Topoisomerase inhibitors exert their function by meddling with trapped topoisomerase with transcription and DNA replication. Etoposide belongs to the family of topoisomerase inhibitors [22, 23]. Platinum-based agents (such as cisplatin) [24], kinase inhibitors (such as imatinib, sorafenib, and gefitinib) [25], and anthracyclines (such as doxorubicin and epirubicin) [26] are other chemotherapeutics (Figure 1).

2.2 *Radiotherapy*

Although chemotherapies suppress molecular mechanisms required for cancer cell progression, as many cells are not relying on these mechanisms for their survival, they can mediate drug resistance. Interestingly, radiation therapy is capable to induce cytotoxic signal pathway activation, thereby promoting cell death. It bears noting that radiotherapy has both cytotoxic and cytostatic effects on cancer cells. Interestingly, although radiotherapy leads to the activation of cytoprotective mechanisms, they can be suppressed by anti-cancer drugs which resulted in enhancing the anti-cancer activity of chemotherapeutic agents [27]. Noteworthy, radiation therapy is applied for the majority of cancer patients as curative or palliative treatment. In 1953,

Robin Mole stated that radiation could be associated with anti-tumor activities outside the radiation region. This finding resulted in increasing the attention to the field of immunotherapy–radiotherapy combination. In this case, different clinical trials also have been designed [28, 29]. Interestingly, the rational combination of radiotherapy with other therapies is proven to be effective. It has been reported that low-dose radiotherapy increases T cells, predominantly $CD4^{+}$ cells with Th1 signature, and penetration in tumor cells with a low rate of T-cell infiltration [30]. Moreover, radiotherapy could enhance locoregional- and distant metastasis-free survival in breast cancer patients and indirectly prevents cancer death via depletion of relapse risk [31]. However, despite the promising results provided by enormous studies carried out in this field, radiotherapy resistance associated with a high risk of locoregional relapse is still one of the obstacles to cancer therapy [32]. Radiotherapy in combination with chemotherapy is also associated with outstanding results. For instance, in a study on prostate cancer, it was revealed that 24 hours after multi-fractioned and 2 months after single-dose irradiation promotes the activation of cell survival–related signaling pathways. Besides, single-dose irradiation increased the activity of VEGFR2, insulin-like growth factor 1 receptor (IGF-1R), and Akt and decreased HDAC. Also, single-dose radiotherapy increases the sensitivity of cells to foretinib (VEGFR2 inhibitor), BMS-754807 (IGF-1R inhibitor), and ipatasertib (Akt inhibitor), but low sensitivity to panobinostat (HDACi). The results of this study indicated the importance of understanding the molecular alteration following irradiation in improving the efficacy of drugs [33]. In addition, chemo-radiotherapy in combination with phytomedicines is studied widely. For example, ellagic acid, a polyphenol compound found in plant foods, has been shown to possess a synergistic impact with chemo-radiotherapy and reduce side effects due to its anti-inflammatory and antioxidant properties [34].

3. miRNAs in chemotherapy

miRNAs differently affect chemotherapies; they could promote [35] or suppress [36] chemo-resistance and act as predictor biomarkers of

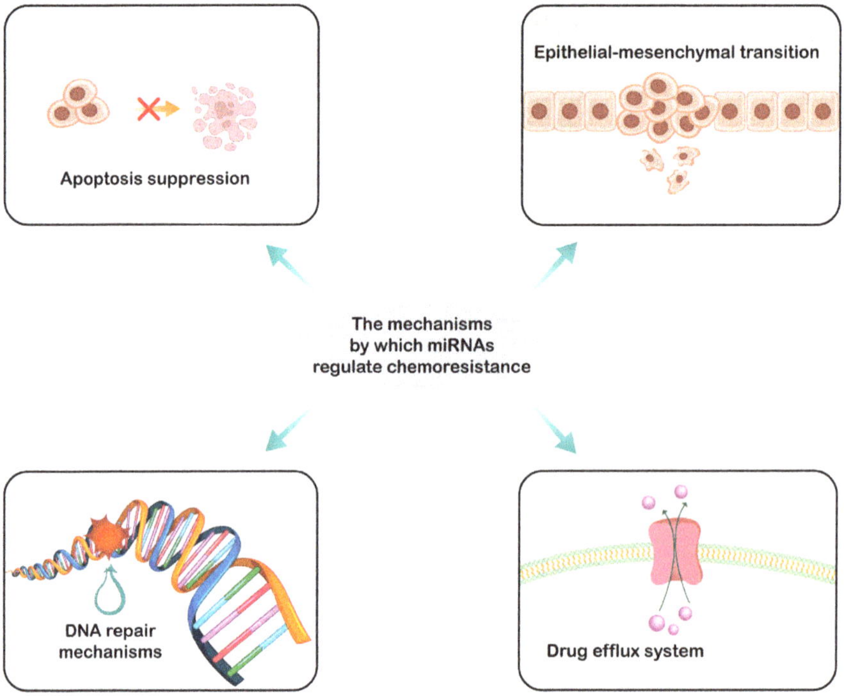

Figure 2. The mechanisms involved in the regulation of chemotherapy resistance and sensitization by miRNAs.

cancer response to chemotherapy [37]. Response to chemotherapy by cells relies on some signaling pathways and miRNAs could target these pathways. DNA repair mechanisms, efflux system for the reduction of drug amount in cells, drug detoxification within cellular environment, apoptosis suppression, epithelial–mesenchymal transition (EMT), β-tubulin or other drug target mutations, alterations in drug structures, and stem cells are among them (Figure 2) [38–40]. The two following parts have been written to detail the role of miRNAs in the regulation of chemotherapy response by cancer cells.

4. miRNAs inducing chemo-resistance

miRNA-363-3p targets dual specificity phosphatase 10 to suppress it and promote the phosphorylation of c-Jun *N*-terminal kinase. This connection is associated with doxorubicin-induced double-strand break repair via affecting ATF2, thereby promoting doxorubicin resistance [41]. Both miRNA-106a and miRNA-19a/b are involved in inducing Adriamycin resistance via increasing drug efflux in gastric cancer. miRNA-106a targets runt-related transcription factor 3 (RUNX3) to induce multi-drug resistance and drug efflux. Furthermore, miRNA-106a suppresses apoptosis induced by chemotherapy [42]. On the other hand, miRNA-19a/b increases Adriamycin efflux via multi-drug resistance mutation 1 (MDR1) and P-glycoprotein (P-gp) upturning. Besides, miRNA-19a/b targets Bax and Bcl-2 to suppress apoptosis and targets PTEN as an Akt inhibitor to mediate multi-drug resistance [43]. Furthermore, it was suggested that oncomiRNA-675-5p expression is increased in colorectal cancer cells during hypoxia and interferes with the apoptotic activity of 5-FU by targeting caspase-3 and poly (ADP-ribose) polymerase (PARP) to increase drug resistance [44]. In addition to hypoxia, cellular stressors could mediate downregulation or upregulation of miRNAs involved in drug resistance mechanisms. For instance, miRNA-301a-3p expression is increased in response to endoplasmic stress in human epidermal growth factor receptor 2–positive gastric cancer cells. Then, the overexpressed miRNA-301a-3p mediates the downturning of leucine-rich repeats and immunoglobulin-like domains containing protein 1 expression to promote the expression of IGF-1R and fibroblast growth factor receptor 1 (FGFR1), thereby increasing trastuzumab resistance [45]. Furthermore, extracellular vesicles derived from highly metastatic tumor cells containing miRNA-1246 could induce drug resistance in tumor endothelial cells by increasing IL-6 via androgen receptor downregulation, and subsequent activation of STAT3 and Akt [46]. Similarly, exosomes derived from the tamoxifen-resistant MCF-7 cells containing miRNA-9-5P negatively regulate ADIPOQ to induce resistance to tamoxifen in breast cancer cells [47]. Moreover, miRNA-93-5p overexpression mediates gemcitabine resistance, promotes cell viability, induces multi-drug resistance via PI3K/Akt pathway, and decreases apoptosis. Besides, miRNA-93-5p suppresses PTEN to increase the phosphorylated form of Akt in pancreatic cancer [48]. Different signaling pathways involved in drug resistance are regulated by miRNAs. For instance, exosomes derived from cancer-associated fibroblasts (CAFs) which contain miRNA-130a are involved in increasing cisplatin-resistant non-small cell lung cancer cells and its packaging is mediated by pumilio homolog 2, a RNA-binding protein [49]. Moreover, miRNAs could mediate drug resistance by regulating cancer cell hallmarks, such as EMT. EMT is characterized by low levels of E-cadherin and high levels of N-cadherin, vimentin, and also loss of apico-basal polarity. In addition, the key EMT-related transcription factors include Snail, Twist, and ZEB [50]. miRNA-125b-5p is one of the examples of EMT-regulating miRNA activity in drug resistance. It was revealed that miRNA-125b-5p overexpression is associated with drug resistance in hepatocellular carcinoma. miRNA-125b-5p induces EMT via down-regulation of E-cadherin and upregulation of vimentin and subsequently induces sorafenib resistance. Furthermore, miRNA-125b-5p targets ataxin-1 to regulate its translation, but not transcription, and subsequently induces the Snail upturning to induce EMT, migration, and invasion [51]. Autophagy is one of the mechanisms that could induce either drug resistance or sensitivity. miRNA-495-3p overexpression leads to the reduction of glucose-regulated protein 78 to inhibit autophagy and mediate sensitivity to Adriamycin, 5-FU, and vincristine. In contrast, miRNA-21 promotes resistance to tamoxifen, doxorubicin, and etoposide by decreasing autophagy by inhibiting PTEN, as an inhibitor of PI3K/Akt/mTOR signaling [40]. Likewise, miRNA-135b-5p exerts drug resistance activity in colorectal cancer cells by inducing protective autophagy. Indeed, miRNA-135b-5p induces oxaliplatin resistance by suppressing MUL1, which is responsible for the degradation of a key molecule of autophagy named ULKl through its degradation to induce protective autophagy in increasing drug resistance [52]. Moreover, miRNAs could affect cancer immune response and surveillance by targeting immune checkpoint inhibitors in the tumor microenvironment. This would modulate drug resistance by cancer cells [53].

5. miRNAs suppressing chemo-resistance

miRNA-197-5p overexpression is associated with inhibiting the resistance of fibrosarcoma cancer cells to doxorubicin via reducing drug efflux. miRNA-197-5p mediates apoptosis and cell cycle arrest at G2/M phase in combination with doxorubicin [54]. Moreover, miRNA-27b is involved in suppressing drug detoxification mediated by CYP1B1. Indeed, miRNA-27b increases the sensitivity of cancer cells to anti-cancer drugs through the activation of p53-dependent apoptosis and suppression of CYP1B1, especially in patients with a high level of CYP1B1 and p53-wild type. In addition, miRNA-27b regulates p-53 by targeting CCNG1. Moreover, in this study, it was additionally revealed that miRNA-27b exerts a synergistic impact with doxorubicin. The authors also demonstrated that drug-sensitizing effect of miRNA-27b does not result from drug efflux mechanisms [55]. In pancreatic ductal adenocarcinoma, miRNA-3662 expression is decreased as a tumor suppressor agent. miRNA-3662 increases the sensitivity to gemcitabine by targeting hypoxia-inducible factor 1α. Besides, miRNA-3662 adversely regulates aerobic glycolysis in cancer cells [56]. Likewise, miRNA-9-3p upregulation is associated with drug sensitivity in breast cancer cells. miRNA-9-3p targets MTDH, a metastatic adhesion protein, to downregulate its expression and mediate gemcitabine sensitivity; induce apoptosis; and suppress tumor cell growth, proliferation, invasion, EMT, and migration [57]. miRNA-200c-3p is another example of miRNAs that regulate drug sensitivity. In a study carried out by Chen *et al.*, the authors reported that miRNA-526b-3p suppresses cisplatin resistance in lung cancer cells via inhibiting STAT3 and subsequently programmed death ligand 1 (PD-L1) suppression. Besides, miRNA-526b-3p overexpression is associated with low cancer cell viability and migration while increasing CD8+ T cell population. Furthermore, miRNA-526b-3p upregulation is accompanied by decreased levels of c-Myc, as oncogenic agent, and MDR1, as multi-drug resistance factor [58]. miRNA-506-3p, an inhibitor of EMT, promotes the sensitivity of high-grade serous ovarian cancer to PARP inhibitors and cisplatin by decreasing the enhancer of zeta homolog 2 and subsequently β-catenin suppression [59]. Interestingly, miRNAs could regulate drug sensitivity by targeting mitochondrial factors involved in apoptosis such as Bcl2. For instance, miRNA-15 and miRNA-16 promote gastric cancer cells' resistance to vincristine, cisplatin, etoposide, and Adriamycin by negatively targeting Bcl-2. Furthermore, in this review Riquelme and colleagues stated that elevation of tumor suppressor miRNAs could induce drug sensitivity in gastric cancer cells through different mechanisms such as suppression of autophagy-specific gene 12 (ATG12), the high mobility group box 2, and microtubule-associated protein tau protein [60]. In another study on miRNA-29a, it was proved that overexpression of miRNA-29a is associated with the increased level of PTEN in colon cancer cells. By suppressing PI3K/Akt pathway, the increased level of PTEN resulted in the inhibition of P-gp and doxorubicin sensitivity. Furthermore, the upregulation of miRNA-29a leads to decreased cell viability, proliferation, multi-drug resistance while increasing apoptosis [61]. As well, miRNA-34c-5p mediates drug sensitivity toward carboplatin and docetaxel by directly targeting amphiregulin/EGFR/ERK signal pathway in ovarian cancer cells. Amphiregulin, a glycoprotein and a ligand for EGFR, augments drug resistance, advanced tumor stage, poor prognosis, and stemness. miRNA-34c-5p functions ultimately resulted in the suppression of tumorigenesis induced by amphiregulin [62].

6. miRNAs in radiotherapy

In addition to chemotherapy, radiotherapy is also one of the common methods in cancer therapy and is used to suppress cancer progression alongside chemotherapy. There are two types of radiotherapy including external and internal radiation therapy. External or internal radiation, the choice is highly dependent on the type and stage of cancer. As a worrying obstacle, radio-resistance may occur following prolonged exposure to radiation, and the role of miRNAs in this event is not ignorable [63]. Interestingly, in a study on miRNAs' role in the regulation of radio-resistance in breast cancer cells, it was demonstrated that single-dose or multi-fraction radiotherapy could induce different responses by miRNAs [64]. Besides, miRNA biogenesis machinery knockdown is used to study miRNAs' regulatory role on radio-resistance. For example, dysfunctional types of Drosha and Dicer would decrease DNA damage response during irradiation. Noteworthy, DNA damage induced by irradiation is recognized by different factors such as ataxia telangiectasia mutated (ATM), which augments DNA repair mechanisms. Interestingly, miRNAs could modulate radio-resistance by targeting these factors [65]. Furthermore, the role of miRNAs in prognosis and prediction of radiotherapy efficacy has been evaluated in different studies [66, 67]. Table 1 provides examples of miRNAs involved in radiotherapy resistance/sensitivity in cancer cells.

7. miRNAs inducing radio-resistance

Different signaling pathways are suggested to be miRNAs' targets that are involved in radio-resistance, such as PI3K/Akt, NF-κB, MAPK, TGF-β, cdc25, p53, and BRCA [74]. Various miRNAs are involved in radio-resistance. For instance, miRNA-144 is an oncomiR whose expression in breast cancer cells is higher than in normal tissue. miRNA-144 promotes invasion and metastasis and also increases EMT by E-cadherin downregulation and Snail upregulation. Besides, miRNA-144 augments Akt signaling via the downregulation of PTEN. Moreover, the upregulation of miRNA-144 has been shown to be associated with radio-resistance and radiotherapy-induced apoptosis in cancer cells [75]. miRNA-622 expression is high in colorectal cancer cells, and its expression is associated with radio-resistance. miRNA-622 suppresses Rb via directly targeting RB1-3′UTR. Rb is involved in inducing pro-apoptotic activation in association with E2F1–P/CAF complex. Furthermore, radiotherapy caused increased miRNA-622 expression, resulting in radio-resistance and poor prognosis [76]. Another tumor-promoting miRNA is miRNA-32 which induces radio-resistance by regulating autophagy. DAB2-interacting protein (DAB2IP), which is the miR-32-dependent tumor inhibitor gene, is downregulated in prostate cancer, and its low expression in cancer cells resulted in autophagy promotion and low rate of radiotherapy-induced apoptosis. miRNA-32 inhibits DAB2IP to mediate tumor cell survival and radio-resistance. In addition to DAB2IP, miRNA-32 also targets other regulators of autophagy, such as LC3B-I/II and beclin-1 [77]. Moreover, miRNA-93 mediates radio-resistance in esophageal squamous carcinoma by negatively regulating mutated B-cell translocation gene 3 [78]. The tumor-promoting

Table 1. miRNAs with radio-resistance/radio-sensitizer activity.

miRNA	Cancer Type	Function	Signaling network	Remark	Ref
miRNA-196a	Head and neck cancer	Radio-resistance	Annexin A1	miRNA-196a overexpression inhibits annexin A1 to induce radio-resistance. miRNA-196a promotes proliferation, invasion, EMT, and migration.	[68]
miRNA-17-5p	Esophageal adenocarcinoma	Radio-resistance	C6orf120	Upregulation of miRNA-17-5p mediates radio-resistance in cancer cells.	[69]
miRNA-208a	Lung cancer cells	Radio-resistance	P21/Akt/mTOR	Radiation therapy induces miRNA-20a expression. miRNA-20a promotes proliferation and radio-resistance by suppressing p21 to increase Akt/mTOR signal pathway.	[70]
miRNA-125b	Oral squamous cell carcinoma	Radio-sensitivity	ICAM2	miRNA-125b suppresses ICAM2 to mediate radio-sensitivity and diminish proliferation.	[71]
miRNA-18a-5p	Lung cancer	Radio-sensitivity	ATM and HIF-1α	miRNA-18a-5p enhances the radio-sensitivity of cancer cells by downregulation of ATM and HIF-1α.	[72]
miRNA-499	Lung cancer	Radio-sensitivity	CK2α/p65	Overexpressed miRNA-499 suppresses cell viability, promotes radio-sensitivity, and enhances cancer cell apoptosis. miRNA-499 suppresses p65 phosphorylation by CK2α expression downturning.	[73]

function of miRNA-21 has been demonstrated in various cancers. Also, its radio-resistance enhancer activity has been proven in non-small cell lung cancer. miRNA-21 targets programmed cell death protein 4 to downregulate its expression and augments PI3K/Akt/mTOR signal pathway, thereby increasing the radiation resistance [79].

8. miRNAs suppressing radio-resistance

In the case of miRNAs with inhibitory function on radio-resistance by cancer cells, miRNA-200c is an example. miRNA-200c, in the form of miRNA-200c-loaded nanoparticles, synergistically acts with radiotherapy in gastric cancer to counteract immune escape mediated by PD-L1 and to reverse EMT and cell proliferation, as well as abrogating cancer stem cell–associated characteristics [80]. In another study, it was revealed that miRNA-200c overexpression could augment radio-sensitivity in esophageal squamous cancer cells by inducing cell cycle arrest in G2/M and sub-G1 phases via targeting cyclin B1, p21, and cdc2 [81]. Another example is miRNA-23b whose overexpression in pancreatic cancer cells is associated with radio-sensitization. To exert its function, miRNA-23b inhibits radiation-induced autophagy by targeting ATG12, LC3-II, and p62. Besides, autophagy suppression by miRNA-23b resulted in the elevation of radiation-induced cytochrome c unleash and activation of caspase-3/9 to instigate apoptosis [82]. Likewise, miRNA-216a upregulation increases the sensitivity of pancreatic cancer cells via targeting autophagy. miRNA-216a suppresses beclin-1, a critical factor of autophagy, to prevent autophagy and sensitize cells to radiotherapy. Besides, miRNA-216a reversely affects tumor cell growth and colony formation while promoting apoptosis [83]. In addition to targeting radiation-induced autophagy, miRNAs could also target apoptosis induced by irradiation in cancer. For example, miRNA-18a impairs DNA damage repair and augments apoptosis in cervical cancer cells to increase their susceptibility to radiotherapy via suppressing ATM, by targeting its 3′UTR site [84]. Similarly, miRNA-451 overexpression mediates sensitivity to radiotherapy by the augmentation of apoptosis. Indeed, miRNA-451 promotes the inhibitory effect of radiation therapy on colony formation of non-small cell lung cancer cells and enhances the instigator effect of radiotherapy on apoptosis and PTEN expression [85]. Besides, miRNA-196b's mechanism for inhibiting radio-resistance in gastric cancer is similar to miRNA-18a and exerted by preventing DNA repair by targeting RAD23B. In fact, miRNA-196b counteracts RAD23B to inhibit its function of repairing DNA after exposure to radiation [86]. Furthermore, miRNA-20b-5p accompanied by pembrolizumab enhanced the sensitization of cancer cells to radiation therapy via targeting PD-L1 and suppression of PD-L1/programmed death-1 [87]. miRNA-29c, which has an inhibitory function on nasopharyngeal carcinoma cells, mediates cancer cells' sensitivity to radiation and cisplatin by promoting apoptosis. Bcl-2 and Mcl-1 are the potential targets of miRNA-29c [88].

9. Conclusion and remarks

Considering the heterogeneous nature of cancer, it is one of the difficult-to-treat diseases. Reverse response to therapy by cells is common in cancer therapy. Different mechanisms and regulators are taking part in resistance to chemotherapies and radiation therapy, and miRNAs are among them. As the master regulators of cellular functions, miRNAs critically regulate the response of cells to therapies. The findings in this field are promising, but further studies are required until bringing cancer under control.

Conflict of interest:

The authors declare no conflict of interest.

References

1. Xia, C., et al., *Cancer statistics in China and United States, 2022: Profiles, trends, and determinants.* Chinese Medical Journal, 2022. **135**(05): p. 584–590.

2. Matthews, H.K., C. Bertoli, and R.A. de Bruin, *Cell cycle control in cancer.* Nature Reviews Molecular Cell Biology, 2022. **23**(1): p. 74–88.
3. Hanahan, D., *Hallmarks of cancer: New dimensions.* Cancer Discovery, 2022. **12**(1): p. 31–46.
4. Entezari, M., et al., *LncRNA-miRNA axis in tumor progression and therapy response: An emphasis on molecular interactions and therapeutic interventions.* Biomedicine & Pharmacotherapy, 2022. **154**: p. 113609.
5. Mirzaei, S., et al., *Regulation of nuclear factor-kappaB (NF-κB) signaling pathway by non-coding RNAs in cancer: Inhibiting or promoting carcinogenesis?* Cancer Letters, 2021. **509**: p. 63–80.
6. Paskeh, M.D.A., et al., *Revealing the role of miRNA-489 as a new onco-suppressor factor in different cancers based on pre-clinical and clinical evidence.* International Journal of Biological Macromolecules, 2021. **191**: p. 727–737.
7. Abadi, A.J., et al., *Small in size, but large in action: MicroRNAs as potential modulators of PTEN in breast and lung cancers.* Biomolecules, 2021. **11**(2): p. 304.
8. Liu, J., et al., *The biogenesis of miRNAs and their role in the development of amyotrophic lateral sclerosis.* Cells, 2022. **11**(3): p. 572.
9. Huang, W., et al., *Regulatory mechanism of miR-20a-5p expression in Cancer.* Cell Death Discovery, 2022. **8**(1): p. 1–10.
10. Uzuner, E., et al., *The role of MiRNA in cancer: Pathogenesis, diagnosis, and treatment*, in *miRNomics.* 2022, Springer. p. 375–422.
11. Rani, V. and R.S. Sengar, *Biogenesis and mechanisms of microRNA-mediated gene regulation.* Biotechnology and Bioengineering, 2022. **119**(3): p. 685–692.
12. Sharma, P., et al., *Innovation in cancer therapeutics and regulatory perspectives.* Medical Oncology, 2022. **39**(5): p. 1–12.
13. Anand, U., et al., *Cancer chemotherapy and beyond: Current status, drug candidates, associated risks and progress in targeted therapeutics.* Genes & Diseases, 2022.
14. Patel, S. and S.K. Sahai, *Traditional cancer therapies and perioperative implications*, in *Perioperative Care of the Cancer Patient.* 2023, Elsevier. p. 46–55.

15. Schirrmacher, V., *From chemotherapy to biological therapy: A review of novel concepts to reduce the side effects of systemic cancer treatment.* International Journal of Oncology, 2019. **54**(2): p. 407–419.
16. Fu, D., J.A. Calvo, and L.D. Samson, *Balancing repair and tolerance of DNA damage caused by alkylating agents.* Nature Reviews Cancer, 2012. **12**(2): p. 104–120.
17. Egea, J., et al., *Alkylating agent-induced toxicity and melatonin-based therapies.* Frontiers in Pharmacology, 2022. **13**: p. 873197.
18. Ralhan, R. and J. Kaur, *Alkylating agents and cancer therapy.* Expert Opinion on Therapeutic Patents, 2007. **17**(9): p. 1061–1075.
19. A'hern, R.P., et al., *Taxane benefit in breast cancer — a role for grade and chromosomal stability.* Nature Reviews Clinical Oncology, 2013. **10**(6): p. 357–364.
20. Fanale, D., et al., *Stabilizing versus destabilizing the microtubules: A double-edge sword for an effective cancer treatment option?* Analytical Cellular Pathology, 2015. **2015**: p. 690916.
21. Eckschlager, T., et al., *Histone deacetylase inhibitors as anticancer drugs.* International Journal of Molecular Sciences, 2017. **18**(7): p. 1414.
22. Pommier, Y., *Topoisomerase I inhibitors: Camptothecins and beyond.* Nature Reviews Cancer, 2006. **6**(10): p. 789–802.
23. Skok, Z.I., et al., *Dual inhibitors of human DNA topoisomerase II and other cancer-related targets.* Journal of Medicinal Chemistry, 2019. **63**(3): p. 884–904.
24. Rottenberg, S., C. Disler, and P. Perego, *The rediscovery of platinum-based cancer therapy.* Nature Reviews Cancer, 2021. **21**(1): p. 37–50.
25. Zhang, J., P.L. Yang, and N.S. Gray, *Targeting cancer with small molecule kinase inhibitors.* Nature Reviews Cancer, 2009. **9**(1): p. 28–39.
26. Ferrero, A., et al., *Predicting response to anthracyclines in ovarian cancer.* International Journal of Environmental Research and Public Health, 2022. **19**(7): p. 4260.
27. Petroni, G., et al., *Radiotherapy as a tool to elicit clinically actionable signalling pathways in cancer.* Nature Reviews Clinical Oncology, 2022. **19**(2): p. 114–131.
28. Kwan, E.M., et al., *Avelumab combined with stereotactic ablative body radiotherapy in metastatic castration-resistant prostate cancer: The phase 2 ICE-PAC clinical trial.* European Urology, 2022. **81**(3): p. 253–262.

29. Pointer, K.B., S.P. Pitroda, and R.R. Weichselbaum, *Radiotherapy and immunotherapy: Open questions and future strategies.* Trends in Cancer, 2022. **8**(1): p. 9–20.
30. Herrera, F.G., et al., *Low-dose radiotherapy reverses tumor immune desertification and resistance to immunotherapy.* Cancer Discovery, 2022. **12**(1): p. 108–133.
31. da Luz, F.A.C., et al., *The effectiveness of radiotherapy in preventing disease recurrence after breast cancer surgery.* Surgical Oncology, 2022. **41**: p. 101709.
32. Larionova, I., et al., *Radiotherapy resistance: Identifying universal biomarkers for various human cancers.* Journal of Cancer Research and Clinical Oncology, 2022. **148**: p. 1–17.
33. Eke, I., et al., *Radiotherapy alters expression of molecular targets in prostate cancer in a fractionation-and time-dependent manner.* Scientific Reports, 2022. **12**(1): p. 1–13.
34. Xue, P., et al., *Synergism of ellagic acid in combination with radiotherapy and chemotherapy for cancer treatment.* Phytomedicine, 2022. **99**: p. 153998.
35. Shi, L., et al., *Cancer-associated fibroblast-derived exosomal microRNA-20a suppresses the PTEN/PI3K-AKT pathway to promote the progression and chemoresistance of non-small cell lung cancer.* Clinical and Translational Medicine, 2022. **12**(7): p. e989.
36. Enkhnaran, B., et al., *MicroRNA-106b-5p promotes cell growth and sensitizes chemosensitivity to sorafenib by targeting the BTG3/Bcl-xL/p27 signaling pathway in hepatocellular carcinoma.* Journal of Oncology, 2022. **2022**: p. 1971559.
37. Konoshenko, M. and P. Laktionov, *The miRNAs involved in prostate cancer chemotherapy response as chemoresistance and chemosensitivity predictors.* Andrology, 2022. **10**(1): p. 51–71.
38. Alharbi, M., et al., *The potential role of miRNAs and exosomes in chemotherapy in ovarian cancer.* Endocrine-Related Cancer, 2018. **25**(12): p. R663–R685.
39. Wang, J., et al., *The role of microRNAs in the chemoresistance of breast cancer.* Drug Development Research, 2015. **76**(7): p. 368–374.
40. Jing, Y., et al., *Autophagy-mediating microRNAs in cancer chemoresistance.* Cell Biology and Toxicology, 2020. **36**(6): p. 517–536.

41. Zhou, W., et al., *MiRNA-363-3p/DUSP10/JNK axis mediates chemoresistance by enhancing DNA damage repair in diffuse large B-cell lymphoma.* Leukemia, 2022. **36**: p. 1–9.
42. Zhang, Y., Q. Lu, and X. Cai, *MicroRNA-106a induces multidrug resistance in gastric cancer by targeting RUNX3.* FEBS Letters, 2013. **587**(18): p. 3069–3075.
43. Wang, F., et al., *MicroRNA-19a/b regulates multidrug resistance in human gastric cancer cells by targeting PTEN.* Biochemical and Biophysical Research Communications, 2013. **434**(3): p. 688–694.
44. Zichittella, C., et al., *Mir-675-5p supports hypoxia-induced drug resistance in colorectal cancer cells.* BMC Cancer, 2022. **22**(1): p. 1–12.
45. Guo, J., et al., *MiR-301a-3p induced by endoplasmic reticulum stress mediates the occurrence and transmission of trastuzumab resistance in HER2-positive gastric cancer.* Cell Death & Disease, 2021. **12**(7): p. 1–14.
46. Torii, C., et al., *MiRNA-1246 in extracellular vesicles secreted from metastatic tumor induces drug resistance in tumor endothelial cells.* Scientific Reports, 2021. **11**(1): p. 1–16.
47. Liu, J., et al., *Exosomes from tamoxifen-resistant breast cancer cells transmit drug resistance partly by delivering miR-9-5p.* Cancer Cell International, 2021. **21**(1): p. 1–15.
48. Wu, Y., et al., *MiRNA-93-5p promotes gemcitabine resistance in pancreatic cancer cells by targeting the PTEN-mediated PI3K/Akt signaling pathway.* Annals of Clinical & Laboratory Science, 2021. **51**(3): p. 310–320.
49. Zhang, T., P. Zhang, and H.-X. Li, *CAFs-derived exosomal miRNA-130a confers cisplatin resistance of NSCLC cells through PUM2-dependent packaging.* International Journal of Nanomedicine, 2021. **16**: p. 561.
50. Sadrkhanloo, M., et al., *STAT3-EMT axis in tumors: Modulation of cancer metastasis, stemness and therapy response.* Pharmacological Research, 2022. **182**: p. 106311.
51. Hirao, A., et al., *MiR-125b-5p is involved in sorafenib resistance through ataxin-1-mediated epithelial-mesenchymal transition in hepatocellular carcinoma.* Cancers, 2021. **13**(19): p. 4917.
52. Zhu, Y., et al., *WTIP upregulates FOXO3a and induces apoptosis through PUMA in acute myeloid leukemia.* Cell Death & Disease, 2021. **13**(1): p. 1–11.

53. Mondal, P., et al. *The emerging role of miRNA in the perturbation of tumor immune microenvironment in chemoresistance: Therapeutic implications*, in *Seminars in Cell & Developmental Biology*. 2021. Elsevier.
54. Jain, N., B. Das, and B. Mallick, *MiR-197-5p increases doxorubicin-mediated anticancer cytotoxicity of HT1080 fibrosarcoma cells by decreasing drug efflux.* DNA Repair, 2022. **109**: p. 103259.
55. Mu, W., et al., *MiR-27b synergizes with anticancer drugs via p53 activation and CYP1B1 suppression.* Cell Research, 2015. **25**(4): p. 477–495.
56. Liu, A., et al., *MiRNA-3662 reverses the gemcitabine resistance in pancreatic cancer through regulating the tumor metabolism.* Cancer Chemotherapy and Pharmacology, 2021. **88**(2): p. 343–357.
57. Wang, Y., et al., *MiR-9-3p regulates the biological functions and drug resistance of gemcitabine-treated breast cancer cells and affects tumor growth through targeting MTDH.* Cell Death & Disease, 2021. **12**(10): p. 1–14.
58. Chen, K.-B., et al., *MiR-526b-3p inhibits lung cancer cisplatin-resistance and metastasis by inhibiting STAT3-promoted PD-L1.* Cell Death & Disease, 2021. **12**(8): p. 1–10.
59. Sun, Y., et al., *MicroRNA-506-3p increases the response to PARP inhibitors and cisplatin by targeting EZH2/β-catenin in serous ovarian cancers.* Translational Oncology, 2021. **14**(2): p. 100987.
60. Riquelme, I., et al., *Emerging role of miRNAs in the drug resistance of gastric cancer.* International Journal of Molecular Sciences, 2016. **17**(3): p. 424.
61. Shi, X., et al., *MiRNA-29a reverses P-glycoprotein-mediated drug resistance and inhibits proliferation via up-regulation of PTEN in colon cancer cells.* European Journal of Pharmacology, 2020. **880**: p. 173138.
62. Tung, S., et al., *MiRNA-34c-5p inhibits amphiregulin-induced ovarian cancer stemness and drug resistance via downregulation of the AREG-EGFR-ERK pathway.* Oncogenesis, 2017. **6**(5): p. e326–e326.
63. Robertson, N.M. and M.V. Yigit, *The role of microRNA in resistance to breast cancer therapy.* Wiley Interdisciplinary Reviews: RNA, 2014. **5**(6): p. 823–833.
64. Leung, C.-M., et al., *MicroRNA expression profiles in human breast cancer cells after multifraction and single-dose radiation treatment.* Oncology Reports, 2014. **31**(5): p. 2147–2156.

65. Korpela, E., D. Vesprini, and S. Liu, *MicroRNA in radiotherapy: MiRage or miRador?* British Journal of Cancer, 2015. **112**(5): p. 777–782.
66. Ahmad, P., et al., *MicroRNA-15b-5p predicts locoregional relapse in head and neck carcinoma patients treated with intensity-modulated radiotherapy.* Cancer Genomics & Proteomics, 2019. **16**(2): p. 139–146.
67. Wei, W. and C. Liu, *Prognostic and predictive roles of microRNA-411 and its target STK17A in evaluating radiotherapy efficacy and their effects on cell migration and invasion via the p53 signaling pathway in cervical cancer.* Molecular Medicine Reports, 2020. **21**(1): p. 267–281.
68. Suh, Y.E., et al., *MicroRNA-196a promotes an oncogenic effect in head and neck cancer cells by suppressing annexin A1 and enhancing radioresistance.* International Journal of Cancer, 2015. **137**(5): p. 1021–1034.
69. Lynam-Lennon, N., et al., *MicroRNA-17 is downregulated in esophageal adenocarcinoma cancer stem-like cells and promotes a radioresistant phenotype.* Oncotarget, 2017. **8**(7): p. 11400.
70. Tang, Y., et al., *Radiation-induced miR-208a increases the proliferation and radioresistance by targeting p21 in human lung cancer cells.* Journal of Experimental & Clinical Cancer Research, 2016. **35**(1): p. 1–14.
71. Shiiba, M., et al., *MicroRNA-125b regulates proliferation and radioresistance of oral squamous cell carcinoma.* British Journal of Cancer, 2013. **108**(9): p. 1817–1821.
72. Chen, X., et al., *Radiosensitizing effects of miR-18a-5p on lung cancer stem-like cells via downregulating both ATM and HIF-1α.* Cancer Medicine, 2018. 7(8): p. 3834–3847.
73. Ma, Y.-S., et al., *MicroRNA-499 serves as a sensitizer for lung cancer cells to radiotherapy by inhibition of CK2α-mediated phosphorylation of p65.* Molecular Therapy-Oncolytics, 2021. **21**: p. 171–182.
74. Nguyen, L., et al., *The emerging role of miRNAs for the radiation treatment of pancreatic cancer.* Cancers, 2020. **12**(12): p. 3703.
75. Yu, L., et al., *MicroRNA-144 affects radiotherapy sensitivity by promoting proliferation, migration and invasion of breast cancer cells.* Oncology Reports, 2015. **34**(4): p. 1845–1852.
76. Ma, W., et al., *Radiation-induced microRNA-622 causes radioresistance in colorectal cancer cells by down-regulating Rb.* Oncotarget, 2015. **6**(18): p. 15984.

77. Liao, H., et al., *microRNA-32 induces radioresistance by targeting DAB2IP and regulating autophagy in prostate cancer cells.* Oncology Letters, 2015. **10**(4): p. 2055–2062.
78. Cui, H., et al., *Direct downregulation of B-cell translocation gene 3 by microRNA-93 is required for desensitizing esophageal cancer to radiotherapy.* Digestive Diseases and Sciences, 2017. **62**(8): p. 1995–2003.
79. Jiang, L.-P., C.-Y. He, and Z.-T. Zhu, *Role of microRNA-21 in radiosensitivity in non-small cell lung cancer cells by targeting PDCD4 gene.* Oncotarget, 2017. **8**(14): p. 23675.
80. Qian, L., et al., *MicroRNA-200c nanoparticles sensitized gastric cancer cells to radiotherapy by regulating PD-L1 expression and EMT.* Cancer Management and Research, 2020. **12**: p. 12215.
81. Zheng, R., et al., *MiRNA-200c enhances radiosensitivity of esophageal cancer by cell cycle arrest and targeting P21.* Biomedicine & Pharmacotherapy, 2017. **90**: p. 517–523.
82. Wang, P., et al., *MicroRNA 23b regulates autophagy associated with radioresistance of pancreatic cancer cells.* Gastroenterology, 2013. **145**(5): p. 1133–1143. e12.
83. Zhang, X., et al., *MicroRNA-216a enhances the radiosensitivity of pancreatic cancer cells by inhibiting beclin-1-mediated autophagy.* Oncology Reports, 2015. **34**(3): p. 1557–1564.
84. Liu, S., et al., *MicroRNA-18a enhances the radiosensitivity of cervical cancer cells by promoting radiation-induced apoptosis.* Oncology Reports, 2015. **33**(6): p. 2853–2862.
85. Tian, F., et al., *Upregulation of microrna-451 increases the sensitivity of A 549 cells to radiotherapy through enhancement of apoptosis.* Thoracic Cancer, 2016. 7(2): p. 226–231.
86. Shen, Y.N., et al., *MicroRNA-196b enhances the radiosensitivity of SNU-638 gastric cancer cells by targeting RAD23B.* Biomedicine & Pharmacotherapy, 2018. **105**: p. 362–369.
87. Jiang, K. and H. Zou, *MicroRNA-20b-5p overexpression combing Pembrolizumab potentiates cancer cells to radiation therapy via repressing programmed death-ligand 1.* Bioengineered, 2022. **13**(1): p. 917–929.
88. Zhang, J.-X., et al., *MicroRNA-29c enhances the sensitivities of human nasopharyngeal carcinoma to cisplatin-based chemotherapy and radiotherapy.* Cancer Letters, 2013. **329**(1): p. 91–98.

https://doi.org/10.1142/9789811267390_0004

Chapter 4

Exosomal miRNAs in cancer progression and diagnosis

Mehrdad Hashemi[1,2], Afshin Taheriazam[2,3], Sepideh Mirzaei[4], Shokooh Salimimoghadam[5]* and Amir Reza Aref[6,7]

[1]*Department of Genetics, Faculty of Advanced Science and Technology, Tehran Medical Sciences, Islamic Azad University, Tehran, Iran*
[2]*Farhikhtegan Medical Convergence Sciences Research Center, Farhikhtegan Hospital Tehran Medical Sciences, Islamic Azad University, Tehran, Iran*
[3]*Department of Orthopedics, Faculty of Medicine, Tehran Medical Sciences, Islamic Azad University, Tehran, Iran*
[4]*Department of Biology, Faculty of Science, Islamic Azad University, Science and Research Branch, Tehran, Iran*
[5]*Department of Biochemistry and Molecular Biology, Faculty of Veterinary Medicine, Shahid Chamran University of Ahvaz, Ahvaz, Iran*
[6]*Belfer Center for Applied Cancer Science, Dana-Farber Cancer Institute, Harvard Medical School, Boston, MA, USA*
[7]*Translational Sciences, Xsphera Biosciences Inc., Boston, MA, USA*

*Corresponding author: Shokooh Salimimoghadam, Department of Biochemistry and Molecular Biology, Faculty of Veterinary Medicine, Shahid Chamran University of Ahvaz, Ahvaz, Iran, Email: Shokoohmoghadam@yahoo.com

Abstract

Cancer is one of the most causes of death in the world, and its treatment still remains as a challenge. Cancer is studied from different aspects, and various factors that target signaling pathways of cancer hallmarks have been identified now. Exosomes are closed membranes of 30–150 nm in diameter, which orchestrate the intercellular interaction and contain a type of nucleic acid called microRNAs (miRNAs). miRNAs belong to the family of non-coding RNAs and regulate vital cell processes including gene expression and protein functions. Exosomal miRNAs have critical roles in cancer progression and therapy, and their expression profiles reflect the cancer cells' response to therapy and the stage of the disease. Regarding the key role of exosomal miRNAs in cancer, this chapter discusses the current knowledge on the effect of exosomal miRNAs on tumor growth, invasion and metastasis, and response to therapies. Besides, exosomal miRNAs' importance as prognostic and diagnostic biomarkers is also addressed.

1. Introduction

Exosomes were initially identified in the in vitro-cultured sheep reticulocyte supernatants in 1983 [1, 2]. Copiously exist in biofluids, exosomes are extracellular vesicles produced by endocytosis from most cell types. Exosomes are lipid bilayer structures with 30- to 150-nm diameter carrying biological signals to regulate cellular interactions, the physiological state of the body, and tumorigenesis. Indeed, these lipid bilayer–closed membranes are useful tools for monitoring the onset and progression of cancer [3, 4]. Extracellular stimuli such as stressors lead to the production of exosomes. Cells responded to these stimuli by the generation of early endosomes at first. Early endosomes are formed by inward endocytosis of the cell membrane. Gradually, this early endosome migrates within the cell and getting mature into the late endosomes. Then, the late endosome encapsulates different elements, such as DNA, RNA, proteins, lipids, amino acids, and metabolites, and forms the intraluminal vesicles (ILVs). Late endosomes with ILVs inside them are called multivesicular bodies (MVBs). If MVBs get fused with the cell membrane, their ILVs are released into the extracellular space. These secreted vesicles are called exosomes (Figure 1) [3, 5, 6].

Exosomes are promising drug delivery tools resulting from their high safety profile, stability, and tissue specificity. Interestingly, they transfer their contents to the exact target to produce the desired response [7–9]. In addition, the internal cargo of exosomes, they have some proteins on their surface such as tetraspanins (CD9, CD81, CD82), and fusion and heat shock proteins (HSP70/90) and MHC. In the case of cancer therapy, exosomes could be loaded with different therapeutic materials such as non-coding RNAs (ncRNAs). Moreover, modification of their surface using chemical and biological matters for targeted therapy is promising. The surface of exosomes could be modified by aptamers, antibodies, peptides, proteins, and antigens, based on the purpose of therapy. Exosome-mediated cell-to-cell interaction could be performed through different mechanisms, such as directly binding exosomes to the receptors on the surface of the cell

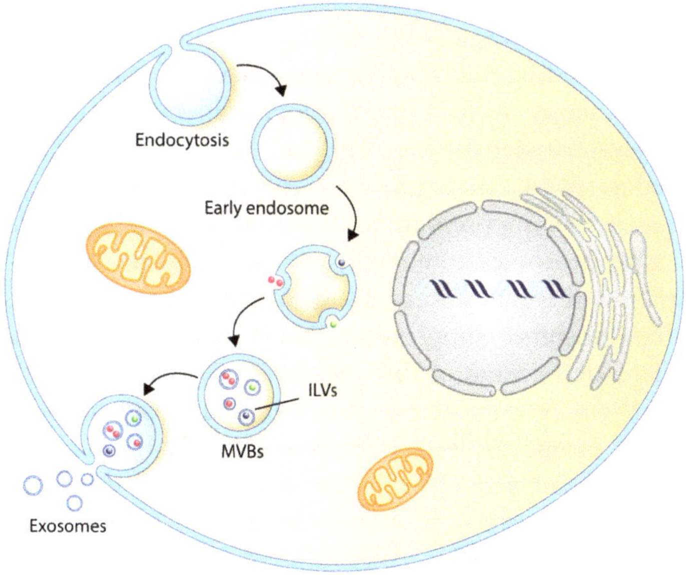

Figure 1. Illustration of the synthesis process of exosomes.

membrane; transferring the content of exosomes directly into the cytoplasm by fusing with the plasma membrane of recipient cells; and internalization of exosomes into the cells, which merged with endosomes to be delivered to neighboring cells or be degraded if endosomes are getting mature into lysosomes. The endocytosis is performed by clathrin-mediated endocytosis and macropinocytosis [10–13].

MicroRNAs (miRNAs) are a highly conserved gene class of ncRNAs with almost 22 nucleotides in length. After generation, miRNAs are loaded into miRNA-induced silencing complex (RISC) to guide it to the binding site on their targets. miRNAs mostly target the 3′ untranslated region (3′UTR) of their targets, and they also target other regions including 5′UTR and promoter of their targets. miRNAs regulate vital processes in cells such as gene expression, translation, and protein functions [14]. miRNAs could mediate the interaction between cells which have high distances with the help of exosomes to regulate gene expression in normal physiological conditions and also in cancer [15–20]. miRNA sorting into exosomes is mainly mediated through five different mechanisms: (1) miRNAs' 3′ ends-associated pathway, (2) the pathway related to the RISC, (3) the pathway mediated by neural sphingomyelinase 2, (4) miRNA motifs and heterogeneous nuclear ribonucleoprotein–related pathway, and (5) ceramide-related pathway [21]. miRNA-based cancer therapies are divided into two classes: therapies with tumor suppressor miRNAs and therapies that suppress tumor-promoting miRNAs (oncomiRs). For instance, exosomes containing miRNA-375 inhibit the invasion and migration of colon cancer cells. Furthermore, miRNA-155 inhibitor-loaded exosomes suppress miRNA-155 in increasing cisplatin sensitivity [10]. The aim of this chapter is to discuss the critical role of exosomal miRNAs in the regulation of cancer hallmarks, including growth and metastasis. Furthermore, their role in cancer therapy response is also detailed.

2. Exosomal miRNAs in cancer progression

A large body of studies has provided strong evidence that exosomal miRNAs have critical roles in cancer functions. For instance, they could be used as promising biomarkers [22]. Besides, their roles involve regulation of cancer progression [23], proliferation [24], apoptosis [25], immune evasion [25], epithelial–mesenchymal transition (EMT), invasion, metastasis [26], and angiogenesis [27]. Different mechanisms have been suggested for exosomal miRNAs' effect on cancer cells, but as the main mechanism, it has been demonstrated that exosomes containing miRNA-21 and miRNA-29a secreted by cancer cells are able to bind to Toll-like receptor 8 as their paracrine agonist and activate it, leading to the activation of nuclear factor kappa B (NF-κB) to unleash pro-metastatic inflammatory cytokines. This process ultimately resulted in tumor progression and metastasis [28]. As mentioned before, exosomes are released in response to stressors. It bears noting that one of the features of the tumor microenvironment (TME) is a low pH level resulting from hypoxia. This low pH level causes an increased exosome release in TME, which represents the critical role of exosomes in cancer [29]. It is well-known and accepted now that the cells placed in the TME are involved in tumor progression through exchanging proteins and nucleic acids. There are two types of macrophages in TME: M1 macrophages with anti-tumorigenic function and M2 macrophages with pro-tumorigenic functions. Tumor-associated macrophages (TAMs, M2 type) are the most important cells in TME; therefore, their interaction with tumor cells is mediated by exosomes and other type of extracellular vesicles in regulating cancer progression [30]. For instance, exosomes derived from M2 macrophages containing miRNA-942 have been shown to be associated with lung adenocarcinoma progression. Indeed, exosomal miRNA-942 targets FOXO1/Wnt/β-catenin signaling pathway to mediate cancer progression, invasion, migration, and angiogenesis [31]. Furthermore, the importance of TAMs in cancer progression is further discussed in a recent published study by Zhu *et al.* They have demonstrated that medulloblastoma-derived exosomal miRNA-221-3p and let-7i-5p mediate M2-like polarization of TAMs through targeting peroxisome proliferator–activated receptor γ (PPARγ) [32]. Table 1 represents an example of exosomal miRNAs with critical functions in cancer. This section is focused on the relationship between exosomal miRNAs and tumor growth, metastasis, and response to therapy.

Table 1. An overview of exosomal miRNAs in carcinogenesis.

miRNA	Cancer Type	Function	Signaling Network	Remark	Ref
miR-23a-3p	Cholangiocarcinoma	Tumor promoting	Dynamin-3	Exosomal miR-23a-3p suppresses Dynamin-3 to increase tumor growth, proliferation, invasion, and metastasis.	[33]
miR-17-5p	Colorectal cancer	Tumor promoting	Speckle-type POZ protein (SPOP)	Exosomal miR-17-5p suppresses SPOP to increase tumor cell growth and inhibits anti-tumor immunity in cancer cells via promoting programmed death-ligand 1. Upregulation of miR-17-5p promotes malignant behaviors of cancer cells.	[34]
miR-19b	Colorectal cancer	Tumor promoting	FBXW7	Colorectal cancer–derived exosomal miR-19b improves the radio-resistance and stemness properties of cancer cells by negatively targeting FBXW7.	[35]
miR-101-3p/ miR-423-5p	Medulloblastoma	Tumor suppressor	*FOXP4*	Exosomal miR-101-3p and miR-423-5p suppress proliferation, colony formation, migration, and invasion of tumor cells and increase cancer cell apoptosis via negatively targeting *FOXP4*. Exosomal miR-101-3p targets both *FOXP4* and *EZH2*.	[36]
miR-7-5p	Acute myeloid leukemia	Tumor suppressor	PI3K/ AKT/ mTOR/ *OSBPL11*	Exosomal miRNA-7-5p derived from bone marrow mesenchymal stem cells inhibits phosphorylation of the PI3K/AKT/mTOR to downregulate *OSBPL11*, induce apoptosis, and inhibit proliferation. Overexpression of miR-7-5p curbed cellular proliferation and promoted apoptosis.	[37]

2.1 *Exosomal miRNAs and cancer growth*

In a study, it has been demonstrated that exosomal mRNA-503-3p derived from human umbilical cord blood mesenchymal stem cells (MSCs) inhibits the growth and biological functions of endometrial cancer cells via targeting mesoderm-specific transcript [38]. Interestingly, in another study it was revealed that exosomal miRNAs could have dual roles. Exosomal miRNA-1298-5p has tumor suppressor activity on glioma cells via targeting SETD7 but improves the immunosuppressive effects of myeloid-derived suppressor cells by affecting MSH2 to accelerate glioma growth and progression. The results of this study have shown that tumor-suppressive miRNAs could be removed from cancer cells through exosomes to target tumor-associated immune cells and induce tumor-promoting phenotypes [39]. Moreover, MSC-derived exosomal miRNA-15a effect on hepatocellular carcinoma cells was assessed in a study by Ma *et al.*, and it was suggested that this exosomal miRNA-15a could reversely affect spalt-like transcription factor 4 expression to suppress tumorigenesis and proliferation of cancer cells [40]. Likewise, human umbilical cord MSC-derived exosomal miRNA-139-5p mediates polycomb repressor complex 1 downregulation to suppress tumor growth and promotes apoptosis in bladder cancer cells [41]. In contrast, the evaluation of macrophage-derived exosomal miR-503-3p role in breast cancer cells has revealed that miRNA-503-3p downregulates disheveled-associated binding antagonist of beta-catenin 2 (DACT2) resulting in enhanced metabolism of cancer cells and tumor growth. Indeed, upregulation of miRNA-503-3p mediates the upregulation of glycolysis via increasing glucose uptake. Besides, Wnt/β-catenin signaling pathway is activated by which the rate of oxygen consumption and ATP level in breast cancer cells are diminished. In fact, this miRNA enhances glycolysis, which represses mitochondrial oxidative phosphorylation via targeting DACT2 and Wnt/β-catenin signaling pathway [42]. Similar to previous examples, MSC-derived exosomal miRNA-181a suppresses nasopharyngeal carcinoma cell growth in vitro and in vivo via negatively regulating lysine-specific demethylase 5C (KDM5C) [43]. In the case of exosomal miRNAs with tumor-promoting functions, exosomal miRNA-19b-3p could be another instance. Bone marrow MSC-derived exosomal miRNA-19b-3p promotes esophageal cancer cells growth, proliferation, invasion, EMT, as well as migration, while suppressing the apoptosis process via reversely targeting suppressor of cytokine signaling 1 (SOCS1) [44].

2.2 *Exosomal miRNAs and cancer metastasis*

Exosomes produced by cancer cells and also TME cells are involved in the regulation of all stages of the metastasis process [45]. EMT is a mechanism that enables cancer cells to migrate to distant tissues and survive. It is characterized by a low expression level of E-cadherin, while high levels of N-cadherin and vimentin resulted from the upregulation of EMT transcription factors, including Slug, Snail, Twist, and ZEB [46]. The role of exosomal miRNAs in the regulation of metastasis through the EMT process is the subject of various studies. For instance, colorectal cancer cell–derived exosomes carrying miRNA-106b-5p are able to induce metastasis by increasing EMT. For this purpose, exosomal miRNA-106b-5p is transferred to macrophages to directly inhibit programmed cell death 4 and mediates PI3K/Akt/mTOR activation resulting in the promotion of M2 polarization of macrophages. This leads to enhancing EMT-mediated invasion, migration, as well as metastasis in colorectal cancer cells [47]. In contrast, MSC-derived exosomal miRNA-3940-5p suppresses these cancer hallmarks. Exosomal miRNA-3940-5p suppresses integrin alpha6 and subsequently transforming growth factor β1 inhibition to decrease EMT, tumor progression, invasion, and metastasis [43]. Wnt/β-catenin is one of the important signaling pathways that influenced EMT process. Interestingly, the alterations that happened during the EMT process, such as depletion of E-cadherin, are highly regulated by Wnt/β-catenin pathway. And more interesting is that miRNAs regulate Wnt/β-catenin signaling by which their expression undergoes up- or downturning during EMT [48]. Cancer-associated fibroblasts (CAFs) are another important cells present in the TME. The results of a study have revealed that CAF-derived exosomal miRNA-148b-3p promotes EMT, metastasis, proliferation, and drug resistance in bladder cancer via upregulation of Wnt/β-catenin signaling and downregulation of PTEN. In fact, the authors have demonstrated that upregulation of β-catenin induced by miRNA-148b-3p could be reversed by PTEN [49]. Moreover, circulating exosomal miRNA-203 derived from colorectal cancer cells' overexpression is associated with a high level of distant metastasis and poor prognosis, via promoting the differentiation of monocytes to M2-type macrophages [50]. Intriguingly, a research was done on the plasma-derived exosomal miRNAs to find their correlation with bone metastasis of non-small cell lung cancer. The authors have reported three consensuses of differentially expressed miRNA clusters, including miRNA-574-5p, which is a Wnt/β-catenin suppressor, and miRNA-328-3p and miRNA-423-3p, which are activators of that pathway in lung cancer patients with developed bone metastasis. Furthermore, they stated that this cluster may be involved in pre-conditioning of the metastatic niche [51]. Interestingly, exosomes are not only vehicles to deliver molecules to another cell but they could also perform other functions. For instance, miRNA-100 has tumor suppressor activity and inhibits migratory and invasive capacities of cancer cells. Cancer cells have been demonstrated to release exosomal miRNA-100 to decrease the levels of this miRNA, which resulted in increasing the rate of migration and invasion. Of note, colorectal cancer cell–derived exosomal miRNA-200c and miRNA-141 are involved in reversing EMT via upregulation of E-cadherin. They could also suppress EMT by directly targeting ZEB [52]. Tropomyosin-1 (TPM1) is a factor where its tumor suppressor activity is studied in different cancers. In prostate cancer, it has been shown that exosomal miRNA-183 could enhance metastasis and invasion via negatively regulating TPM1 [53]. Furthermore, hypoxic lung adenocarcinoma cell–derived exosomal miRNA-31-5p promotes EMT, invasion, and metastasis of normoxic lung adenocarcinoma cells via downregulation of Special AT-Rich Sequence–Binding Protein 2 (SATB2) and upregulation of MEK/

ERK signaling pathway [54]. Furthermore, exosomal miRNAs could mediate distant metastasis by regulating the responsible factors. C-C motif chemokine ligand 2 (CCL2) is crucial for breast cancer cells' organotropic metastases to the lung. Breast cancer cell–derived exosomal miRNA-200b-3p is involved in the formation of a pre-metastatic niche before the metastasis of tumor cells. These exosomes are uptaken by alveolar epithelial type II cells to regulate the micro-environment. Besides, exosomal miRNA-200-b-3p suppresses PTEN to activate Akt/NF-κB/p65 pathway and increase CCL2 secretion, thereby increasing the metastasis of breast cancer cells to the lung [55]. Additionally, exosomal miRNAs could provide a condition for brain metastasis of tumor cells. For example, triple-negative breast cancer cells release exosomal miRNA-181c, which targets PDPK1 to increase abnormal localization of actin and subsequent destruction of blood–brain barriers. These changes ultimately resulted in brain metastasis promotion [56]. Similarly, exosomal miRNA-103 regulates metastasis by targeting vessels. It was found that hepatocellular carcinoma cell–derived exosomal miRNA-103 upsurges the permeability of endothelial monolayers. In fact, this exosomal miRNA could weaken the integration of endothelial cell junction via suppression of zonula occludens 1, VE-cadherin, and p120-catenin expression and increase tumor cell metastasis [57]. Moreover, in a study it was suggested that non-small cell lung cancer cell–derived exosomal miRNA-1260b suppresses homeodomain-interacting protein kinase-2 to promote migration, angiogenesis, distant metastasis, and cisplatin resistance, and to mediate high-grade disease and poor survival rate [58]. It bears noting that studies have shown that certain exosomal miRNAs could be the biomarker for certain cancers. For instance, the analysis of plasma exosomal miRNAs in papillary thyroid carcinoma has revealed that exosomal miRNA-6879-5p and miRNA-6774-3p are highly correlated with lymph node metastasis in this cancer type [59]. Many other studies strongly confirm the critical role of exosomal miRNAs in regulating metastasis of cancer cells (Figure 2) [60–63].

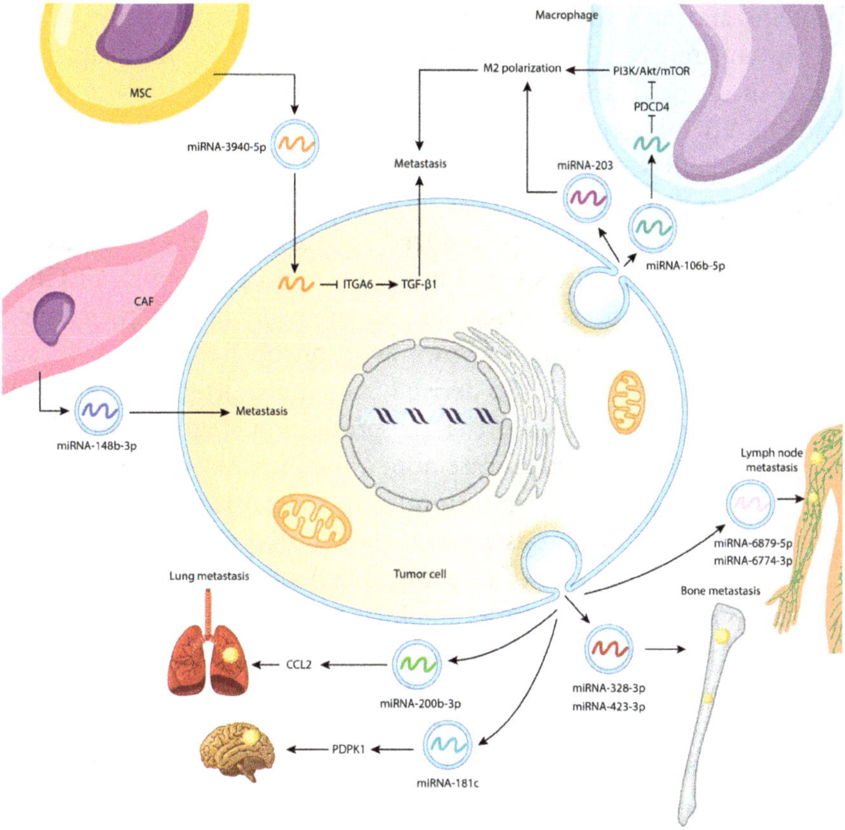

Figure 2. Illustration of exosomal miRNAs involved in metastasis.

2.3 *Exosomal miRNAs and therapy response*

The critical role of exosomal miRNAs in drug resistance/sensitivity of various types of cancers such as colorectal cancer [64], hepatocellular carcinoma [65], osteosarcoma [66], breast cancer [67], and prostate cancer [68] has been elucidated. Exosomal miRNAs are involved in drug resistance through different mechanisms, such as oncogenic pathways, drug efflux, drug target mutation, DNA repair mechanisms, drug detoxification, and modulation of multidrug resistance proteins and apoptosis induction. For instance, exosomal miRNA-21-5p and miRNA-21-3p are responsible for mediating drug resistance in ovarian cancer by affecting the detoxification mechanisms and DNA damage repair processes, respectively [69–71]. Additionally, exosomal miRNAs may target vessels to affect chemo-resistance. Exosomal miRNA-484 mediates normalization of vessels to sensitize cancer cells to chemotherapy-induced apoptosis. In this study, RGD-modified exosomal miRNA-484 has been shown to suppress VEGF-A in cancer cells, and the corresponding receptors in endothelial cells [72]. PI3K/Akt signaling is known as an oncogenic pathway in cancer. Exosomal miRNA-32-5p derived from multi-drug resistance cells is delivered to sensitive cells, thereby promoting chemo-resistance to therapies in hepatocellular carcinoma. Besides, exosomal miRNA-32-5p augments PTEN expression to promote PI3K/Akt activation to further induce drug resistance via modulation of EMT and angiogenesis [73]. In the case of targeting DNA repair mechanisms, exosomal miRNA-151a is an example. Overexpression of exosomal miRNA-151a increases the sensitivity of temozolomide-resistant glioblastoma multiforme to therapy via suppressing XRCC4, which is involved in DNA damage repair produced following cancer therapies [74]. Interestingly, Patel and coworkers have revealed that exosomes containing catalase (CAT) and superoxide dismutase 2 (SOD2) mRNA, and miRNA-155 derived from gemcitabine-treated pancreatic cancer cells could mediate drug resistance. These exosomes promote the expression of reactive oxygen species (ROS)-detoxifying enzymes of CAT and SOD2, while decreasing deoxycytidine kinase (DCK), an enzyme responsible for metabolizing gemcitabine. In fact, the function of CAT and SOD2 protects pancreatic cancer cells from ROS-induced cell death, thereby inducing chemo-resistance in pancreatic cancer cells. Furthermore, exosome-mediated DCK suppression has been proved to be regulated by miRNA-155. miRNA-155 targets the 3′UTR region of DCK to downregulate its expression [75]. Desirable function of exosomal miRNAs in regulating drug resistance induced by multidrug-resistant protein1 (MDR1; also called P-gp) is well addressed [76, 77]. In a study, it was shown that human cerebral endothelial cell-derived exosomal miRNA-214 could promote the efficacy of anti-cancer drugs of sorafenib and oxaliplatin in reducing cancer cells viability and invasion in hepatocellular carcinoma. In fact, exosomal miRNA-214 decreases P-gp and suppresses splicing factor 3B subunit 3 to suppress drug resistance and cancer cell proliferation, respectively [78]. In addition to chemo-resistance, exosomal miRNAs could also be involved in hormonal resistance [79, 80]. For instance, exosomal miRNA-221/222 derived from MCF-7 tamoxifen-resistant cells is entering into MCF-7 tamoxifen-sensitive cells to reduce the expression level of p27 and estrogen receptor α, thereby promoting tamoxifen resistance in recipient cells [81]. Moreover, exosomal miRNAs' role in mediating resistance to immunotherapeutics and human epidermal growth factor receptor 2–targeted therapies has been revealed before [82]. Radiotherapy is another type of cancer therapy, which is used in almost 50% of localized cancer patients. Cancer cells become resistant to radiation therapy via different mechanisms such as modulating DNA damage repair, autophagy, cell cycle checkpoint, apoptosis, and gene mutations. Interestingly, exosomal miRNAs are also involved in regulating response of cancer cells to radiotherapy [80, 83, 84]. An example is exosomal miRNA-590-3p, which induces radio-resistance in colorectal cancer cells. CAF-derived exosomal miRNA-590-3p decreased the sensitivity of colorectal cancer cells to radiation via targeting CLCA4, PI3K/Akt, PARP, caspase-3, and γH2AX. In addition, exosomal miRNA-590-3p promotes tumor growth [85].

3. Exosomal miRNAs and tumor microenvironment

TME is the key player in carcinogenesis and consists of cancer cells, CAFs, immune cells, TAMs, endothelial cells, extracellular matrix (ECM), biomolecules, and microvessels. Heterogeneity in cancers could be induced by transferring primary tumor-derived exosomal miRNAs to non-malignant cells placed in the TME. Interestingly, exosomal miRNAs could also be secreted from non-malignant cells to further mediate tumor cell growth. Exosomal miRNAs affect CAFs and endothelial cells to induce ECM reshaping necessary for the spread of cancer cells and to form an extensive network of blood vessels, respectively. Mediating infiltration of inflammatory cells and immune evasion are among the other regulatory role of exosomal miRNAs on TME [86]. Intriguingly, exosomal miRNAs derived from different cells of TME are responsible for mediating tumor progression and also drug resistance. As an example, CAF cell–derived exosomal miRNA-155 mediates the resistance of breast cancer cells to doxorubicin and paclitaxel. Moreover, gemcitabine-resistant pancreatic cancer stem cell–derived exosomal miRNA-210 transferred the resistant phenotype to drug-sensitive cancer cells to increase proliferation and suppress apoptosis via targeting mTOR signaling pathway [87]. Additionally, cancer cells induce metabolic remodeling in the TME via exosomal miRNAs to mediate their further progression as a feedback loop. For instance, melanoma cell–derived exosomal miRNA-155 and miRNA-210 target fibroblasts to increase their glycolysis and decrease oxidative phosphorylation, thereby producing an acidic environment. This acidification is associated with creating the pre-metastatic niche to accelerate tumor invasion and metastasis [88]. Another interesting example of exosomal miRNAs' role in metabolic reprogramming is cancer cell–derived exosomal miRNA-105, which affects CAFs. Yan *et al.* have revealed that in the condition in which nutrients are sufficient, exosomal miRNA-105 induces glucose and glutamine metabolism in CAFs to provide energy for cancer cells. While in the condition of low nutrient levels, where the level of metabolic by-products is high in the cells, CAFs use these metabolic wastes and detoxify them to convert into high-energy metabolites. Both these ways induced by exosomal miRNA-155 converge at increasing the cancer cell growth. It bears noting that exosomal miRNA-155 activates MYC signaling pathway to exert this metabolic reprogramming [89]. Also, some exosomal miRNAs have tumor suppressor activities. CAF-derived exosomal miRNA-139 has been proven to decrease the levels of matrix metalloproteinase 11 in gastric cancer cells, and subsequently decrease tumor growth, invasion, and metastasis [90]. Cancer cells also affect macrophages and increase their M2 polarization to promote their progression. As a stimulation, endoplasmic reticulum stress leads to exosomal miRNA-23a-3p release from hepatocellular carcinoma, which affects macrophages to increase programmed death ligand 1 via upregulation of STAT3 signaling pathway, resulting in promoting immune evasion capacity of liver cancer cells. In addition, it was found that epithelial ovarian cancer cell–derived exosomal miRNA-21-3p, miRNA-181-5p, and miRNA-125b-5p are released in response to hypoxic condition of TME to mediate macrophage polarization into M2 type via targeting SOCS4-5/STAT3/HIF-1α axis [91–93].

4. Exosomal miRNAs in cancer diagnosis

Cancer diagnosis in the early stages is of great importance for decreasing morbidity and mortality. Exosomal miRNAs are critical diagnostic and prognostic factors in cancer [94]. An example is miRNA-205, where its expression is significantly different in ovarian cancer cells compared to benign and normal cells. It has been elucidated that the plasma level of exosomal miRNA-205 is high in ovarian cancer patients, which represents its important role, especially, in early diagnosis and prognostic evaluation of ovarian cancer [95]. Different exosomal miRNAs are considered as diagnostic and prognostic biomarkers for pancreatic cancer, including miRNA-17-5p, miRNA-21, miRNA-16a, miRNA-23b-3p, miRNA-222, and miRNA-155 [96]. In the case of high-grade glioma cancer, exosomal miRNA-21, miRNA-222, and miRNA-124-3p are valuable biomarkers for complementing clinical evaluation of early tumor progression during post-surgical therapy [97]. Furthermore, microarray analysis of miRNAs in exosome-enriched fractions of colon cancer patient's serum samples has elucidated that exosomal let-7a, miRNA-21, miRNA-150, miRNA-1246, miRNA-223, miRNA-1229, and miRNA-23a levels in serum are notably higher than those in a healthy patient's serum. Hence, these exosomal miRNA signatures represent pathological changes in colorectal cancer patients and are considered as a promising biomarker for non-invasive diagnosis [98]. Furthermore, as its level is significantly high in the serum of patients, exosomal miRNA-19a is another promising prognostic biomarker that could be used for monitoring cancer recurrence in colorectal cancer patients [99]. Interestingly, it has been demonstrated that exosomal miRNA-532-5p present in the urinary of prostate cancer patients is a promising biomarker for the prediction of biochemical recurrence at intermediate risk after radical prostatectomy [100]. Moreover, different exosomal miRNAs are promising for monitoring hepatocellular carcinoma. For instance, exosomal miRNA-665 has a high level of expression in the serum of patients and its expression is related to tumor size, invasion, survival time, and clinical stage. Similar to other cancer types, a high level of expression of exosomal miRNA-21 has been also seen in hepatocellular carcinoma, making this exosomal miRNA as a novel biomarker [101].

5. Conclusion and remarks

Despite the advantageous enhancements in the field of cancer therapy, cancer is still one of the difficult-to-treat diseases. The nature of cancer is complicated, and an extensive network of signaling pathways is involved in its hallmarks. Exosomes are small extracellular vesicles that mediate the interaction of adjacent or distant cells. miRNAs are one of the factors that are carried by exosomes and their critical role in cancer progression and biology is well accepted now. Exosomal miRNAs have been proven to be responsible for regulating various types of cancer cell growth, proliferation, invasion, metastasis, immune evasion, and angiogenesis. Moreover, exosomal miRNAs mediate response to chemotherapy and radiotherapy and are considered as promising diagnostic and prognostic biomarkers for cancer. Despite the enormous studies performed to find different dimensions of exosomal miRNAs' importance and role in cancer, the number of clinical trials conducted using exosomal miRNAs is very low and further studies should address their clinical application and critical role in cancer therapy.

Conflict of interest:

The authors declare no conflict of interest.

References

1. Harding, C. and P. Stahl, *Transferrin recycling in reticulocytes: pH and iron are important determinants of ligand binding and processing.* Biochemical and Biophysical Research Communications, 1983. **113**(2): p. 650–658.
2. Pan, B.-T. and R.M. Johnstone, *Fate of the transferrin receptor during maturation of sheep reticulocytes in vitro: Selective externalization of the receptor.* Cell, 1983. **33**(3): p. 967–978.
3. Chen, J., et al., *Review on strategies and technologies for exosome isolation and purification.* Frontiers in Bioengineering and Biotechnology, 2022. **9**: p. 811971.
4. Paskeh, M.D.A., et al., *Emerging role of exosomes in cancer progression and tumor microenvironment remodeling.* Journal of Hematology & Oncology, 2022. **15**(1): p. 83.
5. Xie, S., Q. Zhang, and L. Jiang, *Current knowledge on exosome biogenesis, cargo-sorting mechanism and therapeutic implications.* Membranes, 2022. **12**(5): p. 498.
6. Xia, X., et al., *Exosome: A novel neurotransmission modulator or non-canonical neurotransmitter?* Ageing Research Reviews, 2022: p. 101558.
7. Moon, B. and S. Chang, *Exosome as a delivery vehicle for cancer therapy.* Cells, 2022. **11**(3): p. 316.
8. Paskeh, M.D.A., et al., *Emerging role of exosomes in cancer progression and tumor microenvironment remodeling.* Journal of Hematology & Oncology, 2022. **15**(1): p. 1–39.
9. Ashrafizadeh, M., et al., *Exosomes as promising nanostructures in diabetes mellitus: From insulin sensitivity to ameliorating diabetic complications.* International Journal of Nanomedicine, 2022. **17**: p. 1229.
10. Zhang, Y., et al., *Recent advances in exosome-mediated nucleic acid delivery for cancer therapy.* Journal of Nanobiotechnology, 2022. **20**(1): p. 1–29.
11. Zhang, Y., et al., *Exosomes: Biogenesis, biologic function and clinical potential.* Cell & Bioscience, 2019. **9**(1): p. 1–18.
12. Zhang, J., et al., *Exosome and exosomal microRNA: Trafficking, sorting, and function.* Genomics, Proteomics & Bioinformatics, 2015. **13**(1): p. 17–24.

13. Tian, T., et al., *Exosome uptake through clathrin-mediated endocytosis and macropinocytosis and mediating miR-21 delivery.* Journal of Biological Chemistry, 2014. **289**(32): p. 22258–22267.
14. Sempere, L.F., A.S. Azmi, and A. Moore, *microRNA-based diagnostic and therapeutic applications in cancer medicine.* Wiley Interdisciplinary Reviews: RNA, 2021. **12**(6): p. e1662.
15. Garcia-Martin, R., et al., *MicroRNA sequence codes for small extracellular vesicle release and cellular retention.* Nature, 2022. **601**(7893): p. 446–451.
16. Thomou, T., et al., *Adipose-derived circulating miRNAs regulate gene expression in other tissues.* Nature, 2017. **542**(7642): p. 450–455.
17. Groot, M. and H. Lee, *Sorting mechanisms for MicroRNAs into extracellular vesicles and their associated diseases.* Cells, 2020. **9**(4): p. 1044.
18. Mirzaei, S., et al., *The long and short non-coding RNAs modulating EZH2 signaling in cancer.* Journal of Hematology & Oncology, 2022. **15**(1): p. 18.
19. Mirzaei, S., et al., *The role of microRNA-338-3p in cancer: Growth, invasion, chemoresistance, and mediators.* Life Sciences, 2021. **268**: p. 119005.
20. Mirzaei, S., et al., *Regulation of Nuclear Factor-KappaB (NF-κB) signaling pathway by non-coding RNAs in cancer: Inhibiting or promoting carcinogenesis?* Cancer Letters, 2021. **509**: p. 63–80.
21. Li, C., et al., *The role of exosomal miRNAs in cancer.* Journal of Translational Medicine, 2022. **20**(1): p. 1–15.
22. Bakhsh, T., et al., *Exosomal miRNAs as a promising source of biomarkers in colorectal cancer progression.* International Journal of Molecular Sciences, 2022. **23**(9): p. 4855.
23. Saliminejad, K., et al., *An overview of microRNAs: Biology, functions, therapeutics, and analysis methods.* Journal of Cellular Physiology, 2019. **234**(5): p. 5451–5465.
24. Zhang, S., et al., *Exosomal miR-543 inhibits the proliferation of ovarian cancer by targeting IGF2.* Journal of Immunology Research, 2022. **2022**.
25. Hosseini, M., et al., *Tumor-derived exosomes encapsulating miR-34a promote apoptosis and inhibit migration and tumor progression of*

colorectal cancer cells under in vitro condition. DARU Journal of Pharmaceutical Sciences, 2021. **29**(2): p. 267–278.

26. Sun, X., et al., *Exosome-transmitted miRNA-335-5p promotes colorectal cancer invasion and metastasis by facilitating EMT via targeting RASA1.* Molecular Therapy-Nucleic Acids, 2021. **24**: p. 164–174.
27. Wang, W., et al., *Tumor-derived exosomal miRNA-141 promote angiogenesis and malignant progression of lung cancer by targeting growth arrest-specific homeobox gene (GAX).* Bioengineered, 2021. **12**(1): p. 821–831.
28. Fabbri, M., et al., *MicroRNAs bind to Toll-like receptors to induce prometastatic inflammatory response.* Proceedings of the National Academy of Sciences, 2012. **109**(31): p. E2110–E2116.
29. Parolini, I., et al., *Microenvironmental pH is a key factor for exosome traffic in tumor cells.* Journal of Biological Chemistry, 2009. **284**(49): p. 34211–34222.
30. Xu, W.-X., et al., *Exosomal microRNAs shuttling between tumor cells and macrophages: cellular interactions and novel therapeutic strategies.* Cancer Cell International, 2022. **22**(1): p. 1–9.
31. Wei, K., et al., *M2 macrophage-derived exosomes promote lung adenocarcinoma progression by delivering miR-942.* Cancer Letters, 2022. **526**: p. 205–216.
32. Zhu, L., et al., *Exosomal microRNAs induce tumor-associated macrophages via PPARγ during tumor progression in SHH medulloblastoma.* Cancer Letters, 2022. **535**: p. 215630.
33. Ni, Q., et al., *Exosomal microRNA-23a-3p contributes to the progression of cholangiocarcinoma by interaction with Dynamin3.* Bioengineered, 2022. **13**(3): p. 6208–6221.
34. Sun, W., et al., *Tumor stem cell-derived exosomal microRNA-17-5p inhibits anti-tumor immunity in colorectal cancer via targeting SPOP and overexpressing PD-L1.* Cell Death Discovery, 2022. **8**(1): p. 1–11.
35. Sun, T., et al., *Exosomal microRNA-19b targets FBXW7 to promote colorectal cancer stem cell stemness and induce resistance to radiotherapy.* The Kaohsiung Journal of Medical Sciences, 2022. **38**(2): p. 108–119.

36. Xue, P., et al., *Exosomal miR-101-3p and miR-423-5p inhibit medulloblastoma tumorigenesis through targeting FOXP4 and EZH2.* Cell Death & Differentiation, 2022. **29**(1): p. 82–95.
37. Jiang, D., et al., *Bone mesenchymal stem cell-derived exosomal microRNA-7-5p inhibits progression of acute myeloid leukemia by targeting OSBPL11.* Journal of Nanobiotechnology, 2022. **20**(1): p. 1–19.
38. Huang, X., et al., *microRNA-16-5p suppresses cell proliferation and angiogenesis in colorectal cancer by negatively regulating forkhead box K1 to block the PI3K/Akt/mTOR pathway.* European Journal of Histochemistry: EJH, 2022. **66**(2).
39. Qi, Y., et al., *The dual role of glioma exosomal microRNAs: Glioma eliminates tumor suppressor miR-1298-5p via exosomes to promote immunosuppressive effects of MDSCs.* Cell Death & Disease, 2022. **13**(5): p. 1–15.
40. Ma, Y.-S., et al., *Exosomal microRNA-15a from mesenchymal stem cells impedes hepatocellular carcinoma progression via downregulation of SALL4.* Cell Death Discovery, 2021. 7(1): p. 1–11.
41. Jia, Y., et al., *Mesenchymal stem cells-derived exosomal microRNA-139-5p restrains tumorigenesis in bladder cancer by targeting PRC1.* Oncogene, 2021. **40**(2): p. 246–261.
42. Huang, S., et al., *Exosomal microRNA-503-3p derived from macrophages represses glycolysis and promotes mitochondrial oxidative phosphorylation in breast cancer cells by elevating DACT2.* Cell Death Discovery, 2021. 7(1): p. 1–13.
43. Liu, J., M. Zhu, and Q. Tang, *Human umbilical cord mesenchymal stem cells-derived exosomal microRNA-181a retards nasopharyngeal carcinoma development by mediating KDM5C.* Journal of Cancer Research and Clinical Oncology, 2021. **147**(10): p. 2867–2877.
44. Deng, Y., et al., *Bone marrow mesenchymal stem cells-derived exosomal microRNA-19b-3p targets SOCS1 to facilitate progression of esophageal cancer.* Life Sciences, 2021. **278**: p. 119491.
45. Tan, Y., et al., *Tumor-derived exosomal components: The multifaceted roles and mechanisms in breast cancer metastasis.* Cell Death & Disease, 2021. **12**(6): p. 1–18.
46. Sadrkhanloo, M., et al., *STAT3-EMT axis in tumors: Modulation of cancer metastasis, stemness and therapy response.* Pharmacological Research, 2022: p. 106311.

47. Yang, C., et al., *Tumor-derived exosomal microRNA-106b-5p activates EMT-cancer cell and M2-subtype TAM interaction to facilitate CRC metastasis.* Molecular Therapy, 2021. **29**(6): p. 2088–2107.
48. Ghahhari, N.M. and S. Babashah, *Interplay between microRNAs and WNT/β-catenin signalling pathway regulates epithelial–mesenchymal transition in cancer.* European Journal of Cancer, 2015. **51**(12): p. 1638–1649.
49. Shan, G., et al., *Downregulated exosomal microRNA-148b-3p in cancer associated fibroblasts enhance chemosensitivity of bladder cancer cells by downregulating the Wnt/β-catenin pathway and upregulating PTEN.* Cellular Oncology, 2021. **44**(1): p. 45–59.
50. Takano, Y., et al., *Circulating exosomal microRNA-203 is associated with metastasis possibly via inducing tumor-associated macrophages in colorectal cancer.* Oncotarget, 2017. **8**(45): p. 78598.
51. Yang, X.-R., et al., *Correlation of exosomal microRNA clusters with bone metastasis in non-small cell lung cancer.* Clinical & Experimental Metastasis, 2021. **38**(1): p. 109–117.
52. Danac, J.M.C., A.G.G. Uy, and R.L. Garcia, *Exosomal microRNAs in colorectal cancer: Overcoming barriers of the metastatic cascade.* International Journal of Molecular Medicine, 2021. **47**(6): p. 1–16.
53. Dai, Y. and X. Gao, *Inhibition of cancer cell-derived exosomal microRNA-183 suppresses cell growth and metastasis in prostate cancer by upregulating TPM1.* Cancer Cell International, 2021. **21**(1): p. 1–15.
54. Zhu, Y., et al., *WTIP upregulates FOXO3a and induces apoptosis through PUMA in acute myeloid leukemia.* Cell Death & Disease, 2021. **13**(1): p. 1–11.
55. Gu, P., et al., *Breast tumor-derived exosomal microRNA-200b-3p promotes specific organ metastasis through regulating CCL2 expression in lung epithelial cells.* Frontiers in Cell and Developmental Biology, 2021. **9**: p. 1572.
56. Wong, G.L., S. Abu Jalboush, and H.-W. Lo, *Exosomal microRNAs and organotropism in breast cancer metastasis.* Cancers, 2020. **12**(7): p. 1827.
57. Fang, J.H., et al., *Hepatoma cell-secreted exosomal microRNA-103 increases vascular permeability and promotes metastasis by targeting junction proteins.* Hepatology, 2018. **68**(4): p. 1459–1475.

58. Kim, D.H., et al., *Exosomal miR-1260b derived from non-small cell lung cancer promotes tumor metastasis through the inhibition of HIPK2.* Cell Death & Disease, 2021. **12**(8): p. 1–10.
59. Chen, W., et al., *Evaluation of plasma exosomal miRNAs as potential diagnostic biomarkers of lymph node metastasis in papillary thyroid carcinoma.* Endocrine, 2022. **75**(3): p. 846–855.
60. Mao, S., et al., *Exosomal miR-375-3p breaks vascular barrier and promotes small cell lung cancer metastasis by targeting claudin-1.* Translational Lung Cancer Research, 2021. **10**(7): p. 3155.
61. Chen, B., et al., *Exosomal miR-500a-5p derived from cancer-associated fibroblasts promotes breast cancer cell proliferation and metastasis through targeting USP28.* Theranostics, 2021. **11**(8): p. 3932.
62. Tian, W., et al., *Exosomal miR-338-3p suppresses non-small-cell lung cancer cells metastasis by inhibiting CHL1 through the MAPK signaling pathway.* Cell Death & Disease, 2021. **12**(11): p. 1–12.
63. You, X., et al., *Exosomal miR-663b exposed to TGF-β1 promotes cervical cancer metastasis and epithelial-mesenchymal transition by targeting MGAT3.* Oncology Reports, 2021. **45**(4): p. 1.
64. Lampropoulou, D.I., et al., *The role of exosomal non-coding RNAs in colorectal cancer drug resistance.* International Journal of Molecular Sciences, 2022. **23**(3): p. 1473.
65. Wang, W., et al., *The potential roles of exosomal non-coding RNAs in hepatocellular carcinoma.* Frontiers in Oncology, 2022. **12**.
66. Yao, P., et al., *Research progress of exosome-loaded miRNA in osteosarcoma.* Cancer Control, 2022. **29**: p. 10732748221076683.
67. Zhong, S., et al., *MicroRNA expression profiles of drug-resistance breast cancer cells and their exosomes.* Oncotarget, 2016. 7(15): p. 19601.
68. Li, J., et al., *Exosome-derived microRNAs contribute to prostate cancer chemoresistance.* International Journal of Oncology, 2016. **49**(2): p. 838–846.
69. Comandatore, A., et al., *Potential role of exosomes in the chemoresistance to gemcitabine and nab-paclitaxel in pancreatic cancer.* Diagnostics, 2022. **12**(2): p. 286.
70. Console, L. and M. Scalise, *Extracellular vesicles and cell pathways involved in cancer chemoresistance.* Life, 2022. **12**(5): p. 618.

71. Guo, Q.-R., et al., *The role of exosomal microRNA in cancer drug resistance.* Frontiers in Oncology, 2020. **10**: p. 472.
72. Zhao, Z., et al., *Targeted delivery of exosomal miR-484 reprograms tumor vasculature for chemotherapy sensitization.* Cancer Letters, 2022. **530**: p. 45–58.
73. Fu, X., et al., *Exosomal microRNA-32-5p induces multidrug resistance in hepatocellular carcinoma via the PI3K/Akt pathway.* Journal of Experimental & Clinical Cancer Research, 2018. **37**(1): p. 1–18.
74. Zeng, A., et al., *Exosomal transfer of miR-151a enhances chemosensitivity to temozolomide in drug-resistant glioblastoma.* Cancer Letters, 2018. **436**: p. 10–21.
75. Patel, G.K., et al., *Exosomes confer chemoresistance to pancreatic cancer cells by promoting ROS detoxification and miR-155-mediated suppression of key gemcitabine-metabolising enzyme, DCK.* British Journal of Cancer, 2017. **116**(5): p. 609–619.
76. Kanlikilicer, P., et al., *Exosomal miRNA confers chemo resistance via targeting Cav1/p-gp/M2-type macrophage axis in ovarian cancer.* EBioMedicine, 2018. **38**: p. 100–112.
77. Jiang, L., et al., *Exosomal microRNA-107 reverses chemotherapeutic drug resistance of gastric cancer cells through HMGA2/mTOR/P-gp pathway.* BMC Cancer, 2021. **21**(1): p. 1–16.
78. Semaan, L., et al., *MicroRNA-214 enriched exosomes from human cerebral endothelial cells (hCEC) sensitize hepatocellular carcinoma to anticancer drugs.* Oncotarget, 2021. **12**(3): p. 185.
79. Andreeva, O.E., et al., *Towards unravelling the role of ERα-targeting miRNAs in the exosome-mediated transferring of the hormone resistance.* Molecules, 2021. **26**(21): p. 6661.
80. Malla, B., et al., *Exosomes and exosomal microRNAs in prostate cancer radiation therapy.* International Journal of Radiation Oncology* Biology* Physics, 2017. **98**(5): p. 982–995.
81. Wei, Y., et al., *Exosomal miR-221/222 enhances tamoxifen resistance in recipient ER-positive breast cancer cells.* Breast Cancer Research and Rreatment, 2014. **147**(2): p. 423–431.
82. Dong, X., et al., *Exosomes and breast cancer drug resistance.* Cell Death & Disease, 2020. **11**(11): p. 1–14.

83. Ni, J., et al., *Exosomes in cancer radioresistance.* Frontiers in Oncology, 2019. **9**: p. 869.
84. Liao, C., H. Liu, and X. Luo, *The emerging roles of exosomal miRNAs in nasopharyngeal carcinoma.* American Journal of Cancer Research, 2021. **11**(6): p. 2508.
85. Chen, X., et al., *Exosomal miR-590-3p derived from cancer-associated fibroblasts confers radioresistance in colorectal cancer.* Molecular Therapy-Nucleic Acids, 2021. **24**: p. 113–126.
86. Tan, S., et al., *Exosomal miRNAs in tumor microenvironment.* Journal of Experimental & Clinical Cancer Research, 2020. **39**(1): p. 1–15.
87. Santos, P. and F. Almeida, *Role of exosomal miRNAs and the tumor microenvironment in drug resistance.* Cells, 2020. **9**(6): p. 1450.
88. Yang, E., et al., *Exosome-mediated metabolic reprogramming: The emerging role in tumor microenvironment remodeling and its influence on cancer progression.* Signal Transduction and Targeted Therapy, 2020. **5**(1): p. 1–13.
89. Yan, W., et al., *Cancer-cell-secreted exosomal miR-105 promotes tumour growth through the MYC-dependent metabolic reprogramming of stromal cells.* Nature Cell Biology, 2018. **20**(5): p. 597–609.
90. Xu, G., et al., *Exosomal miRNA-139 in cancer-associated fibroblasts inhibits gastric cancer progression by repressing MMP11 expression.* International Journal of Biological Sciences, 2019. **15**(11): p. 2320.
91. Han, C., et al., *Exosome-mediated communication between tumor cells and tumor-associated macrophages: Implications for tumor microenvironment.* Oncoimmunology, 2021. **10**(1): p. 1887552.
92. Liu, J., et al., *Endoplasmic reticulum stress causes liver cancer cells to release exosomal miR-23a-3p and up-regulate programmed death ligand 1 expression in macrophages.* Hepatology, 2019. **70**(1): p. 241–258.
93. Chen, X., et al., *Exosomes derived from hypoxic epithelial ovarian cancer cells deliver microRNAs to macrophages and elicit a tumor-promoted phenotype.* Cancer Letters, 2018. **435**: p. 80–91.
94. Preethi, K.A., et al., *Liquid biopsy: Exosomal microRNAs as novel diagnostic and prognostic biomarkers in cancer.* Molecular Cancer, 2022. **21**(1): p. 1–15.

95. Zhu, Z., et al., *Detection of plasma exosomal miRNA-205 as a biomarker for early diagnosis and an adjuvant indicator of ovarian cancer staging*. Journal of Ovarian Research, 2022. **15**(1): p. 1–10.
96. Uddin, M., et al., *Exosomal microRNA in pancreatic cancer diagnosis, prognosis, and treatment: From bench to bedside.* Cancers, 2021. **13**(11): p. 2777.
97. Olioso, D., et al., *Serum exosomal microRNA-21, 222 and 124-3p as noninvasive predictive biomarkers in newly diagnosed high-grade gliomas: A prospective study.* Cancers, 2021. **13**(12): p. 3006.
98. Ogata-Kawata, H., et al., *Circulating exosomal microRNAs as biomarkers of colon cancer.* PloS One, 2014. **9**(4): p. e92921.
99. Matsumura, T., et al., *Exosomal microRNA in serum is a novel biomarker of recurrence in human colorectal cancer.* British Journal of Cancer, 2015. **113**(2): p. 275–281.
100. Kim, M.Y., et al., *Urinary exosomal microRNA profiling in intermediate-risk prostate cancer.* Scientific Reports, 2021. **11**(1): p. 1–7.
101. Li, S., et al., *Exosomal miRNAs in hepatocellular carcinoma development and clinical responses.* Journal of Hematology & Oncology, 2018. **11**(1): p. 1–9.

https://doi.org/10.1142/9789811267390_0005

Chapter 5

Long non-coding RNAs (lncRNAs) in cancer proliferation: Molecular interactions and possible therapeutic targets

Maliheh Entezari[1,2], Afshin Taheriazam[2,3], Sepideh Mirzaei[4], Shokooh Salimimoghadam[5]*, Azuma Kalu[6,7] and Noushin Nabavi[8]

[1]*Department of Genetics, Faculty of Advanced Science and Technology, Tehran Medical Sciences, Islamic Azad University, Tehran, Iran*
[2]*Farhikhtegan Medical Convergence Sciences Research Center, Farhikhtegan Hospital Tehran Medical Sciences, Islamic Azad University, Tehran, Iran*
[3]*Department of Orthopedics, Faculty of Medicine, Tehran Medical Sciences, Islamic Azad University, Tehran, Iran*
[4]*Department of Biology, Faculty of Science, Islamic Azad University, Science and Research Branch, Tehran, Iran*
[5]*Department of Biochemistry and Molecular Biology, Faculty of Veterinary Medicine, Shahid Chamran University of Ahvaz, Ahvaz, Iran*
[6]*School of Life, Health & Chemical Sciences, The Open University, Milton Keynes, United Kingdom*
[7]*Laboratory Medicine Directorate, Sheffield Teaching Hospital, Sheffield, United Kingdom*
[8]*Department of Urologic Sciences and Vancouver Prostate Centre, University of British Columbia, Vancouver, BC, Canada*

---

*Corresponding author: Shokooh Salimimoghadam, Department of Biochemistry and Molecular Biology, Faculty of Veterinary Medicine, Shahid Chamran University of Ahvaz, Ahvaz, Iran, Email: shokoohmoghadam@yahoo.com

Abstract

Long non-coding RNAs (lncRNAs) are a class of non-protein coding RNAs that have more than 200 nucleotides. lncRNAs have been found to be aberrantly expressed in human diseases including cancer. In cancer, lncRNAs exert critical roles and affect all the cancer hallmarks including apoptosis, proliferative capacity, malignancy, invasiveness, immune evasion, angiogenesis, chemo-resistance, and radio-resistance via regulating various factors and signaling pathways. lncRNAs target other non-coding RNAs, commonly miRNAs. lncRNAs are predominantly either tumor suppressors or oncogenic. However, some lncRNAs have both roles based on the cancer type. For instance, MIR31HG exerts tumor suppressor functions in hepatocellular carcinoma while possessing oncogenic roles in non-small cell lung cancer. Cancer cells inhibit apoptosis, increase metabolic pathways such as glycolysis, and promote cell cycle progression to augment their proliferation. Evidence has revealed the critical role of lncRNAs in the regulation of these mechanisms, either by their suppression or by promotion. Thus, the aim of this chapter is to discuss the importance of lncRNAs in the regulation of apoptosis, autophagy, cell cycle progression, and glycolysis in various types of cancer.

1. Introduction

Long non-coding RNAs (lncRNAs) are non-coding RNAs (ncRNAs) that do not have a protein coding function. ncRNAs mainly include RNAs with <200 and >200 nucleotides in length [1, 2]. microRNAs (miRNAs), small interfering RNAs, and PIWI-interacting RNAs are examples of ncRNAs with less than 200 nucleotides, while lncRNAs contain >200 nucleotides. It has been demonstrated that most of the mutations of the genome that occurs during cancer are placed in regions that are not responsible for coding proteins. Interestingly, lncRNAs are transcribed from these regions. In addition, the aberrant expression of lncRNAs has been shown to be associated with cancer progression [3–8]. lncRNAs affect cancer biology by targeting its hallmarks such as metastasis, apoptosis, proliferation, immune evasion, metabolic reprogramming, and therapy resistance [9–13].

lncRNAs have the ability to bind to DNA, RNAs, and proteins as master regulators of gene expression [14, 15]. Intriguingly, it has been shown that although most of the lncRNAs' expression is dysregulated in a cancer-specific manner, they could have aberrant expressions in various cancer tissues [16].

XIST and H19 discovered in the 1990s were the first lncRNAs to be identified [17, 18]. lncRNAs are transcribed via RNA polymerase II and possess a 5′ cap and 3′ polyadenylated tail. There are different types of classifications for lncRNAs such as their site of origin, their function, and their localization in the cell. lncRNAs could be transcribed and named based on various regions of the genome including sense and antisense strands of DNA, transcribed in a bidirectional way, intronic, and intergenic. Moreover, lncRNAs exert their function in the nucleus or travel to other regions such as mitochondria and cytoplasm [7, 8, 19–22]. lncRNAs are also characterized by histone H3 Lys4 trimethylation in the transcription site and histone H3 trimethylated at Lys36 through the body of the responsible gene [23]. Three major functions are defined for lncRNAs in the regulation of transcription and translation: (1) act as a guide, essential for appropriate localization of regulators such as chromatin-modifying complexes; (2) act as dynamic scaffolds, required for the assembly of cofactors; and (3) act as a decoy, to sequester gene's expression regulators such as miRNAs and transcription factors to inhibit their interaction with their targets [24–27]. This chapter intends to discuss the importance of lncRNAs in modulating cancer cells via targeting cellular processes including apoptosis, autophagy, cell cycle progression, and metabolic pathways.

2. lncRNAs in regulating apoptosis

Accumulating data reveals the critical role of lncRNAs in regulating apoptosis. lncRNAs could suppress or provoke apoptosis to regulate cancer progression. For instance, lncRNA MIR17HG is a tumor suppressor factor that sponges miRNA-21 to increase PTEN and subsequently promote apoptosis in acute myeloid leukemia [28]. Furthermore, lncRNA growth arrest–specific transcript 5 (GAS5) triggers apoptosis to suppress tumor cell growth by inducing endoplasmic reticulum stress by targeting CHOP in hepatocellular carcinoma [29]. Similarly, lncRNA loc285194 induces oxidative stress to suppress tumor cell progression via triggering apoptosis in epithelial ovarian cancer [30]. In contrast, lncRNA nuclear-enriched abundant transcript 1 (lnc-NEAT1) is overexpressed in laryngeal papilloma and suppresses apoptosis. lnc-NEAT1 upregulation has been proven to be associated with apoptosis suppression. For this purpose, lnc-NEAT1 sponges miRNA-577/miRNA-1224-5p to upregulate cyclin T2 (CCNT2), thereby inhibiting apoptosis and increasing cell proliferation. Moreover, lnc-NEAT1 suppresses Bax, caspase 3 and 9 to exert its oncogenic functions [31]. lncRNA LOC550643 has also been shown to be an oncogene. lncRNA LOC550643 suppresses miRNA-29b-2-5p to inhibit apoptosis and increase colon cancer cell growth and metastasis [32]. Furthermore, in acute lymphoblastic leukemia, lncRNA plasmacytoma variant translocation 1 gene (PVT1) sponges miRNA-486-5p to increase mastermind-like transcriptional coactivator 3 (MAML3), a factor which suppresses apoptosis and increases tumor cell growth. Thus, lncRNA PVT1 suppresses apoptosis induction via the upregulation of MAML3 [33]. Similarly, lncRNA prostate cancer-associated transcript 1 (PCAT1) acts as a suppressor for miRNA-134-3p to increase the expression level of pituitary homeobox 2 in breast cancer to suppress apoptosis. Moreover, upregulation of PCAT1 is associated with Bcl-2 upregulation, while Bax and caspase 3/9 expression is decreased [34]. LEF1-AS1 is another lncRNA with tumor-promoting function. LEF1-AS1 acts as a sponge for miRNA-5100 to upregulate DEK. DEK is the downstream target of miRNA-5100 and affects AMPK/mTOR axis to suppress apoptosis and induce autophagy in gastric cancer cells, maintaining their growth [35]. Further, CMB9-22P13.1 is a hepatocellular carcinoma-related lncRNA that is upregulated in this cancer type and is associated with poor prognosis and advanced cancer stage. CMB9-22P13.1 acts as a competing endogenous RNA (ceRNA) for various miRNAs including miRNA-6760-5p, miRNA-6512-3p, miRNA-1298-5p, miRNA-6720-5p, miRNA-4516, and miRNA-6782-5p to increase HOTTIP.

This axis ultimately results in promoting tumor cell growth, invasion, and migration, while suppressing apoptosis. On the other hand, CMB9-22P13.1 promotes the recruitment of hypoxia-inducible factor-1 subunit alpha (HIF-1α) for the activation of vascular endothelial growth factor and angiogenesis [36]. Furthermore, lncRNA PCED1B-AS1 suppresses miRNA-633 for increasing the expression level of HOXA9 in colorectal adenocarcinoma. PCED1B-AS1/miRNA-633/HOXA9 axis activation leads to suppression of apoptosis and elevation of proliferation [37]. In colorectal cancer cells, lncRNAs' thymopoietin antisense transcript 1 (TMPO-AS1) is overexpressed and promotes tumor cell proliferation and stemness, while suppressing apoptosis. TMPO-AS1 suppresses miRNA-98-5p. BCAT1 is the downstream target of miRNA-98-5p and TMPO-AS1 increases its level via inhibiting miRNA-98-5p (Figure 1) [38].

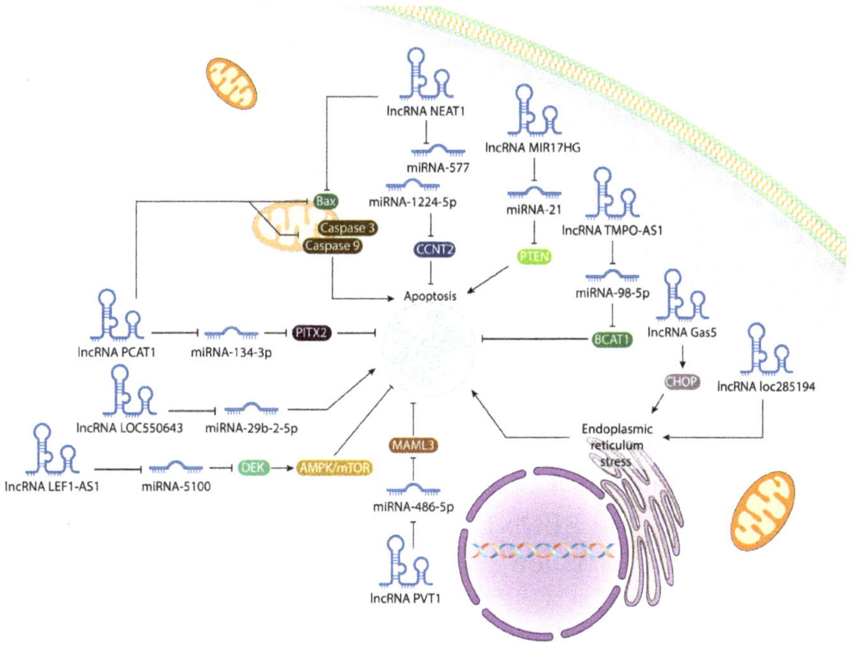

Figure 1. Apoptosis regulation via lncRNAs.

3. lncRNAs in regulating autophagy

Autophagy is a multi-step process, which is carried out by cells for clearing damaged organelles and intracellular proteins. Moreover, autophagy prevents the toxicity of cellular wastes and provides metabolic substrates to be used during starvation by cells as fuels. Autophagy could promote or suppress tumorigenesis. In cancer, autophagy could increase cell viability and survival. One of the important reasons for autophagy in cancer is decreasing the microenvironmental stress [39–44]. Furthermore, the function of autophagy in various cancer hallmarks such as metastasis, response to therapy, and stemness has been previously described [45–48]. The first step of autophagy is the production of a phagophore, a double-layered membrane. Then, this membrane expands to form a vesicle named autophagosome. Being merged with lysosomes, autophagosome turns to autolysosome which degrades its cargo. Various factors target different steps of autophagy to regulate its function. For instance, Unc-51-like autophagy-activating kinase 1 (ULK1) targets phagophore formation, ATG5/ATG12/ATG16 complex targets autophagosome formation, and LC3 II is involved in the selection of substrates to be degraded in autophagy [49–52]. Accumulating evidence shows the critical role of lncRNAs in the regulation of autophagy [53–55]. For instance, exosomal lncRNA H19 derived from tumor-associated macrophages has been demonstrated to induce autophagy via increasing LC3 II and decreasing p26. Moreover, H19 accelerates the stabilization of ULK1 [56]. Similarly, LINC01279 provokes autophagy in lung cancer via targeting FAK and SIN3A [57]. lncRNA Firre intergenic repeating RNA element (FIRRE) increases the translocation of polypyrimidine tract–binding protein (PTBP1) from nucleus to cytoplasm. Furthermore, FIRRE mediates the stabilization of BECN1 via PTBP1 to promote autophagy, thereby increasing tumor growth [58]. LINC01426 suppresses miRNA-143-3p target USP28 to induce autophagy, invasion, and metastasis. In contrast, suppression of LINC01426 leads to the induction of apoptosis in non-small cell lung cancer [58]. In addition, lncRNA colon cancer–associated transcript 1 (lncRNA CCAT1) is another oncogene lncRNA with high expression levels in gastric cancer. CCAT1 promotes autophagy, tumor cell proliferation, invasion, and migration via suppression of miRNA-140-3p and increasing ATG5 [59]. Interestingly, targeting autophagy by lncRNAs could be associated with chemo-resistance. For instance, lncRNA EIF3J-DT inhibits miRNA-188-3p to upregulate ATG14 and promote autophagy, thereby mediating chemo-resistance [60]. Furthermore, lncRNA metastasis–associated lung adenocarcinoma transcript 1 acts as a ceRNA for miRNA-26a-5p to increase Smad1 in colorectal cancer cells. Upregulation of Smad1 is associated with autophagy induction, via targeting ATG5 [61]. Moreover, LINC01559 sponges hsa-miR-1343-3p to promote autophagy, proliferation, and malignancy of lung adenocarcinoma cells [62]. On the other hand, lncRNA DRAIC induces autophagy to suppress tumorigenesis in glioblastoma. DRAIC is a tumor suppressor lncRNA that decreases nuclear factor kappa B (NF-kB) downstream target GLUT1 to increase AMPK. Furthermore, DRAIC suppresses mTOR which ultimately results in the activation of autophagy [63]. Similarly, lncRNA maternally expressed gene 3 (MEG3) induces apoptosis and autophagy in nasopharyngeal carcinoma. To do this, lncRNA MEG3 functions as a sponge for miRNA-21 to increase PTEN. MEG3 is poorly expressed in nasopharyngeal carcinoma, and its overexpression is associated with oncogenic suppression [64].

4. lncRNAs in regulating cell cycle progression

lncRNAs can tightly regulate the expression of cell cycle regulators. Interestingly, dysregulation of lncRNAs which are involved in the regulation of cell cycle progression and genome stability are associated with various human disorders such as cancer [65]. Dysregulation of these lncRNAs could be considered as promising and accurate biomarkers for cancer. An example is lncRNA HOTAIR, which is overexpressed in non-small cell lung cancer cells. HOTAIR upregulation regulates the Rb-E2F pathway to mediate the cell cycle from the restriction point of G1–S phase. In addition, HOTAIR promotes the proliferation of cancer cells, as well as their migration and invasion through epithelial–mesenchymal transition (EMT) and b-catenin pathway. Dysregulation of the cell cycle via HOTAIR also leads to resistance of cancer cells to gefitinib. Overall, in one study it was found that HOTAIR overexpression is a promising indicator for the detection of cell cycle disruption [66]. lncRNA X-inactive-specific transcript (XIST) is upregulated in ovarian cancer cells. XIST overexpression is accompanied by improved cell cycle progression, high proliferation rate, malignancy, invasive capability, and apoptosis suppression. To exert its effect, XIST suppresses miRNA-149-3p, while increasing forkhead box P3 (FOXP3) [67]. In addition, lung cancer–associated transcript 3 (LCAT3) is a novel lncRNA with oncogenic roles in lung adenocarcinoma. LCAT3 stabilization is mediated by N^6-methyladenosine modification. LCAT3 upregulation is associated with cell cycle progression, proliferation, invasion, and metastasis, while its downregulation is accompanied by cell cycle arrest at G1 phase. LCAT3 exerts these functions via activating Myc through recruiting far upstream element–binding protein 1 (FUBP1) [68]. Similarly, LINC00662 enhances proliferation, invasive capacity, and migration in non-small cell lung cancer while suppressing apoptosis. It has been demonstrated that downregulation of LINC00662 is associated with cell cycle arrest at G0/G1 phase. LINC00662 acts as an miRNA-320d sponge to increase E2F1 expression [69]. Likewise, LOXL1-AS1 overexpression in prostate cancer promotes cancer cell cycle progression. LOXL1-AS1 overexpression is associated with increased proliferation and suppressed cell cycle arrest. To exert its function, LOXL1-AS1 inhibits miRNA-541-3p, while increasing CCND1 [70]. lncRNA MINCR is another oncogenic factor that affects cancer hallmarks in non-small cell lung cancer cells. Knockdown of MINCR leads to cell cycle arrest in cancer cells via downregulation of c-Myc. Decreased c-Myc leads to depletion of its downstream targets including cyclin-A and cyclin-D, CD4, CDK2, Bcl-2, and elevation of PARP-1 expression [71].

5. lncRNAs in regulating glycolysis

lncRNAs have been widely studied for their critical role in metabolic reprogramming including regulating glycolysis in cancer [72, 73]. In a study, the results of RNA-Seq assay show that LINC01123 is highly expressed in non-small cell lung cancer cells. There is a positive feedback loop between LINC01123 and c-Myc. Indeed, LINC01123 is directly targeted by c-Myc, via sponging miRNA-199a-5p. More importantly, LINC01123 regulates glycolysis to exert its function [74]. Interestingly, a feedback loop could be existed between c-Myc and a tumor suppressor lncRNAs. For instance, lncRNA FGF13-AS1 expression is decreased in breast cancer cells and its downregulation is associated with poor prognosis. Upregulation of FGF13-AS1 resulted in the suppression of proliferation, migration, and invasive capacity. By exerting its function, FGF13-AS1 impairs glycolysis. Furthermore, FGF13-AS1 suppresses the interaction between c-Myc and insulin-like growth factor 2 mRNA-binding proteins to suppress c-Myc. Moreover, c-Myc has been shown to suppress FGF13-AS1 transcriptionally [75]. As another example, LINC00538 upregulation in breast cancer is associated with high proliferation rate and tumor cell growth. LINC00538 overexpression is associated with an increased phosphorylated form of fructose bisphosphatase PFK2 (PFKFB3) via CDK6. As a result, glucose 6-phosphate is converted into fructose-2,6-bisphosphate [76]. Likewise, lncRNA DLEU2 is overexpressed in endometrial cancer. DLEU2 increases HK2 to promote glycolysis via two distinct pathways: first, suppression of miRNA-455 and second interaction with EZH2 to inhibit miRNA-181a as a direct suppressor of HK2. Upregulation of HK2 further resulted in FAK and subsequent ERK1/2 signaling to promote aerobic glycolysis [77]. In contrast to these examples of oncogenic lncRNAs, lncRNA MEG3 expression in colorectal cancer cells is lower than in normal tissues. Upregulation of MEG3 is associated with glycolysis suppression as well as lactate production. In contrast, these results are reversed following the knockdown of MEG3. MEG3 induces the ubiquitination of c-Myc to increase its degradation and cancer cells [105]. Besides, the inhibitory role of TSLNC8 in glioma cancer hallmarks includes proliferation, metastasis, and apoptosis as previously studied [106]. lncRNA MIR31HG is another example whose overexpression is associated with hepatocellular carcinoma proliferation and metastasis inhibition. MIR31HG suppresses miRNA-575 to increase the expression of suppression of tumorigenicity 7 like (ST7L) [107]. However, some studies have revealed conflicting results in other type of cancers. For instance, Zheng *et al.* has shown that MIR31HG augments non-small cell lung cancer cell proliferation and invasion via targeting Wnt/b-catenin [108]. Furthermore, MIR31HG can target HIF-1α and p21 to promote head and neck cancer cell tumorigenesis and proliferative capacity via enhancing cell cycle progression [109]. Additionally, lncRNA GAS5-AS1 has tumor suppressor activities. It was found that GAS5-AS1 inhibits cervical cancer growth and metastasis by enhancing GAS5 stability [110]. In addition, GAS5-AS1 negatively affects invasion, proliferation, and migration in glioma via targeting miRNA-106b-5p/TUSC2 axis [111] in triple-negative breast cancer via targeting miRNA-196a-5p [112]. In contrast, upregulation of lncRNA GAS5 in gastric cancer is associated with tumorigenesis suppression. To exert its function, GAS5 serves as a sponge for miRNA-106a-5p through the Akt/mTOR signaling pathway [113]. lncRNA XIST, a transcript of chromosome Xq13.2, is placed on the X-inactivation center and mediates the activation of X-linked genes. The tumor suppressor role of XIST is studied in various cancers. For instance, in breast cancer, XIST expression is downregulated and its overexpression is associated with the suppression of miRNA-155. XIST functions as a sponge for miRNA-155 to increase its downstream target, caudal-type homeobox 1 (CDX1), which results in the suppression of breast cancer cell growth, invasion, and migration [114]. Nonetheless, some studies suggest a tumorigenic function for XIST (Figure 2) [115–118].

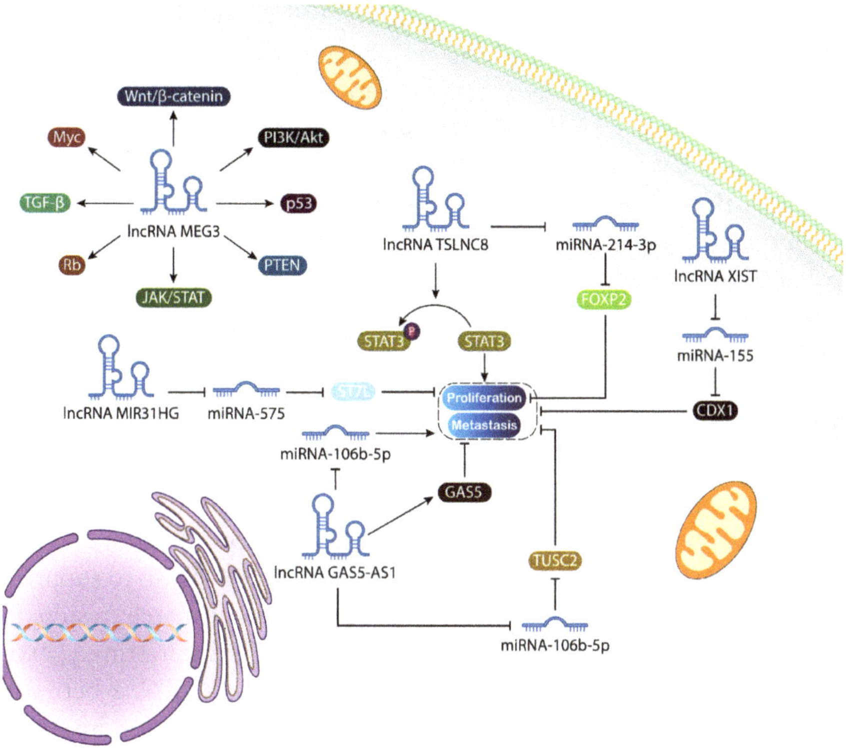

Figure 2. Onco-suppressor lncRNAs.

7. Oncogenic lncRNAs

Similar to tumor suppressor lncRNAs, numerous studies have revealed lncRNAs with oncogenic function [22, 119–123]. As an example, lncRNA RNCR3 targets miRNA-185-5p to enhance prostate cancer progression [124]. Furthermore, lncRNA MIR17HG increases colorectal cancer cell progression by targeting miRNA-17-5p to increase tumor suppressor B-cell linker (BLNK). Elevation of BLNK increases the invasive and migration capacity of cells. Besides,

MIR17HG acts as a sponge for miRNA-375 to upregulate NF-κB/RELA. In addition, MIR17HG upregulates PD-L1 in cancer cells. Overall, MIR17HG act as a tumor promoter by targeting various factors and pathways [125]. Progression-associated lncRNA in breast cancer (PRLB) suppresses miRNA-4766-5p to enhance breast cancer cell growth, proliferation, and metastatic capacity. miRNA-4766-5p is a suppressor of sirtuin 1, and lncRNA PRLB increases its expression by knocking down miRNA-4766-5p. In addition, PRLB functions could result in chemo-resistance [126]. lncRNA EMT-associated lncRNA induced by TGF-β1 (ELIT-1) could be overexpressed via TGF-β/Smad pathway. In fact, TGF-β increases ELIT-1 to elevate Snail via recruiting Smad3 and subsequently promotes EMT. In addition, ELIT-1 increases transforming growth factor β (TGF-β) in a positive feedback loop [127]. In hepatocellular carcinoma, overexpression of BZRAP1-AS1 is associated with high proliferation, metastasis, and invasion. BZRAP1-AS1 interacts with DNMT3b to suppress THBS1 via increasing its methylation. This axis ultimately results in angiogenesis and tumor growth promotion [128]. Interestingly, exosomes have critical roles in transferring oncogenic lncRNAs between cells located in the tumor microenvironment [129]. For instance, exosomal lncRNA CCAL derived from fibroblasts is able to increase chemo-resistance in colorectal cancer cells [130]. Similarly, exosomal lncRNA LNMAT2 enhances lymphatic metastasis of bladder cancer cells [131]. Table 1 provides a list of other lncRNAs with tumor-promoting function in various cancers.

8. Conclusion and remarks

Cancer has remained the most challenging disease for centuries because of its heterogeneous nature, recurrence, and therapy resistance. Cancer is characterized by various hallmarks, including apoptosis suppression, high proliferation rate, invasion, metastasis, immune escape, angiogenesis, and resistance to therapy. Conventional therapies for cancer are surgery, chemotherapy, and radiotherapy. However, targeted therapy has been shown to be a promising method for cancer therapy. lncRNAs belong to a class of ncRNAs

Table 1. Oncogenic lncRNA in different cancers and the underlying mechanisms by which lncRNAs exert their function.

lncRNA	Cancer Type	Signaling Network	Remark	Ref
PVT1	Cholangiocarcinoma	ANGPTL4	Induction of proliferation and migration via ANGPTL4 suppression.	[132]
LncHDAC2	Liver cancer	Hedgehog signaling	Promoting self-renewal capacity of liver cancer stem cells through activation of Hedgehog signaling.	[133]
NONHSAT101069	Breast cancer	miRNA-129-5p/Twist1	Increasing Twist1 via sponging miRNA-129-5p. Increasing epirubicin resistance, EMT, invasion, and migration.	[134]
SNHG14	Breast cancer	PABPC1	Trastuzumab resistance via H3K2 acetylation.	[135]
HCP5	Lung adenocarcinoma	miRNA-203/SNAI	HCP5 upregulation via TGF-β transcriptionally regulation via Smad3. Promotion of metastasis via sponging miRNA-203 and increasing SNAI. Poor prognosis.	[136]
LINC00511	Breast cancer	miRNA-185-3p/E2F1/Nanog	Sponging miRNA-185-3p to increase E2F1. High proliferation rate, tumor growth, and sphere-forming ability. Overexpression of stem factors, including Oct4, Nanog, and SOX2.	[137]
DLGAP1-AS1	Hepatocellular carcinoma	miRNA-486-5p/H3F3B	Sponging miRNA-486-5p to increase H3F3B. Promoting the proliferation.	[138]

that are not responsible for protein coding. lncRNAs affect various cancer hallmarks to regulate their function, and this fact makes them the master regulators of cancer. This chapter discussed the critical role of lncRNAs in cancer progression and suppression. lncRNAs regulate apoptosis by targeting its intrinsic and extrinsic pathways. Furthermore, metabolic reprogramming is the other function of lncRNAs. lncRNAs could affect glycolysis by targeting glucose transporters, and enzymes involved in glycolysis pathways, such as PKM2 and HK2. In addition, cyclins and cyclin-dependent kinases are targeted by lncRNAs in the case of cell cycle arrest and progression. Thus, considering these critical regulators, lncRNAs in cancer therapy are of important, and finding current gaps to overcome obstacles in cancer therapy is crucial.

Conflict of interest:

The authors declare no conflict of interest.

References

1. Mirzaei, S., et al., *The long and short non-coding RNAs modulating EZH2 signaling in cancer.* Journal of Hematology & Oncology, 2022. **15**(1): p. 18.
2. Mirzaei, S., et al., *Molecular landscape of LncRNAs in prostate cancer: A focus on pathways and therapeutic targets for intervention.* Journal of Experimental & Clinical Cancer Research, 2022. **41**(1): p. 214.
3. Huarte, M., *The emerging role of lncRNAs in cancer.* Nature Medicine, 2015. **21**(11): p. 1253–1261.
4. Zhang, R., et al., *LncRNAs and cancer.* Oncology Letters, 2016. **12**(2): p. 1233–1239.
5. Prensner, J.R. and A.M. Chinnaiyan, *The emergence of lncRNAs in cancer biology.* Cancer Discovery, 2011. **1**(5): p. 391–407.
6. Zhang, Y. and L. Tang, *The application of lncRNAs in cancer treatment and diagnosis.* Recent Patents on Anti-Cancer Drug Discovery, 2018. **13**(3): p. 292–301.

7. Hashemi, M., et al., *Long non-coding RNA (lncRNA) H19 in human cancer: From proliferation and metastasis to therapy.* Pharmacological Research, 2022. **184**: p. 106418.
8. Entezari, M., et al., *LncRNA-miRNA axis in tumor progression and therapy response: An emphasis on molecular interactions and therapeutic interventions.* Biomedicine & Pharmacotherapy, 2022. **154**: p. 113609.
9. Jiang, M.-C., et al., *Emerging roles of lncRNA in cancer and therapeutic opportunities.* American Journal of Cancer Research, 2019. **9**(7): p. 1354.
10. Li, J., et al., *Regulation of lncRNA and its role in cancer metastasis.* Oncology Research, 2016. **23**(5): p. 205.
11. Chen, S., et al., *LncRNAs and their role in cancer stem cells.* Oncotarget, 2017. **8**(66): p. 110685.
12. Paskeh, M.D.A., et al., *Emerging role of exosomes in cancer progression and tumor microenvironment remodeling.* Journal of Hematology & Oncology, 2022. **15**(1): p. 83.
13. Mirzaei, S., et al., *Regulation of Nuclear Factor-KappaB (NF-κB) signaling pathway by non-coding RNAs in cancer: Inhibiting or promoting carcinogenesis?* Cancer Letters, 2021. **509**: p. 63–80.
14. Peng, W.-X., P. Koirala, and Y.-Y. Mo, *LncRNA-mediated regulation of cell signaling in cancer.* Oncogene, 2017. **36**(41): p. 5661–5667.
15. Nandwani, A., S. Rathore, and M. Datta, *LncRNAs in cancer: Regulatory and therapeutic implications.* Cancer Letters, 2021. **501**: p. 162–171.
16. Chiu, H.-S., et al., *Pan-cancer analysis of lncRNA regulation supports their targeting of cancer genes in each tumor context.* Cell Reports, 2018. **23**(1): p. 297–312. e12.
17. Bartolomei, M.S., S. Zemel, and S.M. Tilghman, *Parental imprinting of the mouse H19 gene.* Nature, 1991. **351**(6322): p. 153–155.
18. Brown, C.J., et al., *A gene from the region of the human X inactivation centre is expressed exclusively from the inactive X chromosome.* Nature, 1991. **349**(6304): p. 38–44.
19. Liu, Y., et al., *Long non-coding RNAs: Biogenesis, functions, and clinical significance in gastric cancer.* Molecular Therapy-Oncolytics, 2021. **23**: p. 458–476.

20. Fang, Y. and M.J. Fullwood, *Roles, functions, and mechanisms of long non-coding RNAs in cancer.* Genomics, Proteomics & Bioinformatics, 2016. **14**(1): p. 42–54.
21. Bhan, A., M. Soleimani, and S.S. Mandal, *Long noncoding RNA and cancer: A new paradigm.* Cancer Research, 2017. 77(15): p. 3965–3981.
22. Chen, S. and X. Shen, *Long noncoding RNAs: Functions and mechanisms in colon cancer.* Molecular Cancer, 2020. **19**(1): p. 1–13.
23. Mikkelsen, T.S., et al., *Genome-wide maps of chromatin state in pluripotent and lineage-committed cells.* Nature, 2007. **448**(7153): p. 553–560.
24. Balas, M.M. and A.M. Johnson, *Exploring the mechanisms behind long noncoding RNAs and cancer.* Non-Coding RNA Research, 2018. **3**(3): p. 108–117.
25. Gibb, E.A., C.J. Brown, and W.L. Lam, *The functional role of long noncoding RNA in human carcinomas.* Molecular Cancer, 2011. **10**(1): p. 1–17.
26. Zhang, H., et al., *Long non-coding RNA: A new player in cancer.* Journal of Hematology & Oncology, 2013. **6**(1): p. 1–7.
27. Sanchez Calle, A., et al., *Emerging roles of long non-coding RNA in cancer.* Cancer Science, 2018. **109**(7): p. 2093–2100.
28. Huang, X., et al., *microRNA-16-5p suppresses cell proliferation and angiogenesis in colorectal cancer by negatively regulating forkhead box K1 to block the PI3K/Akt/mTOR pathway.* European Journal of Histochemistry: EJH, 2022. **66**(2).
29. Zhang, W.Y., et al., *Long noncoding RNA Gas5 induces cell apoptosis and inhibits tumor growth via activating the CHOP-dependent endoplasmic reticulum stress pathway in human hepatoblastoma HepG2 cells.* Journal of Cellular Biochemistry, 2022. **123**(2): p. 231–247.
30. Yim, G.W., et al., *Long non-coding rna loc285194 promotes epithelial ovarian cancer progression via the apoptosis signaling pathway.* In Vivo, 2022. **36**(1): p. 121–131.
31. Zhao, D. and Y. Hou, *Long non-coding RNA nuclear-enriched abundant transcript 1 (LncRNA NEAT1) upregulates Cyclin T2 (CCNT2) in laryngeal papilloma through sponging miR-577/miR-1224-5p and blocking cell apoptosis.* Bioengineered, 2022. **13**(1): p. 1828–1837.

32. Wu, H.F., et al., *Long noncoding RNA LOC550643 acts as an oncogene in the growth regulation of colorectal cancer cells.* Cells, 2022. **11**(7): p. 1065.
33. Ju, J.-K., W.-N. Han, and C.-L. Shi, *Long non-coding RNA (lncRNA) plasmacytoma variant translocation 1 gene (PVT1) modulates the proliferation and apoptosis of acute lymphoblastic leukemia cells by sponging miR-486-5p.* Bioengineered, 2022. **13**(2): p. 4587–4597.
34. Tang, W., et al., *Long non-coding RNA PCAT1 sponges miR-134-3p to regulate PITX2 expression in breast cancer.* Molecular Medicine Reports, 2022. **25**(3): p. 1–10.
35. Zhang, H., et al., *Long non-coding LEF1-AS1 sponge miR-5100 regulates apoptosis and autophagy in gastric cancer cells via the miR-5100/DEK/AMPK-mTOR axis.* International Journal of Molecular Sciences, 2022. **23**(9): p. 4787.
36. Wei, H., et al., *Long non-coding RNA PAARH promotes hepatocellular carcinoma progression and angiogenesis via upregulating HOTTIP and activating HIF-1α/VEGF signaling.* Cell Death & Sisease, 2022. **13**(2): p. 1–13.
37. Liu, J., et al., *Long non-coding RNA PCED1B-AS1 promotes the proliferation of colorectal adenocarcinoma through regulating the miR-633/HOXA9 axis.* Bioengineered, 2022. **13**(3): p. 5407–5420.
38. Ye, J., et al., *Long non-coding RNA TMPO-AS1 facilitates the progression of colorectal cancer cells via sponging miR-98-5p to upregulate BCAT1 expression.* Journal of Gastroenterology and Hepatology, 2022. **37**(1): p. 144–153.
39. Mathew, R., V. Karantza-Wadsworth, and E. White, *Role of autophagy in cancer.* Nature Reviews Cancer, 2007. 7(12): p. 961–967.
40. White, E., *The role for autophagy in cancer.* The Journal of Clinical Investigation, 2015. **125**(1): p. 42–46.
41. Levy, J.M.M., C.G. Towers, and A. Thorburn, *Targeting autophagy in cancer.* Nature Reviews Cancer, 2017. **17**(9): p. 528–542.
42. Levine, B., *Autophagy and cancer.* Nature, 2007. **446**(7137): p. 745–747.
43. Choi, K.S., *Autophagy and cancer.* Experimental & Molecular Medicine, 2012. **44**(2): p. 109–120.
44. Li, X., S. He, and B. Ma, *Autophagy and autophagy-related proteins in cancer.* Molecular Cancer, 2020. **19**(1): p. 1–16.

45. Yun, C.W. and S.H. Lee, *The roles of autophagy in cancer.* International Journal of Molecular Sciences, 2018. **19**(11): p. 3466.
46. Mowers, E.E., M.N. Sharifi, and K.F. Macleod, *Autophagy in cancer metastasis.* Oncogene, 2017. **36**(12): p. 1619–1630.
47. Rebecca, V. and R. Amaravadi, *Emerging strategies to effectively target autophagy in cancer.* Oncogene, 2016. **35**(1): p. 1–11.
48. Kocaturk, N.M., et al., *Autophagy as a molecular target for cancer treatment.* European Journal of Pharmaceutical Sciences, 2019. **134**: p. 116–137.
49. Sakthivel, K. and R.R. Rasmia, *Role and regulation of autophagy in cancer.* BBA-Molecular Basis of Disease, 2022: p. 1–22.
50. Mizushima, N., *The role of the Atg1/ULK1 complex in autophagy regulation.* Current Opinion in Cell Biology, 2010. **22**(2): p. 132–139.
51. Xie, Z. and D.J. Klionsky, *Autophagosome formation: Core machinery and adaptations.* Nature Cell Biology, 2007. **9**(10): p. 1102–1109.
52. Mizushima, N. and D.J. Klionsky, *Protein turnover via autophagy: Implications for metabolism.* Annual Review of Nutrition, 2007. **27**(1): p. 19–40.
53. Ghafouri-Fard, S., et al., *Exploring the role of non-coding RNAs in autophagy.* Autophagy, 2022. **18**(5): p. 949–970.
54. Jiang, Q., et al., *Prognostic significance of an autophagy-related long non-coding RNA signature in patients with oral and oropharyngeal squamous cell carcinoma.* Oncology Letters, 2021. **21**(1): p. 1.
55. Sun, Y., et al., *The prognostic and molecular landscape of autophagy-related long noncoding RNA in colorectal cancer.* BioMed Research International, 2022. **2022**.
56. Guo, Y., et al., *Long noncoding RNA H19 derived from M2 tumor-associated macrophages promotes bladder cell autophagy via stabilizing ULK1.* Journal of Oncology, 2022. **2022**.
57. Wu, J., et al., *Suppression of the long non-coding RNA LINC01279 triggers autophagy and apoptosis in lung cancer by regulating FAK and SIN3A*, 2022.
58. Wang, Y., et al., *LncRNA FIRRE functions as a tumor promoter by interaction with PTBP1 to stabilize BECN1 mRNA and facilitate autophagy.* Cell Death & Disease, 2022. **13**(2): p. 1–13.

59. Yang, F., et al., *LncRNA CCAT1 upregulates ATG5 to enhance autophagy and promote gastric cancer development by absorbing miR-140-3p.* Digestive Diseases and Sciences, 2022. **67**(8): p. 3725–3741.
60. Luo, Y., et al., *Long noncoding RNA (lncRNA) EIF3J-DT induces chemoresistance of gastric cancer via autophagy activation.* Autophagy, 2021. **17**(12): p. 4083–4101.
61. Zhou, J., et al., *Long noncoding RNA MALAT1 sponging miR-26a-5p to modulate Smad1 contributes to colorectal cancer progression by regulating autophagy.* Carcinogenesis, 2021. **42**(11): p. 1370–1379.
62. Zhao, Z., et al., *Long non-coding RNA LINC01559 exerts oncogenic role via enhancing autophagy in lung adenocarcinoma.* Cancer Cell International, 2021. **21**(1): p. 1–15.
63. Saha, S., et al., *The tumor-suppressive long noncoding RNA DRAIC inhibits protein translation and induces autophagy by activating AMPK.* Journal of Cell Science, 2021. **134**(24): p. jcs259306.
64. Lin, L., X. Liu, and B. Lv, *Long non-coding RNA MEG3 promotes autophagy and apoptosis of nasopharyngeal carcinoma cells via PTEN up-regulation by binding to microRNA-21.* Journal of Cellular and Molecular Medicine, 2021. **25**(1): p. 61–72.
65. Guiducci, G. and L. Stojic, *Long noncoding RNAs at the crossroads of cell cycle and genome integrity.* Trends in Genetics, 2021. **37**(6): p. 528–546.
66. Liu, M., et al., *HOTAIR, a long noncoding RNA, is a marker of abnormal cell cycle regulation in lung cancer.* Cancer Science, 2018. **109**(9): p. 2717–2733.
67. Jiang, R., et al., *Inhibition of long non-coding RNA XIST upregulates microRNA-149-3p to repress ovarian cancer cell progression.* Cell Death & Disease, 2021. **12**(2): p. 1–12.
68. Qian, X., et al., *LCAT3, a novel m6A-regulated long non-coding RNA, plays an oncogenic role in lung cancer via binding with FUBP1 to activate c-MYC.* Journal of Hematology & Oncology, 2021. **14**(1): p. 1–19.
69. Lv, X., et al., *Exosomal long non-coding RNA LINC00662 promotes non-small cell lung cancer progression by miR-320d/E2F1 axis.* Aging (Albany NY), 2021. **13**(4): p. 6010.

70. Long, B., et al., *Long noncoding RNA LOXL1-AS1 regulates prostate cancer cell proliferation and cell cycle progression through miR-541-3p and CCND1.* Biochemical and Biophysical Research Communications, 2018. **505**(2): p. 561–568.
71. Chen, S., et al., *Roles of MYC-targeting long non-coding RNA MINCR in cell cycle regulation and apoptosis in non-small cell lung Cancer.* Respiratory Research, 2019. **20**(1): p. 1–11.
72. Mirzaei, H. and M.R. Hamblin, *Regulation of glycolysis by non-coding RNAs in cancer: Switching on the warburg effect.* Molecular Therapy-Oncolytics, 2020. **19**: p. 218–239.
73. Jiang, Y., et al., *Construction of a glycolysis-related long noncoding RNA signature for predicting survival in endometrial cancer.* Journal of Cancer, 2021. **12**(5): p. 1431.
74. Hua, Q., et al., *LINC01123, a c-Myc-activated long non-coding RNA, promotes proliferation and aerobic glycolysis of non-small cell lung cancer through miR-199a-5p/c-Myc axis.* Journal of Hematology & Oncology, 2019. **12**(1): p. 1–18.
75. Ma, F., et al., *Long non-coding RNA FGF13-AS1 inhibits glycolysis and stemness properties of breast cancer cells through FGF13-AS1/IGF2BPs/Myc feedback loop.* Cancer Letters, 2019. **450**: p. 63–75.
76. Xing, Z., et al., *Expression of long noncoding RNA YIYA promotes glycolysis in breast cancer.* Cancer Research, 2018. **78**(16): p. 4524–4532.
77. Dong, P., et al., *Long non-coding RNA DLEU2 drives EMT and glycolysis in endometrial cancer through HK2 by competitively binding with miR-455 and by modulating the EZH2/miR-181a pathway.* Journal of Experimental & Clinical Cancer Research, 2021. **40**(1): p. 1–16.
78. Zuo, S., et al., *Long non-coding RNA MEG3 activated by vitamin D suppresses glycolysis in colorectal cancer via promoting c-Myc degradation.* Frontiers in Oncology, 2020. **10**: p. 274.
79. Feng, Z., et al., *Long non-coding RNA ASMTL-AS1 inhibits tumor growth and glycolysis by regulating the miR-93-3p/miR-660/FOXO1 axis in papillary thyroid carcinoma.* Life Sciences, 2020. **244**: p. 117298.
80. Liu, J., et al., *Long noncoding RNA AGPG regulates PFKFB3-mediated tumor glycolytic reprogramming.* Nature Communications, 2020. **11**(1): p. 1–16.

81. Shi, J., et al., *Long non-coding RNA HOTTIP promotes hypoxia-induced glycolysis through targeting miR-615-3p/HMGB3 axis in non-small cell lung cancer cells.* European Journal of Pharmacology, 2019. **862**: p. 172615.
82. Lang, N., et al., *Long non-coding RNA BCYRN1 promotes glycolysis and tumor progression by regulating the miR-149/PKM2 axis in non-small-cell lung cancer.* Molecular Medicine Reports, 2020. **21**(3): p. 1509–1516.
83. Liu, Y., et al., *Long noncoding RNA LINC00518 induces radioresistance by regulating glycolysis through an miR-33a-3p/HIF-1α negative feedback loop in melanoma.* Cell Death & Disease, 2021. **12**(3): p. 1–19.
84. Ghafouri-Fard, S. and M. Taheri, *Maternally expressed gene 3 (MEG3): A tumor suppressor long non coding RNA.* Biomedicine & Pharmacotherapy, 2019. **118**: p. 109129.
85. Kruer, T.L., et al., *Expression of the lncRNA maternally expressed gene 3 (MEG3) contributes to the control of lung cancer cell proliferation by the Rb pathway.* PLoS One, 2016. **11**(11): p. e0166363.
86. Sun, Y., et al., *Restoration of miRNA-148a in pancreatic cancer reduces invasion and metastasis by inhibiting the Wnt/β-catenin signaling pathway via downregulating maternally expressed gene-3.* Experimental and Therapeutic Medicine, 2019. **17**(1): p. 639–648.
87. Wang, W., et al., *LncRNA MEG3 acts a biomarker and regulates cell functions by targeting ADAR1 in colorectal cancer.* World Journal of Gastroenterology, 2019. **25**(29): p. 3972.
88. Xu, J., et al., *Paclitaxel promotes lung cancer cell apoptosis via MEG3-P53 pathway activation.* Biochemical and Biophysical Research Communications, 2018. **504**(1): p. 123–128.
89. Al-Rugeebah, A., M. Alanazi, and N.R. Parine, *MEG3: an oncogenic long non-coding RNA in different cancers.* Pathology & Oncology Research, 2019. **25**(3): p. 859–874.
90. Zhu, M., et al., *MEG3 overexpression inhibits the tumorigenesis of breast cancer by downregulating miR-21 through the PI3K/Akt pathway.* Archives of Biochemistry and Biophysics, 2019. **661**: p. 22–30.
91. Lv, D., et al., *Long non-coding RNA MEG3 inhibits cell migration and invasion of non-small cell lung cancer cells by regulating the miR-21-5p/PTEN axis.* Molecular Medicine Reports, 2021. **23**(3): p. 1.
92. Tan, J., L. Xiang, and G. Xu, *LncRNA MEG3 suppresses migration and promotes apoptosis by sponging miR-548d-3p to modulate JAK–STAT*

pathway in oral squamous cell carcinoma. IUBMB Life, 2019. **71**(7): p. 882–890.

93. Wu, D., et al., *Long non-coding RNA maternally expressed gene 3 affects cell proliferation, apoptosis and migration by targeting the microRNA-9-5p/midkine axis and activating the phosphoinositide-dependent kinase/AKT pathway in hepatocellular carcinoma.* Oncology Letters, 2021. **21**(5): p. 1–8.
94. Chen, X. and J. Qu, *Long non-coding RNA MEG3 suppresses survival, migration, and invasion of cervical cancer.* OncoTargets and Therapy, 2018. **11**: p. 4999.
95. Jiao, J. and S. Zhang, *Long non-coding RNA MEG-3 suppresses gastric carcinoma cell growth, invasion and migration via EMT regulation.* Molecular Medicine Reports, 2019. **20**(3): p. 2685–2693.
96. Xu, G., et al., *MEG3/miR-21 axis affects cell mobility by suppressing epithelial-mesenchymal transition in gastric cancer.* Oncology Reports, 2018. **40**(1): p. 39–48.
97. Zhao, Y., et al., *Long non-coding RNA MEG3 regulates migration and invasion of lung cancer stem cells via miR-650/SLC34A2 axis.* Biomedicine & Pharmacotherapy, 2019. **120**: p. 109457.
98. Wang, H., et al., *Overexpression of MEG3 sensitizes colorectal cancer cells to oxaliplatin through regulation of miR-141/PDCD4 axis.* Biomedicine & Pharmacotherapy, 2018. **106**: p. 1607–1615.
99. Zhang, Y., et al., *Long noncoding RNA MEG3 inhibits breast cancer growth via upregulating endoplasmic reticulum stress and activating NF-κB and p53.* Journal of Cellular Biochemistry, 2019. **120**(4): p. 6789–6797.
100. Wang, G., et al., *LncRNA MEG3 promotes endoplasmic reticulum stress and suppresses proliferation and invasion of colorectal carcinoma cells through the MEG3/miR-103a-3p/PDHB ceRNA pathway.* Neoplasma, 2020.
101. Zhang, J., et al., *Long noncoding RNA TSLNC8 is a tumor suppressor that inactivates the interleukin-6/STAT3 signaling pathway.* Hepatology, 2018. **67**(1): p. 171–187.
102. Qin, C., et al., *LncRNA TSLNC8 inhibits proliferation of breast cancer cell through the miR-214-3p/FOXP2 axis.* European Review of Medical and Pharmacological Sciences, 2019. **23**(19): p. 8440–8448.

103. Fan, H., et al., *Long non-coding RNAs (lncRNAs) tumor-suppressive role of lncRNA on chromosome 8p12 (TSLNC8) inhibits tumor metastasis and promotes apoptosis by regulating interleukin 6 (IL-6)/signal transducer and activator of transcription 3 (STAT3)/hypoxia-inducible factor 1-alpha (HIF-1α) signaling pathway in non-small cell lung cancer.* Medical Science Monitor: International Medical Journal of Experimental and Clinical Research, 2019. **25**: p. 7624.
104. Chai, W., et al., *Long noncoding RNA TSLNC8 enhances pancreatic cancer aggressiveness by regulating CTNNB1 expression via association with HuR*. Human Cell, 2021. **34**(1): p. 165–176.
105. Zhou, S.-Z., et al., *LncRNA TSLNC8 synergizes with EGFR inhibitor osimertinib to inhibit lung cancer tumorigenesis by blocking the EGFR-STAT3 pathway.* Cell Cycle, 2020. **19**(21): p. 2776–2792.
106. Chen, D. and X. Yu, *Long noncoding RNA TSLNC8 suppresses cell proliferation and metastasis and promotes cell apoptosis in human glioma.* Molecular Medicine Reports, 2018. **18**(6): p. 5536–5544.
107. Yan, S., et al., *Long noncoding RNA MIR31HG inhibits hepatocellular carcinoma proliferation and metastasis by sponging microRNA-575 to modulate ST7L expression.* Journal of Experimental & Clinical Cancer Research, 2018. **37**(1): p. 1–16.
108. Zheng, S., et al., *MIR31HG promotes cell proliferation and invasion by activating the Wnt/β-catenin signaling pathway in non-small cell lung cancer.* Oncology Letters, 2019. **17**(1): p. 221–229.
109. Wang, R., et al., *LncRNA MIR31HG targets HIF1A and P21 to facilitate head and neck cancer cell proliferation and tumorigenesis by promoting cell-cycle progression.* Molecular Cancer, 2018. **17**(1): p. 1–6.
110. Wang, X., J. Zhang, and Y. Wang, *Long noncoding RNA GAS5-AS1 suppresses growth and metastasis of cervical cancer by increasing GAS5 stability.* American Journal of Translational Research, 2019. **11**(8): p. 4909.
111. Huang, W., et al., *LncRNA GAS5-AS1 inhibits glioma proliferation, migration, and invasion via miR-106b-5p/TUSC2 axis.* Human Cell, 2020. **33**(2): p. 416–426.
112. Li, S., et al., *Long noncoding RNA GAS5 suppresses triple negative breast cancer progression through inhibition of proliferation and invasion by competitively binding miR-196a-5p.* Biomedicine & Pharmacotherapy, 2018. **104**: p. 451–457.

113. Dong, S., X. Zhang, and D. Liu, *Overexpression of long noncoding RNA GAS5 suppresses tumorigenesis and development of gastric cancer by sponging miR-106a-5p through the Akt/mTOR pathway.* Biology Open, 2019. **8**(6): p. bio041343.
114. Zheng, R., et al., *Long non-coding RNA XIST inhibited breast cancer cell growth, migration, and invasion via miR-155/CDX1 axis.* Biochemical and Biophysical Research Communications, 2018. **498**(4): p. 1002–1008.
115. Zhu, H., et al., *LncRNA XIST accelerates cervical cancer progression via upregulating Fus through competitively binding with miR-200a.* Biomedicine & Pharmacotherapy, 2018. **105**: p. 789–797.
116. Chen, X., et al., *Up-regulated lncRNA XIST contributes to progression of cervical cancer via regulating miR-140-5p and ORC1.* Cancer Cell International, 2019. **19**(1): p. 1–19.
117. Zhao, Y., et al., *lncRNA-Xist/miR-101-3p/KLF6/C/EBPα axis promotes TAM polarization to regulate cancer cell proliferation and migration.* Molecular Therapy-Nucleic Acids, 2021. **23**: p. 536–551.
118. Shen, J., et al., *LncRNA XIST promotes pancreatic cancer migration, invasion and EMT by sponging miR-429 to modulate ZEB1 expression.* The International Journal of Biochemistry & Cell Biology, 2019. **113**: p. 17–26.
119. Braicu, C., et al., *The function of non-coding RNAs in lung cancer tumorigenesis.* Cancers, 2019. **11**(5): p. 605.
120. Tornesello, M.L., et al., *The role of microRNAs, long non-coding RNAs, and circular RNAs in cervical cancer.* Frontiers in Oncology, 2020. **10**: p. 150.
121. Chen, Y., et al., *Long non-coding RNA HCG11 modulates glioma progression through cooperating with miR-496/CPEB3 axis.* Cell Proliferation, 2019. **52**(5): p. e12615.
122. Jin, K., et al., *Long non-coding RNA PVT1 interacts with MYC and its downstream molecules to synergistically promote tumorigenesis.* Cellular and Molecular Life Sciences, 2019. **76**(21): p. 4275–4289.
123. Tang, Q. and S.S. Hann, *HOTAIR: An oncogenic long non-coding RNA in human cancer.* Cellular Physiology and Biochemistry, 2018. **47**(3): p. 893–913.

124. Tian, C., et al., *Long non-coding RNA RNCR3 promotes prostate cancer progression through targeting miR-185-5p.* American Journal of Translational Research, 2018. **10**(5): p. 1562.
125. Xu, J., et al., *Long noncoding RNA MIR17HG promotes colorectal cancer progression via miR-17-5pMIR17HG role in colorectal cancer.* Cancer Research, 2019. **79**(19): p. 4882–4895.
126. Liang, Y., et al., *A novel long non-coding RNA-PRLB acts as a tumor promoter through regulating miR-4766-5p/SIRT1 axis in breast cancer.* Cell Death & Disease, 2018. **9**(5): p. 1–16.
127. Sakai, S., et al., *Long noncoding RNA ELIT-1 Acts as a Smad3 cofactor to facilitate TGFβ/Smad signaling and promote Epithelial–mesenchymal TRansition.* Cancer Research, 2019. **79**(11): p. 2821–2838.
128. Wang, W., et al., *Long non-coding RNA BZRAP1-AS1 silencing suppresses tumor angiogenesis in hepatocellular carcinoma by mediating THBS1 methylation.* Journal of Translational Medicine, 2019. **17**(1): p. 1–15.
129. Sun, Z., et al., *Emerging role of exosome-derived long non-coding RNAs in tumor microenvironment.* Molecular Cancer, 2018. **17**(1): p. 1–9.
130. Deng, X., et al., *Long noncoding RNA CCAL transferred from fibroblasts by exosomes promotes chemoresistance of colorectal cancer cells.* International Journal of Cancer, 2020. **146**(6): p. 1700–1716.
131. Chen, C., et al., *Exosomal long noncoding RNA LNMAT2 promotes lymphatic metastasis in bladder cancer.* The Journal of Clinical Investigation, 2020. **130**(1): p. 404–421.
132. Yu, Y., et al., *Long non-coding RNA PVT1 promotes cell proliferation and migration by silencing ANGPTL4 expression in cholangiocarcinoma.* Molecular Therapy-Nucleic Acids, 2018. **13**: p. 503–513.
133. Wu, J., et al., *The long non-coding RNA LncHDAC2 drives the self-renewal of liver cancer stem cells via activation of Hedgehog signaling.* Journal of Hepatology, 2019. **70**(5): p. 918–929.
134. Yao, N., et al., *Long non-coding RNA NONHSAT101069 promotes epirubicin resistance, migration, and invasion of breast cancer cells through NONHSAT101069/miR-129-5p/Twist1 axis.* Oncogene, 2019. **38**(47): p. 7216–7233.
135. Dong, H., et al., *Long non-coding RNA SNHG14 induces trastuzumab resistance of breast cancer via regulating PABPC1 expression through*

H3K27 acetylation. Journal of Cellular and Molecular Medicine, 2018. **22**(10): p. 4935–4947.

136. Jiang, L., et al., *HCP5 is a SMAD3-responsive long non-coding RNA that promotes lung adenocarcinoma metastasis via miR-203/SNAI axis.* Theranostics, 2019. **9**(9): p. 2460.
137. Lu, G., et al., *Long noncoding RNA LINC00511 contributes to breast cancer tumourigenesis and stemness by inducing the miR-185-3p/E2F1/Nanog axis.* Journal of Experimental & Clinical Cancer Research, 2018. **37**(1): p. 1–11.
138. Peng, X., F. Wei, and X. Hu, *Long noncoding RNA DLGAP1-AS1 promotes cell proliferation in hepatocellular carcinoma via sequestering miR-486-5p*. Journal of Cellular Biochemistry, 2020. **121**(2): p. 1953–1962.

https://doi.org/10.1142/9789811267390_0006

Chapter 6

Long non-coding RNAs (lncRNAs) in cancer metastasis: Molecular interactions and possible therapeutic targets

Mehrdad Hashemi[1,2], Shokooh Salimimoghadam[3], Afshin Taheriazam[2,4] and Sepideh Mirzaei[5]*

[1]*Department of Genetics, Faculty of Advanced Science and Technology, Tehran Medical Sciences, Islamic Azad University, Tehran, Iran*
[2]*Farhikhtegan Medical Convergence Sciences Research Center, Farhikhtegan Hospital Tehran Medical Sciences, Islamic Azad University, Tehran, Iran*
[3]*Department of Biochemistry and Molecular Biology, Faculty of Veterinary Medicine, Shahid Chamran University of Ahvaz, Ahvaz, Iran*
[4]*Department of Orthopedics, Faculty of Medicine, Tehran Medical Sciences, Islamic Azad University, Tehran, Iran*
[5]*Department of Biology, Faculty of Science, Islamic Azad University, Science and Research Branch, Tehran, Iran*

Abstract

Although numerous studies have been carried out to find a promising therapy for cancer, this disease still remains one of the most

*Corresponding author: Sepideh Mirzaei, Department of Biology, Faculty of Science, Islamic Azad University, Science and Research Branch, Tehran, Iran, Email: sepidehmirzaei.smv@gmail.com

incurable human disorders. However, the mortality of this disease is significantly decreased compared to the past. The most challenges in the way of cancer therapy are the heterogeneous nature of cancer, recurrence, metastasis to other organs, and resistance to conventional therapies. Thus, targeting certain signaling pathways which are responsible for these events is of great importance. Non-coding RNAs (ncRNAs) contain two main classes based on their length: small ncRNAs such as microRNAs (miRNAs) and long non-coding RNAs (lncRNAs). lncRNAs have more than 200 nucleotides and their critical role in regulating vital cellular processes in cancer has been uncovered years ago. Accumulating evidence has revealed the regulatory role of lncRNAs on cancer hallmarks, such as epithelial–mesenchymal transition, invasion, metastasis, and angiogenesis. lncRNAs act as competing endogenous RNAs or sponges for miRNAs to affect their downstream targets where PI3K/Akt signaling, PTEN, VEGF, β-catenin, and Smad are among them. This chapter intends to discuss the critical role of lncRNAs in the regulation of metastasis.

1. Introduction

Despite the fast advance in science, cancer still remains one of the most challenging diseases for therapy [1–3]. Cancer cells are characterized by their ability in dividing without pause, invasive capacity, metastatic activity, escape from the immune system, metabolic reprogramming, and resistance to therapies [4–9]. Among these factors, metastasis is the major cause of death and cancer cells show distinct metabolic traits compared with the first group of tumor cells that they derived from. Targeting step-dependent metabolic factors or pathways is important for bringing metastasis under control [10]. Long non-coding RNAs (lncRNAs) are a class of non-coding RNAs (ncRNAs) that possess more than 200 nucleotides and are aberrantly expressed in cancer [11–13]. ncRNAs with regulatory roles were initially identified in bacteria and then eukaryotes, and H19 and XIST (X-inactive specific transcript) were the first ones [14, 15]. Interestingly, only 1.2% of the human genome encodes proteins, and the remaining part is counted as the "non-coding" region. lncRNAs are classified based on their length, their origin site in the genome, biogenesis mechanism, subcellular localization, function, and their relation with specific biological mechanisms. In the classification based on their location lncRNAs are named intergenic, anti-sense, bi-directional, and intronic lncRNAs. Furthermore, lncRNA could be classified as scaffold, guide, competing endogenous RNAs (ceRNAs), precursors, decoy (ribo-repressor), and ribo-activator lncRNAs according to their function in cells. Moreover, some lncRNAs are involved in biological processes such as hypoxia, senescence, and stress [16].

RNA-sequencing technologies and computational biology are widely used to identify and characterize lncRNA. Regarding their critical role in the modulation of vital physiological and pathological processes via affecting important mechanisms at the epigenetic, transcriptional, and post-transcriptional levels and targeting various molecules such as RNAs, chromatin, and proteins, lncRNAs are considered master regulators [17–21]. Intriguingly, lncRNAs are implicated in cancer hallmarks including apoptotic pathways, proliferative and invasive capacity, epithelial–mesenchymal transition (EMT), malignancy, immune escape, angiogenic activity, response to therapy, as well as diagnosis and prognosis [22–25]. Furthermore, lncRNAs also regulate cancer cell processes via modulating metabolic pathways of energy metabolism and their reprogramming [26, 27]. It bears noting that lncRNAs act as tumor suppressors or oncogenic factors. However, some of them are playing roles of both oncogene and onco-suppressor based on cancer type. For instance, lncRNA terminal differentiation–induced ncRNA has been shown to be an onco-suppressor or oncogene in various cancers based on the distinct signaling and factors which are prominent in different tissue and are targeted by this lncRNA [28]. Similarly, lncRNA cancer susceptibility candidate 15 (CASC15) is another lncRNA with opposite roles in various cancers which has high expression and oncogenic role in hepatocellular carcinoma, colorectal cancer, and breast cancer, while its expression is low and exerts tumor suppressor function in ovarian cancer and neuroblastoma [29]. This chapter intends to discuss the critical role of lncRNAs in the regulation of cancer metastasis by focusing on their impacts on EMT, matrix metalloproteinases (MMPs), and angiogenesis. Furthermore, the importance of the lncRNA/miRNA axis in the regulation of metastasis is uncovered in the last section.

2. What is the definition of cancer metastasis?

As the primary cause of death in cancer, metastasis comprised complex cellular processes and also the interaction between cancer cells and other cells located in the tumor microenvironment. Metastasis is characterized by four properties: motility and invasion, modified microenvironment, plasticity, and colonization. By growing the neoplastic mass, inflammatory cells are gradually attracted to the site of the tumor, angiogenesis is increased, and mutant variants are highly generated. In the next step, neoplastic cells invade in stroma via various mechanisms including EMT. The cells entered into the vasculature (intravasation) are then rolling along the endothelium. Furthermore, the extracellular matrix (ECM) is re-organized to accelerate invasion. On exiting from the vessels (extravasation), tumor cells interact with a new niche which is appropriate for the colonization of the second tumor mass. Several mechanisms and factors are involved in the activation of metastasis where MMPs, Ras, interleukin 8 (IL-8), PI3K, p53, PTEN, CDKN2A, VEGF, and EGFR are among them [30–32]. Various determinants are considered for the activation of invasion and metastasis such as epigenetic factors, ECM-derived signals and mechanical pressures, the interactions between cells of the tumor microenvironment, soluble signals, and tumor microbiome. EMT occurs via a single cell or through collective dissemination and consists of several steps between epithelial cells and mesenchymal cells with invasive phenotype. These steps are controlled by some factors such as growth factors. Although there is debate on whether EMT is crucial for tumor metastasis, it has been proven that mesenchymal–epithelial transition is critical for the progression of metastasis [33–35].

EMT could also protect cancer cells from the immune system. Neoplastic cells that are in EMT stages express transforming growth factor-β (TGF-β), thrombospondin1, and IL-10 which are involved in immunosuppression. Furthermore, EMT disrupts immunological synapses, resulting in resistance of cancer cells against cytotoxic T cells. EMT is induced by various factors such as TGF-β, growth factors, cytokines, Wingless/integrated, hedgehog and Notch signaling pathways. Interestingly, the interaction between tumor cells and ECM components such as collagens is capable of triggering EMT. EMT-related transcription factors (EMT-TFs) are activated following these stimuli. EMT-TFs are included Snail, Slug, Twist, PRRX1, and ZEB1/2. Activation of EMT-TFs leads to increased mesenchymal phenotypes while decreasing the epithelial properties. Thus, N-cadherin, fibronectin, vimentin, and FSP1 are increased, whereas E-cadherin is decreased. Various mechanisms are involved in the suppression of E-cadherin such as DNA methylation of E-cadherin promoter (CDH1) via the interaction of ZEB1 and DNMT1 and recruiting histone-modifying enzymes [36–42].

3. lncRNAs in regulating EMT

Accumulating evidence has shown that lncRNAs are governed by the metastasis in cancer via regulating EMT [43–48]. For instance, lncRNA NR2F1-AS1 has been demonstrated to be positively related to the malignancy degree and represents a poor prognosis of gastric cancer. Furthermore, it was found that lncRNA NR2F1-AS1 expression is increased in gastric cancer cells after receiving TGF-β, which means that NR2F1-AS1 is responding to EMT activator signaling. Besides, suppression of NR2F1-AS1 was demonstrated to be associated with low proliferation rate, migration, invasiveness, and also G1/S phase cell cycle arrest. More importantly, NR2F1-AS1 targets miRNA-29a-3p/VAMP7 axis to exert its functions. Moreover, the authors stated that the aberrant expression of NR2F1-AS1 may be because of the abnormal EMT signaling in gastric cancer [49]. In addition, lncRNA CYTOR interacts with glycolytic enzyme enolase 2 to prevent the phosphorylation of Yes-associated protein 1, and its activation, followed by increased EMT and metastasis in colorectal cancer [50]. Another example is CASC15, which was found to be involved in the poor prognosis of ovarian cancer patients. In vitro and in vivo, CASC15 promotes metastasis via inducing EMT by increasing TGF-β. CASC15 acts as an inhibitor of miRNA-23b cluster which consists of miRNA-23b-3p and miRNA-24-3p to upregulate SMAD3 expression, which resulted in increased CASC15 mRNA in a positive feedback loop [51]. Furthermore, the knocking down of lncRNA SNHG16 in colorectal cancer leads to poor proliferation, tumor growth, EMT, invasion, and migration of colorectal cancer cells. In fact, lncRNA SNHG16 downregulation resulted in the upregulation of E-cadherin and decreased N-cadherin, vimentin, and Snail-1. lncRNA SNHG16 suppresses miRNA-124-3p to increase MCP-1 expression and subsequently mediates the aforementioned hallmarks [52]. Furthermore, lncRNA PNUTS expression is upregulated in hepatocellular carcinoma. PNUTS increases ZEB1 to promote EMT and enhances invasion and metastasis [53]. It bears noting that cells located in the tumor microenvironment could induce EMT in cancer cells. For instance, lncRNA HISLA derived from M2 tumor-associated macrophages augments EMT in bladder cancer by inhibiting the interaction between GSK3β and β-catenin and increasing the stability of β-catenin [54]. In vitro and in vivo, lncRNA SNHG17 was found to upregulate esophageal squamous cell carcinoma and its overexpression is associated with poor survival. SNHG17 expression is induced by TGF-β which leads to the activation of c-Myc and PI3K/Akt pathway in promoting EMT. SNHG17 directly regulates c-Myc transcription by binding to c-Jun protein and increases the recruiting of a complex to bind to specific sequences in c-Myc promoter, which resulted in the upregulation of c-Myc expression [55]. Targeting PI3K/Akt axis by lncRNAs for increasing EMT is also evaluated in distinct studies. In osteosarcoma, lncRNA NDRG1 inhibits miRNA-96-5p to activate PI3K/Akt signaling pathways and promote EMT [56]. It has been also observed that lncRNA DLEU2 expression upturns in gastric cancer, and its upregulation is associated with tumor differentiation. Furthermore, DLEU2 silencing increases apoptosis, while suppresses tumor cell viability, invasion, and migration. DLEU2 activates PI3K/Akt axis to induce EMT via upregulation of N-cadherin and vimentin and declining E-cadherin expression

[57]. Similarly, lncRNA SNHG6 works as ceRNA for miRNA-944 to inhibit repression of RAB11A by miRNA-944 in pituitary adenoma. This axis consequently resulted in the promotion of cancer cell viability, EMT, invasion, and migration [58]. In addition, lncRNA human leukocyte antigen complex group 18 (HCG18) suppresses miRNA-29a/b to increase TRAF4/TRAF5 to promote EMT and progression of epithelial ovarian cancer cells [59]. In another study, it was demonstrated that lncRNA SND1-IT1 is upregulated via TGF-β1 in gastric cancer in vitro and in vivo. Overexpression of SND1-IT1 via TGF-β1 resulted in increased cancer cell viability, EMT, invasion, and migration. For this purpose, SND1-IT1 functioned as a sponge for miRNA-124 to increase COL4A1. Moreover, the upregulation of miRNA-124 mitigates TGF-β1-induced EMT [60]. In addition, lncRNA Opa-interacting protein 5-antisense RNA 1 (OIP5-AS1) inhibits miRNA-1477a to upregulate IGF1R in increasing EMT of cervical cancer cells [61]. NR2F1-AS1 also is an oncogenic lncRNA with a high expression level in breast cancer. NR2F1-AS1 works as a ceRNA for miRNA-25-3p to increase ZEB2, which consequently resulted in the activation of EMT [62]. Furthermore, lncRNA GATA2-AS1 promotes GATA2 expression levels in colorectal cancer cells to enhance tumor progression. lncRNA GATA2-AS1/GATA2 induces EMT via downregulation of E-cadherin and upregulation of vimentin and N-cadherin, induces stemness via elevation of Oct4 and Nanog. Interestingly, lncRNA GATA2-AS1 recruits DDX3X to increases the stability of GATA2, thereby promoting its expression. More importantly, GATA2 promotes lncRNA GATA2-AS1 expression in a positive feedback loop. In addition to EMT, lncRNA GATA2-AS1 also enhances proliferation and suppresses apoptosis by targeting GATA2 [63]. In contrast, ZNF674-AS1 is an onco-suppressor lncRNA with a low expression level in thyroid carcinoma. Upregulation of ZNF674-AS1 attenuates EMT and metastasis. ZNF674-AS1 acts as ceRNA for miRNA-181a to suppress its function and increase SOCS4 in turn. Thus, ZNF674-AS1 overexpression is in favor of thyroid cancer EMT suppression via targeting miR-181a/SOCS4 axis [64]. Similarly, LINC00244 suppresses programmed cell death ligand 1 to inhibit EMT, metastasis, and tumor progression in hepatocellular

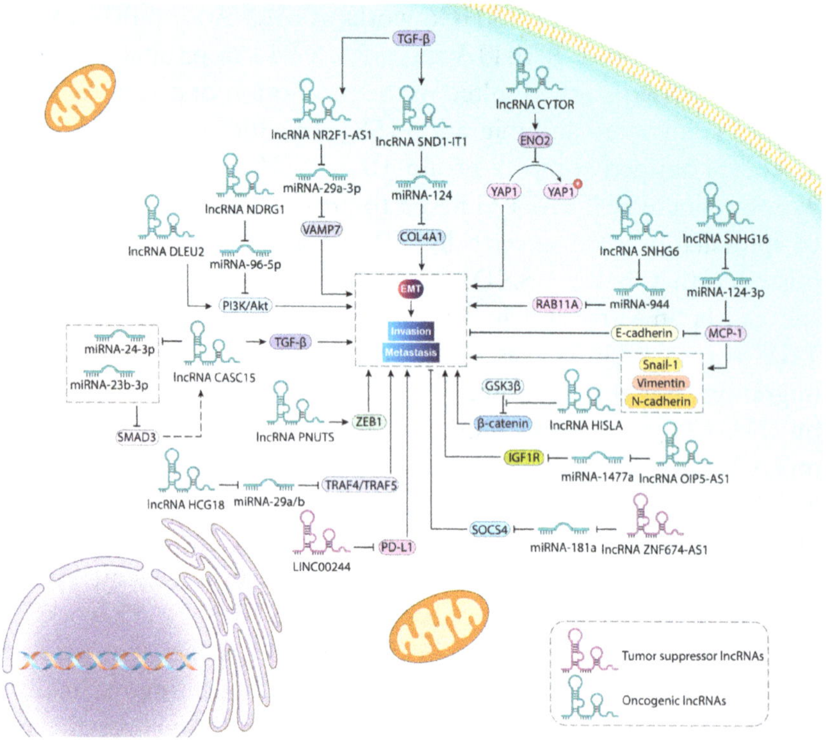

Figure 1. lncRNAs in regulating EMT.

carcinoma [65]. Figure 1 demonstrates the role of lncRNAs in regulating EMT in cancers.

4. lncRNAs in regulating MMPs

lncRNA SCIRT is upregulated in cervical cancer, and its expression is associated with clinical and pathological characteristics of patients, tumor size, and lymph node metastasis. lncRNA SCIRT increases proliferation, colony formation, and invasion via upregulation of MMP-2 and MMP-9, vimentin, as well as N-cadherin, and decreasing E-cadherin [66]. HOXC cluster antisense RNA 1 (HOXC-AS1) overexpression in gastric cancer has been suggested to be associated with poor prognosis. HOXC-AS1 binds to miRNA-99a-3p to mediate its suppression and increase MMP-8. HOXC-AS1/miRNA-99a-3p/MMP-8 axis was observed to promote gastric cancer cells' progression [67]. In a study, it was found that lncRNA BRD3OS (LINC00094) expression is increased in cutaneous squamous cell carcinoma. Furthermore, LINC00094 has high expression level in metastatic cells than in non-metastatic cells. LINC00094 increases the expression of MMP-1, MMP-10, and MMP-13 and elevates collagen I to promote invasion. Furthermore, LINC00094 promotes tumor growth. More importantly, the expression of LINC00094 is regulated by a superenhancer. Also, ERK1/2 pathway suppresses the LINC00094 expression [68]. Furthermore, upregulation of lncRNA GHET1 was observed in triple-negative breast cancer cell lines and tissues. Overexpression of lncRNA GHET1 is associated with a high proliferation rate and migration capacity while decreasing apoptosis. In addition, overexpression of GHET1 increases MMP-9 and MMP-2 expression levels. GHET1 serves as a sponge for miRNA-377-3p to increase GRSF1, and consequently increase tumor cell progression [69]. The results of a study have shown high expression levels of lncRNA CRNDE in ovarian cancer cells. Overexpression of CRNDE is associated with proliferation, invasion, and migration through upregulation of MMP-2 and MMP-9. In addition, CRNDE inhibits miRNA-423-5p to increase its downstream target, FSCN1 [70]. lncRNA-XLOC_006390 is another lncRNA that has been revealed to promote metastasis in colorectal cancer via increasing N-cadherin, MMP-2, and MMP-9 and decreasing E-cadherin. In addition, lncRNA-XLOC_006390 sponges miRNA-296-3p to increase ONECUT2 to exert its functions [71]. Interestingly, a study revealed a type of interaction between miRNAs and lncRNAs in which both of them acts synergistically in increasing tumor metastasis. The results of this study have shown that lncRNA MIR210HG and miRNA-210 are both overexpressed in gastric cancer, and their overexpression results in the invasion and migration of cancer cells in vitro, and lung metastasis in vivo. Promoting metastasis by lncRNA MIR210HG is mediated by increasing MMPs. For increasing MMPs, MIR210HG interacts with DExH-box helicase 9 (DHX9) to upregulate occupancy of DHX9/c-Jun complex on the promoter region of MMPs.

In addition, miRNA-210 inhibits the expression level of dopamine receptor D5, MAX network transcriptional repressor, and serine/threonine kinase 24 for augmenting metastasis in gastric cancer cells. More importantly, MIR210HG and miRNA-210 are both activated via c-Myc synergistically to promote metastasis [72]. Also, there are lncRNAs with onco-suppressor functions, which inhibit metastasis via targeting MMPs. For instance, a pseudogene-derived lncRNA named LPAL2 is decreased in hepatocellular carcinoma and its overexpression is associated with good survival outcomes. Overexpression of LPAL2 suppresses invasion, migration, sphere formation, and tumor formation, as well drug resistance. To exert its functions, LPAL2 decreases the expression level of MMP-9 [73]. Similarly, lncRNA *Homo sapiens* HCG18 is downregulated in papillary thyroid cancer and its overexpression is associated with low tumor cell viability, EMT, invasion, and migration, whereas induces apoptosis. HCG18 upregulation inhibits miRNA-106a-5p to increase protein phosphatase 2 regulatory subunit B and consequently suppress N-cadherin, vimentin, and MMP-2 and MMP-9 expression, and increasing E-cadherin [74].

5. lncRNAs in regulating angiogenesis

Similar to other hallmarks of cancer, lncRNAs could also promote or attenuate angiogenesis [75–81]. In the study of Wang *et al.*, they observed that lncRNA MAGI2-AS3 is downregulated in the most common type of renal cancer, clear cell renal cell carcinoma. lncRNA MAGI2-AS3 overexpression is in favor of suppressing tumor cell viability, migration, vessel-like tube formation (in vitro), and tumor angiogenesis (in vivo). To act in this way, MAGI2-AS3 increases ACY1 transcription by preventing the interaction of HEY1 with ACY1 promoter. Thus, lncRNA MAGI2-AS3 suppresses angiogenesis by regulating HEY1/ACY1 pathway [82]. Similarly, lncRNA ZNF667-AS1 was found to be decreased in gastric cancer samples. It was also demonstrated that hyperregulation of ZNF667-AS1 decreases proliferation, migration, and angiogenesis in vitro. ZNF667-AS1 increases E-cadherin while decreasing N-cadherin and VEGFA [83]. Furthermore, lncRNA H22954 suppresses angiogenesis in acute myeloid leukemia in vitro and in vivo via targeting platelet-derived growth factor subunit A (PDGFA) gene [84]. In contrast, lncRNA CRART16 is overexpressed as an oncogene in gastric cancer and its upregulation is associated with advanced tumor stage and poor prognosis. In vitro, CRART16 increases tumor proliferation, colony formation, resistance to bevacizumab, and angiogenesis. Moreover, increased tumor size has been seen following the upregulation of CRART16 in vivo. For exerting its functions, CRART16 works as a sponge for miRNA-122-5p to upregulate FOS, which in turn, increases VEGFD [85]. In addition, exosomes containing lncRNA ATB derived from ovarian cancer cells have been shown to increase angiogenesis, migration, and tumor cell viability by targeting miRNA-204-3p/TGF-βR2 axis. Furthermore, upregulation of metastasis is mediated by increased levels of N-cadherin and Smad2, while decreasing E-cadherin levels [86]. In colorectal cancer, the expression level of lncRNA OGFRP1 is increased which is correlated with high proliferation, EMT, angiogenesis, invasion and migration, and suppressed apoptosis. OGFRP1 suppresses miRNA-423-5p to upregulate CTCF for exerting its functions [87]. Furthermore, it was revealed that lncRNA DMDRMR increases EZH2 and SMURF1 expression via suppression of miRNA-378a-5p. Upregulation of EZH2 results in the suppression of DAB2IP and its subsequent degradation by SMURF1. This axis subsequently increases the activation of VEGFA/VEGFR2 signaling pathway to promote angiogenesis and sunitinib resistance [88]. In addition, lncRNA KCNQ1OT1 is overexpressed in pituitary adenoma. KCNQ1OT1 augments angiogenesis, stemness, colony formation, and invasiveness by inhibiting miRNA-140-5p. RAB11A is a downstream target of miRNA-140-5p, and its expression is increased following miRNA-140-5p suppression [89]. LINC00467 is another oncogenic lncRNA with high expression level in colorectal cancer. LINC00467 suppresses miRNA-128-3p to increase VEGFC and consequently promoting angiogenesis (Figure 2) [90].

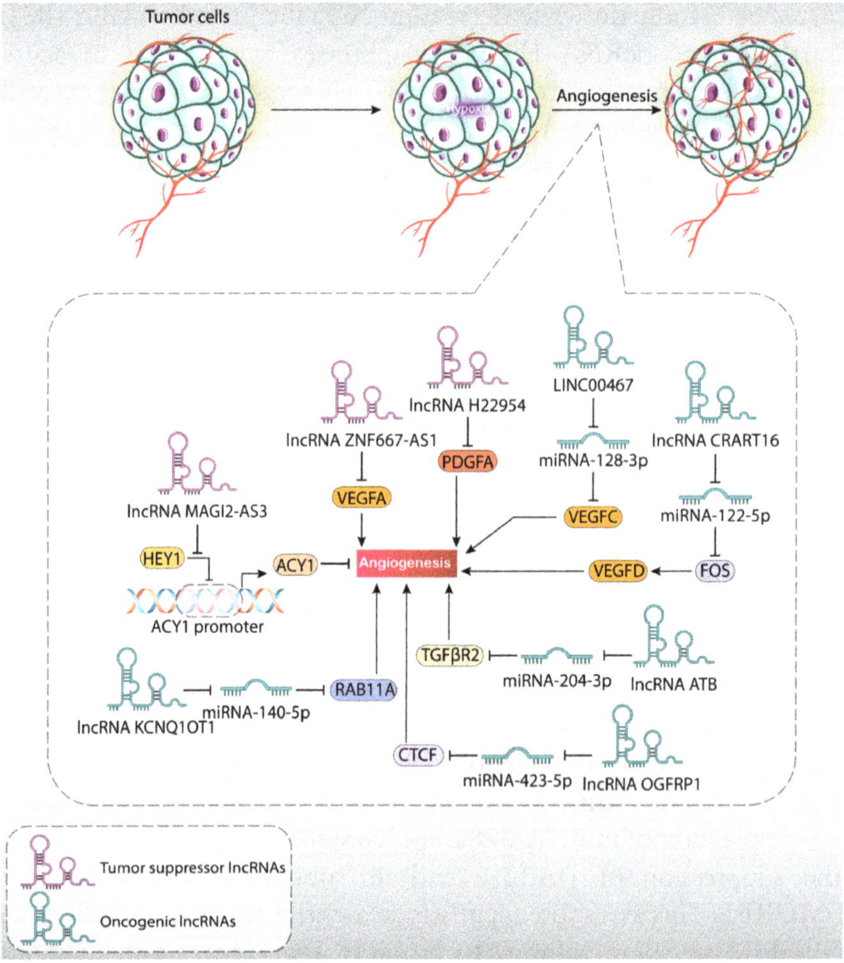

Figure 2. lncRNAs in regulating angiogenesis.

6. lncRNA/miRNA axis in cancer metastasis

As mentioned in previous sections, lncRNAs are one of the important upstream regulators of miRNAs. lncRNAs tumor suppressor or oncogene thereby suppresses oncogenic or tumor suppressor factors to exert their functions, respectively. Meanwhile, there are also synergistic interactions between lncRNAs and miRNAs. The effect of lncRNA/miRNA axis is widely studied in various cancer types [2, 91–96]. lncRNA SNHG16 is an oncogenic factor that suppresses miRNA-205-5p, a tumor suppressor miRNA, to increase its downstream target P21-activated kinases 2 to promote melanoma cancer cell metastasis [97]. Similarly, lncRNA CASC20 is overexpressed in gastric cancer which suppresses miRNA-143-5p to increase MEMO1. This axis ultimately results in enhancing EMT and metastasis [98]. LINC00649 is also overexpressed in cervical cancer, and it suppresses miRNA-216a in increasing proliferation, metastasis, and invasion [99]. Interestingly, exosomes containing lncRNA taurine upregulated gene 1 (TUG1) derived from cancer-associated fibroblasts are enhancers of metastasis in hepatocellular carcinoma cells. TUG1 needs to increase SIX1 to enhance metastasis and for this purpose, it suppresses miRNA-524-5p to prevent its inhibitory role on SIX1 [100]. In contrast, lncRNA SBF2-AS1 is downregulated in laryngeal squamous cell carcinoma. It was found that upregulation of SBF2-AS1 is associated with decreased EMT phenotype and metastasis. SBF2-AS1 serves as a ceRNA for miRNA-302b-3p to increase TGFBR2 [101]. Table 1 provided a list of lncRNA/miRNA axis, which are governed metastasis in various cancers.

7. Conclusion and remarks

As cancer is a disease with high morbidity in the world, finding a promising and certain therapy is important. Cancer is characterized by various hallmarks and metastasis is one of them. Metastasis helps cancer cells to survive and spread to another region. A complex of mechanisms is involved in metastasis and EMT is among them. During EMT, cancer cells lose their epithelial phenotype such as E-cadherin, while gaining mesenchymal properties including N-cadherin, vimentin, and fibronectin. For metastasis, it is required for the cells to have the space for invasion. Thus, ECM is also involved in metastasis. After entering cancer cells with mesenchymal-like phenotype into the bloodstream, they spread to other parts of the body and colonize. It bears noting that each cancer has mainly metastasis to certain organs.

Table 1. lncRNA/miRNA axis in regulating cancer metastasis.

lncRNA	miRNA	Cancer type	Remark	Ref
HCG11	miRNA-490-3p	Nasopharyngeal carcinoma	Upregulation of HCG11 is associated with tumor stage, lymphatic metastasis, poor prognosis, proliferation, and metastasis while suppressing apoptosis. Downregulation of miRNA-490-3p occurs by HCG11 to increase MAP3K9.	[102]
HCP5	miRNA-216a-5p	Cervical cancer	HCP5 is overexpressed in cervical cancer. HCP5 increased proliferation and metastasis via targeting miRNA-216a-5p/CDC42 axis.	[103]
LINC01232	miRNA-506-5p	Gastric cancer	LINC01232 is upregulated in gastric cancer. LINC01232 enhances metastasis and EMT by targeting miRNA-506-5p/PAK1 axis.	[104]
LINC00667	miRNA-200b-3p	Esophageal cancer	LINC00667 expression is increased in esophageal cancer. LINC00667 promotes proliferation, invasion, and metastasis by suppressing miRNA-200b-3p and increasing SLC2A3.	[105]
LINC00511	miRNA-126-5p/ miRNA-218-5p	Lung adenocarcinoma	LINC00511 is upregulated in lung adenocarcinoma. LINC00511 works as a sponge for miRNA-126-5p and miRNA-218-5p to promote COL1A1. COL1A1 overexpression is associated with proliferation and metastasis.	[106]

(*Continued*)

Table 1. (*Continued*)

SNHG1	miRNA-128-3p	Glioblastoma multiforme	SNHG1 is upregulated in glioblastoma. SNHG1 suppresses miRNA-128-3p to increase RRAS2. Activation of RRAS2 is in favor of the promotion of EMT and invasion.	[107]
LINC00483	miRNA-19a-3p	Pancreatic ductal adenocarcinoma	LINC00483 is increased in pancreatic ductal adenocarcinoma. LINC00483 inhibits miRNA-19a-3p to upregulate the TBK1/MAPK pathway. LINC00483 increases EMT, metastasis, and proliferation via upregulation of N-cadherin, c-Myc, and ZEB1.	[108]
PART1	miRNA-374b	Glioma	PART1 is decreased in glioma. PART1 suppresses miRNA-34b to increase SALL1. PART1 upregulation is associated with EMT, proliferation, and metastasis suppression.	[109]
LINC02362	miRNA-516b-5p	Hepatocellular carcinoma	LINC02362 is downregulated in hepatocellular carcinoma. LINC02362 suppresses tumor cell survival, invasion, migration, and EMT via suppressing miRNA-516b-5p and increasing SOSC2.	[110]
NBAT1	miRNA-21-5p	Endometrial cancer	NBAT1 is downregulated in endometrial cancer. NBAT1 increases PTEN via suppression of miRNA-21-5p to inhibit tumor cell proliferation, migration, and invasion.	[111]

Regarding the critical role of lncRNAs in the regulation of cancer hallmarks, this chapter focuses on their function in controlling metastasis. lncRNAs act as tumor suppressors or oncogenes in cancer. Various studies have revealed the interaction between lncRNAs and TGF-β in cancer metastasis. Most of the lncRNAs affect miRNAs as their downstream target to exert their functions. In addition, lncRNAs target EMT-TFs and also factors involved in EMT phenotypes such as N-cadherin, E-cadherin, vimentin, and fibronectin to affect EMT. Besides, signaling pathways such as PI3K/Akt, β-catenin, and tumor suppressor factors including PTEN are the downstream targets of lncRNAs in cancer metastasis. More importantly, lncRNAs affect MMPs in enhancing metastasis. Angiogenesis is also another hallmark of cancer which could be regulated by tumor suppressors or oncogenic lncRNAs. VEGFA, VEGFC, and VEGFD are among the factors that lncRNAs regulate angiogenesis through them. It is worth noting that as lncRNAs are widely regulated metastasis, designing a promising therapy using lncRNAs to overcome cancer metastasis and prevent the malignancy of cancer should be the subject of future clinical trials and studies.

Conflict of interest:

The authors declare no conflict of interest.

References

1. Hashemi, M., et al., *Curcumin in the treatment of urological cancers: Therapeutic targets, challenges and prospects.* Life Sciences, 2022. **309**: p. 120984.
2. Entezari, M., et al., *LncRNA-miRNA axis in tumor progression and therapy response: An emphasis on molecular interactions and therapeutic interventions.* Biomedicine & Pharmacotherapy, 2022. **154**: p. 113609.
3. Mirzaei, S., et al., *Caffeic acid and its derivatives as potential modulators of oncogenic molecular pathways: New hope in the fight against cancer.* Pharmacological Research, 2021. **171**: p. 105759.

4. Hanahan, D., *Hallmarks of cancer: New dimensions.* Cancer Discovery, 2022. **12**(1): p. 31–46.
5. Hegde, P.S. and D.S. Chen, *Top 10 challenges in cancer immunotherapy.* Immunity, 2020. **52**(1): p. 17–35.
6. Huang, T., et al., *Autophagy and hallmarks of cancer.* Critical Reviews™ in Oncogenesis, 2018. **23**(5–6).
7. Ashrafizadeh, M., et al., *Targeting autophagy in prostate cancer: Preclinical and clinical evidence for therapeutic response.* Journal of Experimental & Clinical Cancer Research, 2022. **41**(1): p. 105.
8. Mirzaei, S., et al., *Long non-coding RNAs as new players in bladder cancer: Lessons from pre-clinical and clinical studies.* Life Sciences, 2022. **288**: p. 119948.
9. Mirzaei, S., et al., *Advances in understanding the role of P-gp in doxorubicin resistance: Molecular pathways, therapeutic strategies, and prospects.* Drug Discovery Today, 2022. **27**(2): p. 436–455.
10. Bergers, G. and S.-M. Fendt, *The metabolism of cancer cells during metastasis.* Nature Reviews Cancer, 2021. **21**(3): p. 162–180.
11. Huarte, M., *The emerging role of lncRNAs in cancer.* Nature Medicine, 2015. **21**(11): p. 1253–1261.
12. Prensner, J.R. and A.M. Chinnaiyan, *The emergence of lncRNAs in cancer biology.* Cancer Discovery, 2011. **1**(5): p. 391–407.
13. Liz, J. and M. Esteller, *lncRNAs and microRNAs with a role in cancer development.* Biochimica et Biophysica Acta (BBA)-Gene Regulatory Mechanisms, 2016. **1859**(1): p. 169–176.
14. Bartolomei, M.S., S. Zemel, and S.M. Tilghman, *Parental imprinting of the mouse H19 gene.* Nature, 1991. **351**(6322): p. 153–155.
15. Brown, C.J., et al., *A gene from the region of the human X inactivation centre is expressed exclusively from the inactive X chromosome.* Nature, 1991. **349**(6304): p. 38–44.
16. Jarroux, J., A. Morillon, and M. Pinskaya, *History, discovery, and classification of lncRNAs.* Long Non Coding RNA Biology, 2017: p. 1–46.
17. Zhang, Y. and L. Tang, *The application of lncRNAs in cancer treatment and diagnosis.* Recent Patents on Anti-Cancer Drug Discovery, 2018. **13**(3): p. 292–301.
18. Peng, W.-X., P. Koirala, and Y.-Y. Mo, *LncRNA-mediated regulation of cell signaling in cancer.* Oncogene, 2017. **36**(41): p. 5661–5667.

19. Yang, G., X. Lu, and L. Yuan, *LncRNA: A link between RNA and cancer.* Biochimica et Biophysica Acta (BBA)-Gene Regulatory Mechanisms, 2014. **1839**(11): p. 1097–1109.
20. Dinescu, S., et al., *Epitranscriptomic signatures in lncRNAs and their possible roles in cancer.* Genes, 2019. **10**(1): p. 52.
21. He, R.-Z., D.-X. Luo, and Y.-Y. Mo, *Emerging roles of lncRNAs in the post-transcriptional regulation in cancer.* Genes & Diseases, 2019. **6**(1): p. 6–15.
22. Nandwani, A., S. Rathore, and M. Datta, *LncRNAs in cancer: Regulatory and therapeutic implications.* Cancer Letters, 2021. **501**: p. 162–171.
23. Taniue, K. and N. Akimitsu, *The functions and unique features of LncRNAs in cancer development and tumorigenesis.* International Journal of Molecular Sciences, 2021. **22**(2): p. 632.
24. Wang, J., et al., *Regulatory roles of long noncoding RNAs implicated in cancer hallmarks.* International Journal of Cancer, 2020. **146**(4): p. 906–916.
25. Suman, P., et al., *Long non-coding RNAs involved in different steps of cancer metastasis.* Clinical and Translational Oncology, 2022: p. 1–17.
26. Tan, Y.T., et al., *LncRNA-mediated posttranslational modifications and reprogramming of energy metabolism in cancer.* Cancer Communications, 2021. **41**(2): p. 109–120.
27. Lin, Y.-H., *Crosstalk of lncRNA and cellular metabolism and their regulatory mechanism in cancer.* International Journal of Molecular Sciences, 2020. **21**(8): p. 2947.
28. Ghafouri-Fard, S., et al., *TINCR: An lncRNA with dual functions in the carcinogenesis process.* Non-coding RNA Research, 2020. **5**(3): p. 109–115.
29. Gu, X., et al., *The dual functions of the long noncoding RNA CASC15 in malignancy.* Biomedicine & Pharmacotherapy, 2021. **135**: p. 111212.
30. Welch, D.R. and D.R. Hurst, *Defining the hallmarks of metastasis.* Cancer Research, 2019. **79**(12): p. 3011–3027.
31. Robinson, D.R., et al., *Integrative clinical genomics of metastatic cancer.* Nature, 2017. **548**(7667): p. 297–303.

32. Birkbak, N.J. and N. McGranahan, *Cancer genome evolutionary trajectories in metastasis.* Cancer Cell, 2020. **37**(1): p. 8–19.
33. Fares, J., et al., *Molecular principles of metastasis: A hallmark of cancer revisited.* Signal Transduction and Targeted Therapy, 2020. **5**(1): p. 1–17.
34. Suhail, Y., et al., *Systems biology of cancer metastasis.* Cell Systems, 2019. **9**(2): p. 109–127.
35. Weiss, F., D. Lauffenburger, and P. Friedl, *Towards targeting of shared mechanisms of cancer metastasis and therapy resistance.* Nature Reviews Cancer, 2022. **22**(3): p. 157–173.
36. Yaguchi, T., et al., *The mechanisms of cancer immunoescape and development of overcoming strategies.* International Journal of Hematology, 2011. **93**(3): p. 294–300.
37. Akalay, I., et al., *Epithelial-to-mesenchymal transition and autophagy induction in breast carcinoma promote escape from T-cell–mediated lysis.* Cancer Research, 2013. **73**(8): p. 2418–2427.
38. Cheng, J.-C. and P.C. Leung, *Type I collagen down-regulates E-cadherin expression by increasing PI3KCA in cancer cells.* Cancer Letters, 2011. **304**(2): p. 107–116.
39. Sadrkhanloo, M., et al., *STAT3-EMT axis in tumors: Modulation of cancer metastasis, stemness and therapy response.* Pharmacological Research, 2022: p. 106311.
40. Sadrkhanloo, M., et al., *Non-coding RNAs in EMT regulation: Association with tumor progression and therapy response.* European Journal of Pharmacology, 2022: p. 175212.
41. Fukagawa, A., et al., *δEF1 associates with DNMT1 and maintains DNA methylation of the E-cadherin promoter in breast cancer cells.* Cancer Medicine, 2015. **4**(1): p. 125–135.
42. Aiello, N.M. and Y. Kang, *Context-dependent EMT programs in cancer metastasis.* Journal of Experimental Medicine, 2019. **216**(5): p. 1016–1026.
43. Hamidi, A.A., et al., *Long non-coding RNAs as the critical regulators of epithelial mesenchymal transition in colorectal tumor cells: an overview.* Cancer Cell International, 2022. **22**(1): p. 1–15.
44. Ashrafizadeh, M., et al., *Long noncoding RNAs (lncRNAs) in pancreatic cancer progression.* Drug Discovery Today, 2022.

45. Singh, A., et al., *Role of various non-coding RNAs in EMT, cancer, and metastasis: Recent trends and future perspective.* Advances in Cancer Biology-Metastasis, 2022: p. 100039.
46. Zhou, Y., et al., *Identification of Epithelial Mesenchymal Transition-Related lncRNAs Associated with Prognosis and Tumor Immune Microenvironment of Hepatocellular Carcinoma.* Disease Markers, 2022. **2022**.
47. Yang, X., et al., *Non-coding RNAs regulating epithelial-mesenchymal transition: Research progress in liver disease.* Biomedicine & Pharmacotherapy, 2022. **150**: p. 112972.
48. Sadrkhanloo, M., et al., *Non-coding RNAs in EMT regulation: Association with tumor progression and therapy response.* European Journal of Pharmacology, 2022. **932**: p. 175212.
49. Sheng, S., et al., *MicroRNA-21 induces cisplatin resistance in head and neck squamous cell carcinoma.* PloS One, 2022. **17**(4): p. e0267017.
50. Lv, C., et al., *ENO2 promotes colorectal cancer metastasis by interacting with the LncRNA CYTOR and activating YAP1-induced EMT.* Cells, 2022. **11**(15): p. 2363.
51. Lin, H., et al., *LncRNA CASC15, MiR-23b cluster and SMAD3 form a novel positive feedback loop to promote epithelial-mesenchymal transition and metastasis in ovarian cancer.* International Journal of Biological Sciences, 2022. **18**(5): p. 1989.
52. Li, X., et al., *MicroRNA-486–3p promotes the proliferation and metastasis of cutaneous squamous cell carcinoma by suppressing flotillin-2.* Journal of Dermatological Science, 2022. **105**(1): p. 18–26.
53. Zhao, H., et al., *Alternatively-spliced lncRNA-PNUTS promotes HCC cell EMT via regulating ZEB1 expression.* Tumori Journal, 2022: p. 03008916211072585.
54. Guo, Y., et al., *M2 Tumor Associate Macrophage-(TAM-) Derived lncRNA HISLA Promotes EMT Potential in Bladder Cancer.* Journal of Oncology, 2022. **2022**.
55. Shen, S., et al., *SNHG17, as an EMT-related lncRNA, promotes the expression of c-Myc by binding to c-Jun in esophageal squamous cell carcinoma.* Cancer Science, 2022. **113**(1): p. 319.

56. Wang, Z., et al., *LncRNA NDRG1 aggravates progression and EMT of osteosarcoma by sponging miR-96-5p through the PI3K/AKT pathway.* BMC Cancer, 2022. **22**(1):728
57. Hu, J., et al., *LncRNA DLEU2 silencing impedes the migration, invasion and EMT in gastric cancer cell by suppressing PI3K/AKT signaling pathway.* Immunopharmacology and Immunotoxicology, 2022. **44**(5): p. 1–13.
58. Mao, D., Y. Jie, and Y. Lv, *LncRNA SNHG6 induces epithelial–mesenchymal transition of pituitary adenoma via suppressing miR-944.* Cancer Biotherapy & Radiopharmaceuticals, 2022. **37**(4): p. 246–255.
59. Zhang, F., et al., *LncRNA HCG18 upregulates TRAF4/TRAF5 to facilitate proliferation, migration and EMT of epithelial ovarian cancer by targeting miR-29a/b.* Molecular Medicine, 2022. **28**(1): p. 1–16.
60. Hu, Y.-Z., et al., *LncRNA SND1-IT1 facilitates TGF-β1-induced epithelial-to-mesenchymal transition via miR-124/COL4A1 axis in gastric cancer.* Cell Death Discovery, 2022. **8**(1): p. 1–12.
61. Zhang, L., et al., *LncRNA Opa interacting protein 5-antisense RNA 1 (OIP5-AS1) promotes the migration, invasion and epithelial-mesenchymal transition (EMT) through targeting miR-147a/insulin-like growth factor 1 receptor (IGF1R) pathway in cervical cancer tissues and cell model.* Journal of Obstetrics and Gynaecology Research, 2022. **48**(5): p. 1222–1232.
62. Zhou, Y., et al., *Lnc NR2F1-AS1 promotes breast cancer metastasis by targeting miR-25-3p/ZEB2 axis.* 2022.
63. Pan, Y., et al., *A feedback loop between GATA2-AS1 and GATA2 promotes colorectal cancer cell proliferation, invasion, epithelial-mesenchymal transition and stemness via recruiting DDX3X.* Journal of Translational Medicine, 2022. **20**(1): p. 1–16.
64. Le, F., et al., *lncRNA ZNF674-AS1 inhibits the migration, invasion and epithelial-mesenchymal transition of thyroid cancer cells by modulating the miR-181a/SOCS4 axis.* Molecular and Cellular Endocrinology, 2022. **544**: p. 111551.
65. Sun, Z., et al., *LINC00244 suppresses cell growth and metastasis in hepatocellular carcinoma by downregulating programmed cell death ligand 1.* Bioengineered, 2022. **13**(3): p. 7635–7647.

66. Guan, C., B. Wang, and Q. Dong, *The IncRNA SCIRT promotes the proliferative, migratory, and invasive properties of cervical cancer cells by upregulating MMP-2/-9.* Journal of Oncology, 2022. **2022**.
67. Jiang, Y., et al., *LncRNA HOXC-AS1 Sponges miR-99a-3p and Upregulates MMP8, Ultimately Promoting Gastric Cancer.* Cancers, 2022. **14**(14): p. 3534.
68. Piipponen, M., et al., *Super enhancer-regulated LINC00094 (SERLOC) upregulates the expression of MMP-1 and MMP-13 and promotes invasion of cutaneous squamous cell carcinoma.* Cancers, 2022. **14**(16): p. 3980.
69. Wang, Y. and C. Li, *lncRNA GHET1 Promotes the progression of triple-negative breast cancer via regulation of miR-377-3p/GRSF1 signaling axis.* Computational and Mathematical Methods in Medicine, 2022. **2022**.
70. Wang, Q., et al., *LncRNA CRNDE promotes cell proliferation, migration and invasion of ovarian cancer via miR-423-5p/FSCN1 axis.* Molecular and Cellular Biochemistry, 2022. **477**(5): p. 1477–1488.
71. Ma, T., et al., *Long noncoding XLOC_006390 regulates the proliferation and metastasis of human colorectal cancer via miR-296/ONECUT2 axis.* Journal of Oncology, 2022. **2022**.
72. Li, Z.-Y., et al., *c-Myc-activated intronic miR-210 and lncRNA MIR210HG synergistically promote the metastasis of gastric cancer.* Cancer Letters, 2022. **526**: p. 322–334.
73. Lin, Y.-H., et al., *LPAL2 suppresses tumor growth and metastasis of hepatocellular carcinoma by modulating MMP9 expression.* Cells, 2022. **11**(16): p. 2610.
74. Zhu, Y., et al., *LncRNA-HCG18 regulates the viability, apoptosis, migration, invasion and epithelial-mesenchymal transition of papillary thyroid cancer cells via regulating the miR-106a-5p/PPP2R2A axis.* Pathology-Research and Practice, 2021. **221**: p. 153395.
75. Mabeta, P., R. Hull, and Z. Dlamini, *LncRNAs and the angiogenic switch in cancer: Clinical significance and therapeutic opportunities.* Genes, 2022. **13**(1): p. 152.
76. Liu, J., et al., *The role of long non-coding RNAs in angiogenesis and anti-angiogenic therapy resistance in cancer.* Molecular Therapy-Nucleic Acids, 2022.

77. Liao, Y., et al., *Non-coding RNAs in lung cancer: Emerging regulators of angiogenesis.* Journal of Translational Medicine, 2022. **20**(1): p. 1–11.
78. Golhani, V., S.K. Ray, and S. Mukherjee, *Role of microRNAs and long non-coding RNAs in regulating angiogenesis in human breast cancer: A molecular medicine perspective.* Current Molecular Medicine, 2022.
79. Yang, K., et al., *Exosome-derived noncoding RNAs: Function, mechanism and application in tumour angiogenesis.* Molecular Therapy-Nucleic Acids, 2022.
80. Matthews, H.K., C. Bertoli, and R.A. de Bruin, *Cell cycle control in cancer.* Nature Reviews Molecular Cell Biology, 2022. **23**(1): p. 74–88.
81. Hu, M., et al., *Noncoding RNAs of extracellular vesicles in tumor angiogenesis: From biological functions to clinical significance.* Cells, 2022. **11**(6): p. 947.
82. Wang, G., H. Li, and Y. Hou, *LncRNA MAGI2-AS3 inhibits tumor progression and angiogenesis by regulating ACY1 via interacting with transcription factor HEY1 in clear cell renal cell carcinoma.* Cancer Gene Therapy, 2022. **29**(5): p. 585–596.
83. Yu, C., et al., *The lncRNA ZNF667-AS1 inhibits propagation, invasion, and angiogenesis of gastric cancer by silencing the expression of N-Cadherin and VEGFA.* Journal of Oncology, 2022. **2022**.
84. Li, X., et al., *LncRNA H22954 inhibits angiogenesis in acute myeloid leukemia through a PDGFA-dependent mechanism.* Recent Patents on Anti-Cancer Drug Discovery, 2022. **17**(4): p. 427–434.
85. Zhang, J., et al., *LncRNA CRART16/miR-122-5p/FOS axis promotes angiogenesis of gastric cancer by upregulating VEGFD expression.* Aging (Albany NY), 2022. **14**(9): p. 4137.
86. Yuan, D., et al., *Exosomal lncRNA ATB derived from ovarian cancer cells promotes angiogenesis via regulating miR-204-3p/TGFβR2 axis.* Cancer Management and Research, 2022. **14**: p. 327.
87. Dong, H., et al., *LncRNA OGFRP1 promotes angiogenesis and epithelial-mesenchymal transition in colorectal cancer cells through miR-423-5p/CTCF axis.* Immunobiology, 2022. **227**(2): p. 152176.
88. Zhu, Y., et al., *DMDRMR promotes angiogenesis via antagonizing DAB2IP in clear cell renal cell carcinoma.* Cell Death & Disease, 2022. **13**(5): p. 1–12.

89. Li, Z., et al., *lncRNA KCNQ1OT1 Promotes EMT, angiogenesis, and stemness of pituitary adenoma by upregulation of RAB11A*. Journal of Oncology, 2022. **2022**.
90. Chang, L., et al., *Long intergenic non-protein-coding RNA 467 promotes tumor progression and angiogenesis via the microRNA-128-3p/vascular endothelial growth factor C axis in colorectal cancer.* Bioengineered, 2022. **13**(5): p. 12392–12408.
91. Shetty, A., et al., *LncRNA–miRNA–mRNA regulatory axes in endometrial cancer: A comprehensive overview.* Archives of Gynecology and Obstetrics, 2022: p. 1–17.
92. Zeng, X., et al., *Research progress on the circRNA/lncRNA–miRNA–mRNA axis in gastric cancer.* Pathology-Research and Practice, 2022: p. 154030.
93. Malakoti, F., et al., *Long noncoding RNA SNHG7-miRNA-mRNA axes crosstalk with oncogenic signaling pathways in human cancers.* Chemical Biology & Drug Design, 2022.
94. Pronina, I.V., et al., *Dysregulation of lncRNA–miRNA–mRNA interactome as a marker of metastatic process in ovarian cancer.* Biomedicines, 2022. **10**(4): p. 824.
95. Xu, J., et al., *The role of lncRNA-mediated ceRNA regulatory networks in pancreatic cancer.* Cell Death Discovery, 2022. **8**(1): p. 1–11.
96. Lin, C., et al., *The regulatory mechanism of LncRNA-mediated ceRNA network in osteosarcoma.* Scientific Reports, 2022. **12**(1): p. 1–12.
97. Xia, Y., et al., *Novel lncRNA SNHG16 promotes the growth and metastasis of malignant melanoma by regulating miR-205-5p/PAK2 axis.* Clinical, Cosmetic and Investigational Dermatology, 2022. **15**: p. 1615.
98. Shan, K.-S., et al., *LncRNA cancer susceptibility 20 regulates the metastasis of human gastric cancer cells via the miR-143-5p/MEMO1 molecular axis.* World Journal of Gastroenterology, 2022. **28**(16): p. 1656.
99. Si, C., L. Yang, and X. Cai, *LncRNA LINC00649 aggravates the progression of cervical cancer through sponging miR-216a-3p.* Journal of Obstetrics and Gynaecology Research, 2022.
100. Lu, L., et al., *Exosomal lncRNA TUG1 from cancer-associated fibroblasts promotes liver cancer cell migration, invasion, and glycolysis by regulating the miR-524-5p/SIX1 axis.* Cellular & Molecular Biology Letters, 2022. **27**(1): p. 1–17.

101. Li, Y., et al., *Low expression of lncRNA SBF2-AS1 regulates the miR-302b-3p/TGFBR2 axis, promoting metastasis in laryngeal cancer.* Molecular Carcinogenesis, 2022. **61**(1): p. 45–58.
102. Zheng, J., et al., *LncRNA HCG11 facilitates nasopharyngeal carcinoma progression through miRNA-490-3p/MAP3K9 axis.* Frontiers in Oncology, 2022: p. 1208.
103. Li, X., et al., *LncRNA HCP5 enhances the proliferation and migration of cervical cancer via miR-216a-5p/CDC42 axis.* Journal of Cancer, 2022. **13**(6): p. 1882.
104. Chen, G., et al., *LINC01232 Promotes metastasis and EMT by regulating miR-506-5p/PAK1 axis in gastric cancer.* Cancer Management and Research, 2022. **14**: p. 1729.
105. Pan, J. and Y. Zang, *LINC00667 promotes progression of esophageal cancer cells by regulating miR-200b-3p/SLC2A3 axis.* Digestive Diseases and Sciences, 2022. **67**(7): p. 2936–2947.
106. Wang, Y., et al., *LncRNA LINC00511 promotes COL1A1-mediated proliferation and metastasis by sponging miR-126-5p/miR-218-5p in lung adenocarcinoma.* BMC Pulmonary Medicine, 2022. **22**(1): p. 1–15.
107. Wang, Y., et al., *LncRNA SNHG1 facilitates the epithelial-mesenchymal transition and invasiveness in glioblastoma multiforme via regulation of the miR-128-3p/RRAS2 axis.* 2022.
108. Ni, C., et al., *LINC00483 promotes proliferation and metastasis through the miR-19a-3p/TBK1/MAPK axis in pancreatic ductal adenocarcinoma (PDAC).* Annals of Translational Medicine, 2022. **10**(6).
109. Deng, Y.-W., Y.-G. Shu, and S.-L. Sun, *LncRNA PART1 inhibits glioma proliferation and migration via miR-374b/SALL1 axis.* Neurochemistry International, 2022. **157**: p. 105347.
110. Entezari, M., et al., *LncRNA-miRNA axis in tumor progression and therapy response: An emphasis on molecular interactions and therapeutic interventions.* 2022. **154**: p. 113609.
111. Tian, C., et al., *lncRNA NBAT1 inhibits cell metastasis and promotes apoptosis in endometrial cancer by sponging miR-21-5p to regulate PTEN.* Computational and Mathematical Methods in Medicine, 2022. **2022**.

https://doi.org/10.1142/9789811267390_0007

Chapter 7

Long non-coding RNAs (lncRNAs) in cancer therapy response: Biological aspects

Mohammad Hossein Gholami[1], Alireza Abbaspour[2], Fatemeh Tajik[3], Amirhossein Zabolian[4] and Zhaowu Ma[5]*

[1]*Faculty of Veterinary Medicine, Kazerun Branch, Islamic Azad University, Kazerun, Iran*
[2]*Cellular and Molecular Research Center, Qazvin University of Medical Sciences, Qazvin, Iran*
[3]*Oncopathology Research Center, Iran University of Medical Sciences, Tehran, Iran*
[4]*Resident of Orthopedics, Department of Orthopedics, School of Medicine, 5th Azar Hospital, Golestan University of Medical Sciences, Golestan, Iran*
[5]*School of Basic Medicine, Health Science Center, Yangtze University, Nanhuan Road 1, Jingzhou, Hubei 434023, China*

*Corresponding author: Zhaowu Ma, School of Basic Medicine, Health Science Center, Yangtze University, Nanhuan Road 1, Jingzhou, Hubei 434023, China, Email: mazw@yangtzeu.edu.cn

Abstract

Two major arms for the treatment of cancer include chemotherapy and radiotherapy, and they have been used for a long time in patients to improve survival rates. However, physicians should deal with a new type of challenge, known as therapy resistance that adds more difficulty to cancer treatment. Among different factors involved in cancer therapy resistance, long non-coding RNAs (lncRNAs) have demonstrated high potential. Oncogenic lncRNAs participate in the induction of drug resistance, while onco-suppressor lncRNAs prevent drug resistance. Furthermore, lncRNAs are involved in regulating apoptosis and cell cycle progression that can indirectly affect the response of tumor cells to chemotherapy. In addition, radiotherapy induces apoptosis and DNA damage in impairing tumor progression. Overexpression of oncogenic lncRNAs can induce radio-resistance, leading to therapy failure in patients. This chapter focuses on understanding the role of lncRNAs in regulating drug resistance and radio-resistance in cancer and related signaling networks to pave the way for developing novel therapeutics in near future.

1. Introduction

Both developing and developed countries are facing challenges in the treatment of cancer patients that emanate from different reasons such as inability in early diagnosis of patients and lack of effective treatments. The reason for focusing on cancer treatment is that it is the second leading cause of death after cardiovascular diseases [1, 2]. Cancer has a multi-factorial origin, and a certain reason or factor is not considered for its initiation and development. In fact, a set of reasons including family history, environmental factors such as exposure to toxic agents, living in industrial places as there are more toxic and damaging compounds, lifestyle, smoking, alcohol consumption, and genetic materials are among the reasons for developing cancer in patients. There are different kinds of cancers, such as brain tumors, gynecologic tumors, reproductive tumors, and thoracic tumors. Each cancer demonstrates specific mortality and morbidity, but lung and breast tumors are the most malignant cancers [3]. The geographical distribution of cancers is also different and overall, cancer shows lower incidence rate in developed countries compared to developing countries. There are a number of reasons for this fact. For instance, infection with the hepatitis virus can lead to hepatocellular carcinoma (HCC) development, and in developed countries, there has been an effort in vaccination to reduce the number of HCC cases, while developing countries suffer from funds and budgets for these purposes [4].

In recent years, the field of oncology has witnessed a revolution, and researchers from around the world have focused on understanding the reasons for the progression of cancer cells and their ability in therapy resistance development. Along with these efforts, some new strategies such as the use of anti-cancer agents, gene therapy, and use of nanostructures for targeted delivery of chemotherapy agents and small molecules have been recommended. In the first strategy, researchers use anti-cancer agents to increase the sensitivity of tumor cells to chemotherapy. For instance, cancer cells demonstrate resistance to apoptosis and they increase cell cycle progression in spite of the exposure to chemotherapy agents. This is known as drug resistance, which is common in recent years. The use of other anti-cancer agents can stimulate apoptosis and cell cycle arrest by increasing the chemosensitivity of tumor cells [5]. In the strategy of using nanostructures, two important reasons are followed. At first, since tumor cells are exposed to chemotherapy agents for long term and frequent applications are favored, nanoparticles allow the use of a low concentration of chemotherapy agents to prevent the development of drug resistance. In the second step, nanoparticles can increase internalization of anti-cancer drugs in tumor cells to promote their cytotoxicity [6–8]. In the strategy of gene therapy, which is a new emerging therapeutic strategy and is potential in the field of cancer therapy, biological and molecular mechanisms responsible for cancer progression and drug resistance are understood. Then, genetic tools are used in affecting molecular pathways, cancer progression, and increasing chemosensitivity [9–11]. In addition to chemotherapy resistance, tumor cells have been able to prevent cell death and DNA damage to induce radio-resistance [12].

Thanks to new experiments evaluating the role of molecular pathways in the development of drug resistance and radio-resistance. It has been shown that a wide variety of molecular pathways can involve in therapy resistance in cancer. For instance, exposure of colorectal tumor cells to radiation leads to the overexpression of TGF-β and PODXL, which are responsible for the increase in the invasion of cancer cells and stimulation of radio-resistance [13]. On down-regulation of SFRP2, stimulation of Wnt/β-catenin occurs to increase the stemness of glioma cells and to mediate radio-resistance [14]. By induction of YAP signaling, CD155 is involved in triggering radio-resistance in esophageal cancer [15]. The interesting point regarding experiments is that activation of oncogenic signaling pathways can prevent apoptosis and increase stemness, invasion, and proliferation of tumor cells to mediate radio-resistance [16–20].

Similar to radio-resistance, a number of molecular pathways are involved in drug resistance development. Cancer-associated mesothelial cells are involved in the induction of osteopontin signaling to induce drug resistance in ovarian cancer [21]. SIRT3 promotes the expression level of SOD2 to prevent apoptosis and to mediate chemoresistance in colorectal cancer [22]. Pharmacological inhibition of PTK6 results in the inhibition of JAK2/STAT3 axis to reduce the stemness of colorectal tumor cells and to increase their sensitivity to chemotherapy [23]. Furthermore, FAM49B increases the stability of ELAVL1 to enhance growth and invasion of tumor cells in triggering chemo-resistance [24]. Therefore, molecular pathways affecting the growth and invasion of cancer cells can influence chemosensitivity [25–27]. The aim of this chapter is to focus on the role of long non-coding RNAs (lncRNAs) in regulating chemo-resistance and radio-resistance in cancers. Figure 1 shows an overview of the traditional and new therapies for cancer treatment.

2. lncRNAs: Overview and role in oncology

Protein-coding sequences comprise a small fraction of the human genome, and most of the genome is constituted by non-coding protein sequences [28]. These non-coding transcripts were first

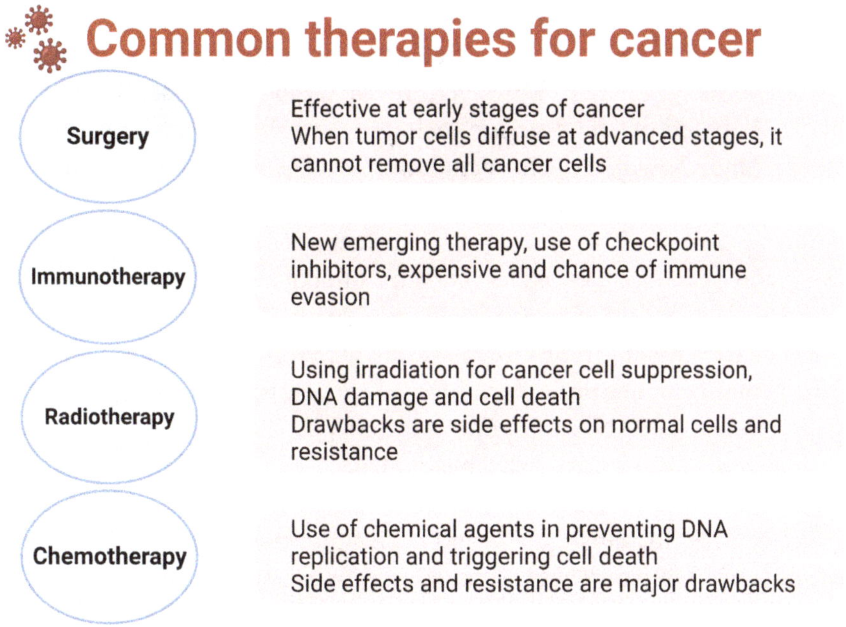

Figure 1. Common therapies for cancer, benefits, and drawbacks for clinical course.

considered as transcriptional noises, but their function was shown to be vital in biological processes occurring in cells [29]. A major class of non-coding transcripts is lncRNAs that identification of a large number of these RNA transcripts, their complexity and function have resulted in their categorization into different groups. Genomic localization and function of lncRNAs are considered for their categorization [30]. Intronic, intergenic, enhancer, bi-directional, sense-overlapping and anti-sense lncRNAs are different types of these non-coding RNA transcripts. Introns of protein-coding genes are responsible for the generation of intronic lncRNAs; intergenic lncRNAs derived from two protein-coding genes; enhancer lncRNAs result from promoter enhancer regions; bi-directional lncRNAs are positioned near a coding transcript of the opposite strand; sense-overlapping lncRNAs demonstrate overlap with one or more than one introns and exons of protein-coding genes in the sense strand of

DNA; and anti-sense lncRNAs result from anti-sense strand of DNA. These were the categorizations of lncRNAs based on their location in the genome [31, 32]. However, there is another classification of lncRNAs based on the function including signaling, decoy, guide, and scaffold lncRNAs [33]. The signaling lncRNAs show interaction with a certain and specific molecular pathways such as lncRNA XIST that demonstrates the inactivation of X in females [34]. Decoy lncRNAs are involved in the process of silencing or activation of genes, such as lncRNA GAS5 and TERRA [33]. Guide lncRNAs are involved in binding to regulatory or enzymatically active protein complexes and direct them to genomic locations or promoters of genes such as CCND1 and lincRNA-21, among others [32, 33].

As RNA transcripts with more than 200 nucleotides, lncRNAs have been shown to be important players in different cancers. They affect various proteins, genes, and even other non-coding RNAs such as microRNAs (miRNAs) via sponging and regulate chromatin remodeling [35–37]. The role of lncRNAs in cancer is regulating hallmarks including proliferation, metastasis, and therapy resistance [38–40]. The overexpression of oncogenic lncRNAs has been implicated in increasing the stemness of tumor cells. lncRNA PKMYT1AR stimulates Wnt signaling to increase stemness and to mediate the progression of lung tumor cells [41]. Overexpression of VEGF has been shown to increase the progression of tumor cells. lncRNA TUSC8 downregulates VEGF expression to inhibit the growth and metastasis of cancer cells [42]. The increase in proliferation of ovarian cancer cells can be obtained by lncRNA OR3A4 by upregulating the expression level of KLF6 [43]. On the other hand, KLF5 promotes the expression level of lncRNA DANCR to inhibit autophagy in facilitating gastric cancer progression [44]. Based on these studies, lncRNAs are closely associated with the progression of tumor cells and regulating their growth and invasion [45, 46]. Furthermore, lncRNAs can be considered as biomarkers for the prognosis of cancer patients [47]. The most important aspect is the involvement of lncRNAs in regulating therapy response [48, 49] which is the focus of this chapter and will be discussed in the following sections.

3. lncRNAs regulating drug resistance

3.1 *Tumor suppressor lncRNAs*

In cancer drug resistance, lncRNAs are categorized into two major kinds including tumor suppressor and tumor-promoting lncRNAs. Although the number of tumor-promoting lncRNAs is higher compared to tumor suppressor lncRNAs, it would be beneficial to show how these onco-suppressor factors regulate drug resistance in cancers and their expression is lower or higher in tumor tissues compared to adjacent tissues. For instance, in gastric cancer, lncRNA ADAMTS9-AS2 has onco-suppressor function and its expression level undergoes downregulation in tumor tissues. Restoring the expression level of ADAMTS9-AS2 is associated with cisplatin sensitivity of gastric cancer cells. ADAMTS9-AS2 promotes NLRP3 expression via miR-223-3p inhibition to induce pyroptosis in gastric cancer cells for their cisplatin sensitivity [50]. Therefore, prevention of cell death and increased proliferation rate are two major factors responsible for drug resistance in cancer. lncRNA ADAMTS9-AS2 induces chemosensitivity in the renal cancer cells. The ability of ADAMTS9-AS2 in mediating drug sensitivity is attributed to the inhibition of renal cancer cell proliferation. ADAMTS9-AS2 promotes FOXO1 expression via miR-27a-3p sponging to suppress growth rate and increase drug sensitivity in renal cancer [51]. It appears that proliferation is a vital element in regulating the drug sensitivity of cancer cells. lncRNA SNHG16 demonstrates low expression levels in hepatocellular carcinoma and by mediating hsa-miR-93 sponging, it can suppress the proliferation rate of cancer cells by providing drug sensitivity [52].

One of the most common malignancies around the world is colorectal cancer which ranks third in terms of morbidity and mortality [53]. Surgery, radiotherapy, chemotherapy, and immunotherapy are major arms in the treatment of colorectal cancer. However, most of the colorectal cancer patients are diagnosed at advanced stages and chemotherapy is not a gold option at this step. Furthermore, colorectal cancer patients receiving chemotherapy have a poor prognosis [54]. Oxaliplatin is commonly used in colorectal cancer treatment that suppresses DNA replication via creating cross-links [55]. lncRNAs have been shown to regulate oxaliplatin sensitivity in colorectal cancer. Lnc-AP downregulates the expression level of a protein, known as TALDO1 to inhibit the pentose phosphate pathway for enhancing oxaliplatin sensitivity of colorectal cancer cells [56]. In addition to the pentose phosphate pathway, which is responsible for the proliferation and metabolism of cancer cells, glycolysis is also involved in this mechanism and can induce chemo-resistance. lncRNA SARCC is involved in increasing the cisplatin sensitivity of osteosarcoma cells. For this purpose, lncRNA SARCC increases the expression level of miR-143 to downregulate HK2 for inhibiting glycolysis and increasing cisplatin sensitivity of osteosarcoma cells [57].

For exerting anti-cancer activity, high levels of anti-tumor agents and drugs should accumulate in tumor cells. However, there are some drug efflux transporters on the surface of cancer cells that show hyperactivity in removing drugs from tumor cells and pumping them out. ATP-binding cassette (ABC) transporters are the most well-known transporters responsible for drug efflux in cancers that can induce drug resistance and their targeting is of importance in reversing chemo-resistance [58–60]. lncRNA FENDRR has been implicated in providing drug sensitivity in osteosarcoma. FENDRR reduces expression levels of ABCB1 and ABCC1 to increase doxorubicin sensitivity of osteosarcoma cells [61]. Therefore, tumor suppressor lncRNAs demonstrate downregulation in tumor cells, and restoring their expression can mediate drug sensitivity via inhibition of oncogenic pathways or upregulation of onco-suppressor factors. Inhibition of proliferation, migration, and metabolism and induction of apoptosis are the major pathways followed by tumor suppressor lncRNAs in mediating drug sensitivity in cancers [62–65].

3.2 *Tumor-promoting lncRNAs*

Most of the studies have shown the role of oncogenic lncRNAs in regulating drug resistance in cancer. The function of these kinds of lncRNAs is to increase the stability and expression of tumor-promoting factors as downstream targets. LINC00943 has been implicated in increasing the stability of c-Myc at the mRNA level by preventing the degradation of MSI2 that are beneficial in preventing apoptosis and increasing stemness of tumor cells in mediating chemo-resistance [66]. Among the different kinds of downstream targets of lncRNAs, miRNAs are the most important and well-known ones. lncRNA ANRIL has been associated with gemcitabine resistance in pancreatic cancer, and by reducing the expression level of miR-181a, ANRIL upregulates HMGB1 to induce autophagy as a pro-survival mechanism in triggering drug resistance [67]. The autophagy mechanism is important in the process of chemo-resistance, as it can have both pro-survival and pro-death functions, and it has been shown that induction of pro-survival mechanism can lead to chemo-resistance, while pro-death autophagy enhances the sensitivity of tumor cells to chemotherapy. Therefore, the regulatory impact of lncRNAs on autophagy in drug resistance should be carefully investigated.

One of the hallmarks of the tumor microenvironment (TME) is hypoxia, which is responsible for increasing the plasticity and heterogeneity of a tumor. Hypoxia accounts for creating a condition that accelerates the development of drug resistance in cancer and is associated with a poor prognosis [68, 69]. Furthermore, hypoxia can induce angiogenesis and vasculogenic mimicry in enhancing tumor progression [70]. Overexpression of lncRNA NORAD has been shown in colorectal cancer that can mediate drug resistance. NORAD reduces the expression level of miR-495-3p via sponging to upregulate HIF-1α in potentiating tumor progression during hypoxia and enhancing drug resistance [71]. However, NORAD is not the only lncRNA that can undergo overexpression during hypoxia to mediate drug resistance in cancer. It has been shown that during stress, an increase occurs in the expression level of lncRNA PVT1 that enhances proliferation, invasion, and survival rate of ovarian cancer cells. Silencing PVT1 impairs tumor progression in vitro and in vivo. As an oncogenic factor, overexpression of PVT1 induces chemo-resistance in ovarian cancer during stress conditions and is responsible for their abnormal progression [72].

Although lncRNAs are master regulators in cancer and are considered as main upstream regulators of molecular pathways involved in tumor progression, there has been an effort in understanding how the expression level of lncRNAs can be affected by other molecular pathways and factors in cancer therapy. SOX transcription factors are a large family of proteins; their role in cancer progression is under evolution; and their members demonstrate similarity in structure. SOX family members can have both oncogenic and onco-suppressor functions and by preventing apoptosis and increasing migration and invasion of cancer cells, they can participate in the development of drug resistance and provide cancer progression [73–75]. SOX12 is one of the important members of SOX family that is involved in drug resistance in cervical cancer. SOX12 can increase the expression level of lncRNA SNHG15 to mediate carcinogenesis and chemo-resistance. Overexpressed SNHG15 promotes HIF-1α expression via miR-4735-3p inhibition to induce chemo-resistance [76]. Due to the role of oncogenic lncRNAs in mediating drug resistance and preventing cytotoxicity of chemotherapy drugs, there have been efforts in silencing such non-coding RNAs to increase the capacity of drugs in cancer therapy and improve the prognosis of patients. lncRNA KCNQ1OT1 is involved in triggering drug resistance in lung cancer and improving tumor progression. In contrast, silencing KCNQ1OT1 prevents metastasis of lung tumor cells via inhibition of the epithelial–mesenchymal transition (EMT) mechanism to drug sensitivity and is associated with favorable prognosis in patients [77].

Among the different kinds of chemotherapy agents used for the treatment of colorectal cancer, oxaliplatin is a common one. However, malignant behavior and abnormal progression of colorectal tumor cells have resulted in the development of oxaliplatin resistance, requiring experiments to highlight molecular pathways involved in this case. lncRNA MCF2L-AS1 shows overexpression in colorectal cancer and is associated with oxaliplatin resistance. MCF2L-AS1 promotes expression level of IL-1β via miR-105 inhibition to induce oxaliplatin resistance in colorectal tumor cells [78]. Another important factor in triggering drug resistance is the activation of glycolysis. Briefly, tumor cells change their metabolic action from oxidative phosphorylation in mitochondria to glycolysis to increase energy generation. This process requires activity of several enzymes including HK2 and G6PD, and glucose uptake by cancer cells should be enhanced by triggering glycolysis and ensuring the proliferation of cancer cells. Increasing evidence has shown the association of glycolysis with drug resistance development in cancers [79–83]. Linc00173 stimulates multi-drug resistance in small-cell lung cancer, and its inhibition is a promising option in cancer therapy and reversing chemo-resistance. The translation of YB1 undergoes induction by linc00173 to increase the activity of HK2 and G6PD by triggering glycolysis and pentose phosphate pathway in mediating chemo-resistance in small-cell lung cancer [84].

Based on these studies, it can be concluded that apoptosis, autophagy, glucose metabolism, proliferation, and metastasis of cancer cells are regulated by lncRNAs. The regulation of these important biological mechanisms is important in affecting therapy response in cancer. Oncogenic lncRNAs prevent apoptosis and pro-death autophagy, while they induce glycolysis, proliferation, and invasion of tumor cells to mediate drug resistance in cancer. Therefore, silencing such tumor-promoting lncRNAs is associated with increased sensitivity of cancer cells to chemotherapy by inducing apoptosis and reducing tumor progression (Table 1) [85–92].

4. lncRNAs regulating radio-resistance

4.1 *Tumor suppressor lncRNAs*

DNA damage repair is vital for the process of radio-resistance in cancers. Several signal transduction mechanisms such as ATM-CHK2 and ATR-CHK1 are involved in DNA damage response. Stimulation of the aforementioned pathways is necessary for the coordination of checkpoint and DNA repair processes [102]. ATM activation is mediated by the MRN complex by recruiting ATM to DNA lesions and inducing kinase activity [103]. For ATM activation, its phosphorylation on Ser1981 is vital and leads to the dissociation of dimer ATM into monomers [104]. Upregulation of linc00312 has been associated with radio-sensitivity in cancer due to preventing DNA damage repair. Linc00312 reduces the expression level of MRN to downregulate ATM-CHK2 and ATR-CHK1 in providing radio-sensitivity

Table 1. The role of lncRNAs in regulating drug resistance in cancer.

Cancer Type	Molecular Pathway	Drug Resistance Drug Sensitivity	Remarks	Ref
Breast cancer	NEAT1/miR-23a-3p/FOXA1	Drug resistance	NEAT1 sponges miR-23a-3p to increase FOXA1 expression in enhancing tumor progression. Stimulation of taxol resistance.	[93]
Breast cancer	AFAP1-AS1/miR-195/545	Drug resistance	AFAP1-AS1 induces drug resistance in breast cancer via sponging miR-195 and miR-545. Formononetin decreases the expression level of AFAP1-AS1 in providing chemosensitivity.	[94]
Gastric cancer	FEZF1-AS1/ATG5	Drug resistance	Induction of multi-drug resistance in gastric cancer by FEZF1-AS1 via overexpression of ATG5.	[95]
Head and neck squamous cell carcinoma	PVT1/miR-124-3p	Drug resistance	PVT1 induces cetuximab resistance via downregulation of miR-124-3p.	[96]
Small-cell lung cancer	MEG3/miR-15a-5p/CCNE1	Drug resistance	Exosomal MEG3 is involved in cisplatin resistance by miR-15a-5p sponging and subsequent upregulation of CCNE1.	[97]
Prostate cancer	PCAT1/c-Myc/miR-25-3p/SLC7A11	Drug resistance	TFAP2C increases the expression level of PCAT1 to mediate miR-25-3p sponging via c-Myc upregulation, resulting in increased SLC7A11 stability. Ferroptosis inhibition and subsequent induction of docetaxel resistance.	[98]
Colon cancer	HCG11/miR-144-3p/PDK4	Drug resistance	HCG11 promotes PDK4 expression via miR-144-3p sponging to induce glycolysis and to mediate 5-flourouracil resistance.	[99]
Pancreatic cancer	UPK1A-AS1	Drug resistance	UPK1A-AS1 participates in DNA damage repair to mediate platinum resistance.	[100]
Ovarian cancer	ACTA2-AS1/miR-378a-3p/Wnt5a	Drug resistance	ACTA2-AS1 induces Wnt5a expression via miR-378a-3p inhibition to induce cisplatin resistance in ovarian cancer.	[101]

[105]. The interesting point is that overexpression of tumor suppressor lncRNAs such as GAS5 can induce G2/M cell cycle arrest and prevents DNA damage repair for radio-sensitivity of cancer cells [106]. lncRNA/miRNA axis has been shown to be involved in regulating radio-sensitivity of lung cancer cells [107]. lncRNAs are promising targets for cancer diagnosis and treatment, and they demonstrate both carcinogenic and anti-tumoral impacts [108]. lncRNA CYTOR undergoes overexpression in non-small cell lung cancer and is associated with undesirable prognosis [109]. By increasing cancer motility, metastasis, and EMT induction, CYTOR participates in the aggressive behavior of tumor cells and mediates poor prognosis [110, 111]. lncRNA CYTOR stimulates prothymosin α via miR-206 downregulation to induce radio-sensitivity in lung cancer in vitro and in vivo [112]. A number of proteins have the capacity of binding to promoter region in regulating the expression level of genes. EZH2 protein is such a factor that its recruitment to the promoter region can decrease gene expression levels. Restoring the expression level of lncRNA MAGI2-AS3 is associated with irradiation sensitivity in esophageal cancer. MAGI2-AS3 recruits EZH2 to the promoter of HOXB7 to reduce its expression in reducing proliferation, inducing apoptosis, and mediating radio-sensitivity [113].

An aggressive and common type of brain tumor in the central nervous system is glioblastoma (GBM) [114]. Diffuse infiltration and local metastasis into surrounding brain tissues, abnormal proliferation, angiogenesis, genomic instability, and resistance to apoptosis are some of the characteristics of GBM cells [115]. Due to such aggressive features of GBM cells, they can obtain resistance to radiotherapy. Upregulation of NRGN by lncRNA RBPMS-AS1 has been considered as a pivotal way of providing radio-sensitivity in GBM. By proliferation, inhibition, and apoptosis induction, RBPMS-AS1 increases the radio-sensitivity of GBM cells. For this purpose, RBPMS-AS1 increases CAMTA1 expression via miR-301a-3p inhibition to upregulate NRGN in mediating radio-resistance in GBM [116]. In brain tumors, cancer stem cells (CSCs) are considered as the main reasons for recurrence, and similar to other types of tumors such as breast and liver cancers, CSCs increase the survival rate for mediating radio-resistance and drug resistance [117–120]. Increased population of

CSCs leads to the stemness of glioma cells. lncRNA TPTEP1 stimulates p38 MAPK signaling via miR-106a-5p downregulation to suppress stemness and CSCs in glioma for enhancing their radio-sensitivity [121]. Therefore, targeting lncRNAs is important for the process of radio-sensitivity in cancers.

4.2 *Tumor-promoting lncRNAs*

The main way for oncogenic lncRNAs in triggering radio-resistance is by enhancing tumorigenesis and malignant behavior of cancer cells. LINC00963 contributes to carcinogenesis and proliferation of breast tumor cells to mediate radiation resistance. LINC00963 prevents DNA damage and oxidative stress by providing radio-resistance in breast cancer. Mechanistically, LINC00963 promotes ACK1 expression via miR-324-3p sponging by providing radio-resistance in breast cancer [122]. Therefore, preventing DNA damage and oxidative stress are factors that can lead to radio-resistance. Under irradiation, tumor cells prefer to preserve their proliferation rate and this is provided by preventing apoptosis. Therefore, molecular pathways and signaling networks that lead to apoptosis inhibition can provide radio-resistance. p53 is one of the factors that is involved in cell death along with Bax and caspase cascade. lncRNA CCAT2 is implicated in triggering radio-resistance in esophageal carcinoma. CCAT2 reduces the expression level of miR-145 and its downstream target p70S6K1 to induce radio-resistance in esophageal cancer. Furthermore, CCAT2 downregulates p53 expression in preventing apoptosis. Silencing CCAT2 promotes Bax/Bcl-2 ratio and activates caspase-3 in triggering apoptosis and inducing radio-sensitivity [123].

The ideal concept regarding to targeting lncRNAs is that these non-coding RNA transcripts can regulate apoptosis, DNA damage, and cell cycle progression during radiotherapy. Therefore, if they are affected, a significant increase in radio-sensitivity is provided. Overexpression of BLACAT1 is observed in head and neck squamous cell carcinoma and is responsible for poor prognosis of patients. BLACAT1 increases the expression level of PSEN1 to prevent DNA damage, cell cycle arrest, and apoptosis in triggering radio-resistance

[124]. Enhanced proliferation is the most important hallmark of different cancers. When growth rate of cancer cells enhances, they can easily obtain resistance to apoptosis and cytotoxic impact of drugs. SBF2-AS1 and MBLN3 show overexpression in lung cancer, while the expression level of miR-302a decreases to induce radio-resistance. SBF2-AS1 increases MBLN3 expression via miR-302a sponging to increase proliferation and to inhibit apoptosis in radio-resistance feature of lung cancer cells [125]. Silencing oncogenic lncRNAs such as XIST and UCA1 has been ideal in enhancing radio-sensitivity by triggering apoptosis and reducing proliferation [126, 127]. Overall, it can be concluded that oncogenic lncRNAs are master regulators of molecular pathways in cancers, and by inducing tumor-promoting pathways such as Akt signaling, they can mediate radio-resistance. The molecular mechanisms that are tightly affected by lncRNAs in regulating radio-resistance are apoptosis, DNA damage, and cell cycle progression. Furthermore, they increase migration and growth of cancer cells by triggering radio-resistance (Table 2) [128–130]. Figure 2 schematically demonstrates the role of lncRNAs in regulating drug resistance and radio-resistance in different cancers.

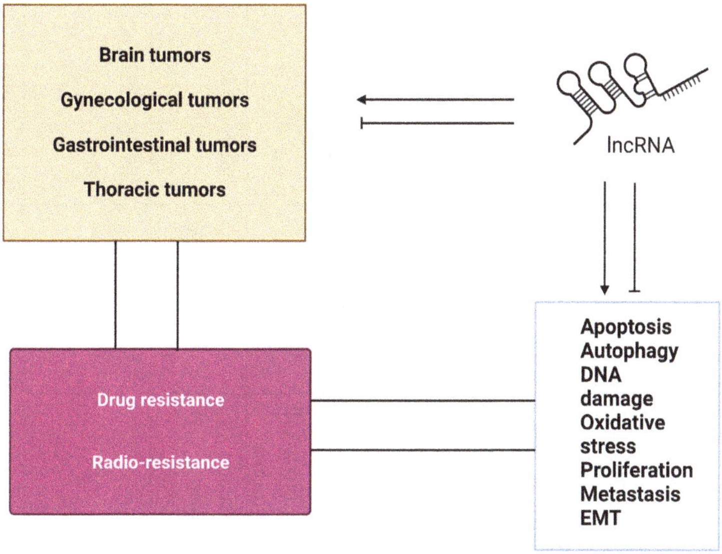

Figure 2. lncRNAs regulate therapy response in different cancers.

Table 2. The role of lncRNAs in regulating radio-resistance in cancer.

Cancer type	Molecular pathway	Radio-resistance Radio-sensitivity	Remark(s)	Ref
Ovarian cancer	FAM83H-AS1/ HuR	Radio-resistance	FAM83H-AS1 is involved in tumor progression and resistance to therapy via stabilizing HuR protein.	[131]
Cervical cancer	SNHG6/ miR-485-3p	Radio-resistance	Overexpression of SNHG6 in cervical cancer. SNHG6 sponges miR-485-3p in mediating radio-resistance.	[132]
Nasopharyngeal carcinoma	CASC19/ AMPK/ mTOR	Radio-resistance	Autophagy induction. Stimulating radio-resistance. Inhibition of AMPK/mTOR axis by CASC19. Silencing CASC19 triggers apoptosis in tumor cells.	[133]
Osteosarcoma	LINC00210/ miR-342-3p/ GFRA1	Radio-resistance	Overexpression of LINC00210 in tumor tissues. LINC00210 promotes GFRA1 expression via miR-342-3p downregulation.	[134]
Head and neck squamous cell carcinoma	LINC00473/ Wnt/β-catenin	Radio-resistance	LINC00473 stimulates Wnt signaling as an oncogenic pathway to increase tumor progression and to mediate radio-resistance.	[135]
Colorectal cancer	OIP5-AS1/ miR-396-3p/ DYRK1A	Radio-sensitivity	OIP5-AS1 promotes the expression level of DYRK1A via miR-396-3p sponging to suppress tumor survival and induce apoptosis.	[136]
Cervical cancer	NEAT1/ miR-193b-3p/ CCND1	Radio-resistance	Silencing NEAT1 stimulates apoptosis and G0/G1 cell cycle arrest. NEAT1 promotes CCND1 expression via miR-193b-3p sponging.	[137]
Neuroblastoma	XIST/miR-375/L1CAM	Radio-resistance	Silencing XIST impairs tumorigenesis and increases radio-sensitivity. XIST promotes L1CAM expression via miR-375 sponging.	[138]

(*Continued*)

Table 2. (*Continued*)

Rectal cancer	EGOT/ miR-211-5p/ ErbB4	Radio-resistance	Increased cancer colony formation and prevention of apoptosis by EGOT in cancer cells. EGOT promotes ErB4 expression via miR-211-5p sponging.	[139]
Nasopharyngeal carcinoma	XIST/miR-29c	Radio-resistance	Silencing XIST suppresses proliferation and enhances radio-sensitivity of tumor cells via upregulation of miR-29c.	[140]
Non-small cell lung cancer	CCAT1/MAPK	Radio-resistance	Silencing CCAT1 enhances radio-sensitivity, stimulates apoptosis and G2/M cell cycle arrest. CCAT1 downregulation leads to the inhibition of p38 and ERK, and the induction of JNK signaling pathway.	[141]
Cervical cancer	PCAT1/ miR-128/ GOLM1	Radio-resistance	Association of PCAT1 with migration and proliferation rates of tumor cells. PCAT1 promotes GOLM1 expression via miR-128 downregulation.	[142]
Gastric cancer	OGFRP1/ miR-149-5p/ MAP3K3	Radio-resistance	Increased proliferation. Apoptosis inhibition. OGFRP1 promotes MAP3K3 expression via miR-149-5p inhibition.	[143]
Colon cancer	ANRIL/ miR-181a-5p	Radio-resistance	ANRIL sponges miR-181a-5p to prevent chito-oligosaccharide-mediated radio-sensitivity in tumor cells.	[144]
Triple-negative breast cancer	PCAT6/ miR-185-5p/ TPD52	Radio-resistance	PCAT6 is involved in radio-resistance, increasing tumor proliferation, and inhibiting apoptosis via miR-185-5p sponging and subsequent upregulation of TPD52.	[145]
Breast cancer	CCAT1/ miR-148b	Radio-resistance	CCAT1 promotes the survival of cancer cells under irradiation via downregulation of miR-148b.	[146]
Nasopharyngeal carcinoma	ANCR/PTEN	Radio-resistance	Inhibition of PTEN signaling by ANCR is involved in tumorigenesis, increasing proliferation and mediating therapy resistance.	[147]

5. Conclusion and remarks

Different challenges are faced in cancer treatment that therapy resistance is far most challenging problem that physicians have ever observed. Chemotherapy and radiotherapy are the conventional methods in treatment of cancer and due to their frequent and long-term application, tumor cells have demonstrated resistance to these kinds of therapies. Among the different factors that can lead to development of drug resistance and radio-resistance in cancer, epigenetic factors of interest and in recent years, a high number of laboratories around the world have focused on revealing role of underlying molecular mechanisms that are affected by epigenetic factors in cancers. lncRNAs are a member of epigenetic factor and belong to large family of non-coding RNAs that can regulate tumor progression and are reliable biomarkers. The current chapter revealed role of lncRNAs in regulating drug resistance and radio-resistance. Although multiple types of lncRNAs regulating therapy response in cancers have been identified, their mechanism of action in providing therapy resistance/sensitivity is similar. There are two categories of lncRNAs including tumor suppressor and tumor-promoting lncRNAs. Overexpression of oncogenic lncRNAs occurs in radio-resistance and drug resistance, while onco-suppressor lncRNAs demonstrate a decrease in expression level. lncRNAs inducing therapy resistance prevent apoptosis and pro-death autophagy, induce DNA damage repair, cell cycle progression, proliferation and metastasis of tumor cells. Therefore, lncRNAs increase malignancy of tumor cells in triggering radio-resistance and drug resistance. On the other hand, lncRNAs inducing therapy sensitivity mainly stimulate apoptosis and G2/M cell cycle arrest as well as DNA damage. Since expression level of lncRNAs is detectable in serum of patients, they can be used for predicting response of cancer patients to therapy.

Conflict of interest:

The authors declare no conflict of interest.

References

1. Foo, M.A., et al., *Clinical translation of patient-derived tumour organoids- bottlenecks and strategies.* Biomarker Research, 2022. **10**(1): p. 10.
2. Jayasinghe, M.K., et al., *New approaches in extracellular vesicle engineering for improving the efficacy of anti-cancer therapies.* Seminars in Cancer Biology, 2021. **74**: p. 62–78.
3. Siegel, R.L., et al., *Cancer statistics, 2021.* 2021. **71**(1): p. 7–33.
4. Deldar Abad Paskeh, M., et al., *Wnt/β-Catenin signaling as a driver of hepatocellular carcinoma progression: An emphasis on molecular pathways.* 2021.
5. Ashrafizadeh, M., et al., *Curcumin in cancer therapy: A novel adjunct for combination chemotherapy with paclitaxel and alleviation of its adverse effects.* 2020. **256**: p. 117984.
6. Xie, R., et al., *Furin-instructed aggregated gold nanoparticles for re-educating tumor associated macrophages and overcoming breast cancer chemoresistance.* Biomaterials, 2021. **275**: p. 120891.
7. García-Garrido, E., M. Cordani, and Á. Somoza, *Modified gold nanoparticles to overcome the chemoresistance to gemcitabine in mutant p53 cancer cells.* Pharmaceutics, 2021. **13**(12).
8. Chen, Q., et al., *Dual-pH responsive chitosan nanoparticles for improving in vivo drugs delivery and chemoresistance in breast cancer.* Carbohydrate Polymers, 2022. **290**: p. 119518.
9. Tang, S., et al., *Intraperitoneal siRNA nanoparticles for augmentation of gemcitabine efficacy in the treatment of pancreatic cancer.* Molecular Pharmaceutics, 2021. **18**(12): p. 4448–4458.
10. Fujii, K., et al., *Functional depletion of HSP72 by siRNA and quercetin enhances vorinostat-induced apoptosis in an HSP72-overexpressing cutaneous T-cell lymphoma cell line, Hut78.* International Journal of Molecular Sciences, 2021. **22**(20).
11. Sritharan, S., et al., *Meta analysis of bioactive compounds, miRNA, siRNA and cell death regulators as sensitizers to doxorubicin induced chemoresistance.* Apoptosis, 2022. 27(9–10): p. 622–646.
12. Li, Z., et al., *Long noncoding RNAs regulate the radioresistance of breast cancer.* Analytical Cellular Pathology (Amsterdam), 2021. **2021**: p. 9005073.

13. Lee, H., et al., *Radiation-induced overexpression of TGFβ and PODXL contributes to colorectal cancer cell radioresistance through enhanced motility.* Cells, 2021. **10**(8).
14. Wu, Q., et al., *Downregulation of SFRP2 facilitates cancer stemness and radioresistance of glioma cells via activating Wnt/β-catenin signaling.* PLoS One, 2021. **16**(12): p. e0260864.
15. Xin, H., et al., *CD155 promotes radioresistance and malignancy of esophageal cancer by regulating Hippo-YAP pathway.* Discover Oncology, 2022. **13**(1): p. 53.
16. Zhang, Z., et al., *Circ_0011058 facilitates proliferation, angiogenesis and radioresistance in papillary thyroid cancer cells by positively regulating YAP1 via acting as miR-335-5p sponge.* Cell Signal, 2021. **88**: p. 110155.
17. Zhou, S., et al., *KLK5 is associated with the radioresistance, aggression, and progression of cervical cancer.* Gynecologic Oncology, 2022. **166**(1): p. 138–147.
18. Lin, J.C., et al., *miR-671-5p inhibition by MSI1 promotes glioblastoma tumorigenesis via radioresistance, tumor motility and cancer stem-like cell properties.* Biomedicines, 2021. **10**(1).
19. Chuang, P.C., et al., *MicroRNA-29a manifests multifaceted features to intensify radiosensitivity, escalate apoptosis, and revoke cell migration for palliating radioresistance-enhanced cervical cancer progression.* International Journal of Molecular Sciences, 2022. **23**(10).
20. Zhong, X., et al., *RNF6 enhances radioresistance in colorectal cancer via activating the Wnt pathway.* JBUON, 2021. **26**(5): p. 1925–1930.
21. Qian, J., et al., *Cancer-associated mesothelial cells promote ovarian cancer chemoresistance through paracrine osteopontin signaling.* The Journal of Clinical Investigation, 2021. **131**(16).
22. Paku, M., et al., *SIRT3-mediated SOD2 and PGC-1α contribute to chemoresistance in colorectal cancer cells.* Annals of Surgical Oncology, 2021. **28**(8): p. 4720–4732.
23. Liu, C., et al., *Pharmacological targeting PTK6 inhibits the JAK2/STAT3 sustained stemness and reverses chemoresistance of colorectal cancer.* Journal of Experimental & Clinical Cancer Research, 2021. **40**(1): p. 297.

24. Li, Y., et al., *FAM49B promotes breast cancer proliferation, metastasis, and chemoresistance by stabilizing ELAVL1 protein and regulating downstream Rab10/TLR4 pathway.* Cancer Cell International, 2021. **21**(1): p. 534.
25. Li, J., R. Mo, and L. Zheng, *Inhibition of the cell migration, invasion and chemoresistance of colorectal cancer cells through targeting KLF3 by miR-365a-3p.* Journal of Cancer, 2021. **12**(20): p. 6155–6164.
26. Yuan, L., et al., *EBV infection-induced GPX4 promotes chemoresistance and tumor progression in nasopharyngeal carcinoma.* Cell Death Differ, 2022.
27. Zhao, T., et al., *Knockdown of OLR1 weakens glycolytic metabolism to repress colon cancer cell proliferation and chemoresistance by downregulating SULT2B1 via c-MYC.* Cell Death & Disease, 2021. **13**(1): p. 4.
28. Peng, W.X., P. Koirala, and Y.Y. Mo, *LncRNA-mediated regulation of cell signaling in cancer.* Oncogene, 2017. **36**(41): p. 5661–5667.
29. Entezari, M., et al., *Long non-coding RNAs and exosomal lncRNAs: Potential functions in lung cancer progression, drug resistance and tumor microenvironment remodeling.* Biomedicine & Pharmacotherapy, 2022. **150**: p. 112963.
30. Bhan, A., M. Soleimani, and S.S. Mandal, *Long noncoding RNA and cancer: A new paradigm.* Cancer Research, 2017. 77(15): p. 3965–3981.
31. Bhan, A. and S.S. Mandal, *Long noncoding RNAs: Emerging stars in gene regulation, epigenetics and human disease.* ChemMedChem, 2014. **9**(9): p. 1932–1956.
32. Ma, L., V.B. Bajic, and Z. Zhang, *On the classification of long non-coding RNAs.* RNA Biology, 2013. **10**(6): p. 924–933.
33. Wang, K.C. and H.Y. Chang, *Molecular mechanisms of long noncoding RNAs.* Molecular Cell, 2011. **43**(6): p. 904–914.
34. Pontier, D.B. and J.J. Gribnau, *Xist regulation and function explored.* Human Genetics, 2011. **130**(2): p. 223–236.
35. Mirzaei, S., et al., *Molecular landscape of LncRNAs in prostate cancer: A focus on pathways and therapeutic targets for intervention.* Journal of Experimental & Clinical Cancer Research, 2022. **41**(1): p. 1–26.
36. Mirzaei, S., et al., *The long and short non-coding RNAs modulating EZH2 signaling in cancer.* Journal of Hematology & Oncology, 2022. **15**(1): p. 1–34.

37. Paskeh, M.D.A., et al., *Emerging role of exosomes in cancer progression and tumor microenvironment remodeling.* Journal of Hematology & Oncology, 2022. **15**(1): p. 1–39.
38. Ashrafizadeh, M., et al., *Crosstalk of long non-coding RNAs and EMT: Searching the missing pieces of an incomplete puzzle for lung cancer therapy.* Current Cancer Drug Targets, 2021. **21**(8): p. 640–665.
39. Mirzaei, S., et al., *Regulation of Nuclear Factor-KappaB (NF-κB) signaling pathway by non-coding RNAs in cancer: Inhibiting or promoting carcinogenesis?* Cancer Letters, 2021. **509**: p. 63–80.
40. Ashrafizaveh, S., et al., *Long non-coding RNAs in the doxorubicin resistance of cancer cells.* Cancer Letters, 2021. **508**: p. 104–114.
41. Schiliro, C. and B.L. Firestein, *Mechanisms of metabolic reprogramming in cancer cells supporting enhanced growth and proliferation.* Cells, 2021. **10**(5): p. 1056.
42. Hu, R., et al., *LncRNA TUSC8 suppresses the proliferation and migration of esophageal cancer cells by downregulation of VEGFA.* Journal of Cancer, 2021. **12**(21): p. 6393–6400.
43. Guo, F., et al., *lncRNA OR3A4 promotes the proliferation and metastasis of ovarian cancer through KLF6 pathway.* Frontiers in Pharmacology, 2021. **12**: p. 727876.
44. Cheng, Z., et al., *KLF5 activates lncRNA DANCR and inhibits cancer cell autophagy accelerating gastric cancer progression.* NPJ Genomic Medine, 2021. **6**(1): p. 75.
45. Kanabe, B.O., et al., *Expression patterns of LncRNA-GAS5 and its target APOBEC3C gene through miR-103 in breast cancer patients.* Cellular & Molecular Biology (Noisy-le-grand), 2021. **67**(3): p. 5–10.
46. Xin, L., et al., *Transfer of LncRNA CRNDE in TAM-derived exosomes is linked with cisplatin resistance in gastric cancer.* EMBO Reports, 2021. **22**(12): p. e52124.
47. Wang, L.F., L.P. Wu, and J.D. Wen, *LncRNA AC079630.4 expression associated with the progression and prognosis in lung cancer.* Aging (Albany NY), 2021. **13**(14): p. 18658–18668.
48. Zhang, M., et al., *LncRNA SNHG1 promotes tumor progression and cisplatin resistance through epigenetically silencing miR-381 in breast cancer.* Bioengineered, 2021. **12**(2): p. 9239–9250.

49. Sun, J., et al., *lncRNA TUG1 Facilitates colorectal cancer stem cell characteristics and chemoresistance by enhancing GATA6 protein stability.* Stem Cells International, 2021. **2021**: p. 1075481.
50. Ren, N., et al., *LncRNA ADAMTS9-AS2 inhibits gastric cancer (GC) development and sensitizes chemoresistant GC cells to cisplatin by regulating miR-223-3p/NLRP3 axis.* Aging (Albany NY), 2020. **12**(11): p. 11025–11041.
51. Song, E.L., et al., *LncRNA ADAMTS9-AS2 inhibits cell proliferation and decreases chemoresistance in clear cell renal cell carcinoma via the miR-27a-3p/FOXO1 axis.* Aging (Albany NY), 2019. **11**(15): p. 5705–5725.
52. Xu, F., et al., *Overexpressing lncRNA SNHG16 inhibited HCC proliferation and chemoresistance by functionally sponging hsa-miR-93.* Onco Targets and Therapy, 2018. **11**: p. 8855–8863.
53. Siegel, R.L., K.D. Miller, and A. Jemal, *Cancer statistics, 2019.* CA: A Cancer Journal for Clinicians, 2019. **69**(1): p. 7–34.
54. Van der Jeught, K., et al., *Drug resistance and new therapies in colorectal cancer.* World Journal of Gastroenterology, 2018. **24**(34): p. 3834.
55. Slyskova, J., et al., *Base and nucleotide excision repair facilitate resolution of platinum drugs-induced transcription blockage.* Nucleic Acids Research, 2018. **46**(18): p. 9537–9549.
56. Wang, X., et al., *lncRNA-encoded pep-AP attenuates the pentose phosphate pathway and sensitizes colorectal cancer cells to Oxaliplatin.* EMBO Reports, 2022. **23**(1): p. e53140.
57. Wen, J.F., et al., *LncRNA-SARCC sensitizes osteosarcoma to cisplatin through the miR-143-mediated glycolysis inhibition by targeting Hexokinase 2.* Cancer Biomarkers, 2020. **28**(2): p. 231–246.
58. Wang, Y., et al., *The role of non-coding RNAs in ABC transporters regulation and their clinical implications of multidrug resistance in cancer.* Expert Opinion on Drug Metabolism & Toxicology, 2021. **17**(3): p. 291–306.
59. Ween, M.P., et al., *The role of ABC transporters in ovarian cancer progression and chemoresistance.* Critical Reviews in Oncology/Hematology, 2015. **96**(2): p. 220–256.
60. Dauer, P., et al., *GRP78-mediated antioxidant response and ABC transporter activity confers chemoresistance to pancreatic cancer cells.* Molecular Oncology, 2018. **12**(9): p. 1498–1512.

61. Kun-Peng, Z., M. Xiao-Long, and Z. Chun-Lin, *LncRNA FENDRR sensitizes doxorubicin-resistance of osteosarcoma cells through down-regulating ABCB1 and ABCC1.* Oncotarget, 2017. **8**(42): p. 71881–71893.
62. Zhang, M., et al., *LncRNA KB-1471A8.2 Overexpression suppresses cell proliferation and migration and antagonizes the paclitaxel resistance of ovarian cancer cells.* Cancer Biotherapy and Radiopharmaceuticals, 2019. **34**(5): p. 316–324.
63. Zhang, F., et al., *LncRNA CRNDE attenuates chemoresistance in gastric cancer via SRSF6-regulated alternative splicing of PICALM.* Molecular Cancer, 2021. **20**(1): p. 6.
64. Zheng, B., et al., *lncRNA RP11-147L13.8 suppresses metastasis and chemo-resistance by modulating the phosphorylation of c-Jun protein in GBC.* Molecular Therapy Oncolytics, 2021. **23**: p. 124–137.
65. Ye, X., et al., *Increased m(6)A modification of lncRNA DBH-AS1 suppresses pancreatic cancer growth and gemcitabine resistance via the miR-3163/USP44 axis.* Annals of Translational Medicine, 2022. **10**(6): p. 304.
66. Zhu, Y., et al., *LncRNA LINC00942 promotes chemoresistance in gastric cancer by suppressing MSI2 degradation to enhance c-Myc mRNA stability.* Clinical and Translational Medicine, 2022. **12**(1): p. e703.
67. Wang, L., et al., *lncRNA ANRIL aggravates the chemoresistance of pancreatic cancer cells to gemcitabine by targeting inhibition of miR-181a and targeting HMGB1-induced autophagy.* Aging (Albany NY), 2021. **13**(15): p. 19272–19281.
68. Jing, X., et al., *Role of hypoxia in cancer therapy by regulating the tumor microenvironment.* Molecular Cancer, 2019. **18**(1): p. 1–15.
69. Wilson, W.R. and M.P. Hay, *Targeting hypoxia in cancer therapy.* Nature Reviews. Cancer, 2011. **11**(6): p. 393–410.
70. Wei, X., et al., *Mechanisms of vasculogenic mimicry in hypoxic tumor microenvironments.* Molecular Cancer, 2021. **20**(1): p. 1–18.
71. Zhang, L., et al., *Induction of lncRNA NORAD accounts for hypoxia-induced chemoresistance and vasculogenic mimicry in colorectal cancer by sponging the miR-495-3p/ hypoxia-inducible factor-1α (HIF-1α).* Bioengineered, 2022. **13**(1): p. 950–962.

72. Tabury, K., et al., *PVT1 is a stress-responsive lncRNA that drives ovarian cancer metastasis and chemoresistance.* Life Science Alliance, 2022. **5**(11).
73. Abadi, A.J., et al., *The role of SOX family transcription factors in gastric cancer.* International Journal of Biological Macromolecules, 2021. **180**: p. 608–624.
74. Ashrafizadeh, M., et al., *Interplay between SOX9 transcription factor and microRNAs in cancer.* International Journal of Biological Macromolecules, 2021. **183**: p. 681–694.
75. Ashrafizadeh, M., et al., *Cancer and SOX proteins: New insight into their role in ovarian cancer progression/inhibition.* Pharmacological Research, 2020. **161**: p. 105159.
76. Yang, J., et al., *lncRNA SNHG15 induced by SOX12 promotes the tumorigenic properties and chemoresistance in cervical cancer via the miR-4735-3p/HIF1a pathway.* Oxidative Medicine and Cell Longevity, 2022. **2022**: p. 8548461.
77. Li, D., et al., *Inhibition of lncRNA KCNQ1OT1 improves apoptosis and chemotherapy drug response in small cell lung cancer by TGF-β1 mediated epithelial-to-mesenchymal transition.* Cancer Research and Treatment, 2021. **53**(4): p. 1042–1056.
78. Cai, M., et al., *lncRNA MCF2L-AS1/miR-105/ IL-1β axis regulates colorectal cancer cell oxaliplatin resistance.* Cancer Management and Research, 2021. **13**: p. 8685–8694.
79. Zhang, C. and N. Liu, *Noncoding RNAs in the glycolysis of ovarian cancer.* Frontiers in Pharmacology, 2022. **13**: p. 855488.
80. Zhao, N., et al., *Mechanisms of long non-coding RNAs in biological characteristics and aerobic glycolysis of glioma.* International Journal of Molecular Sciences, 2021. **22**(20).
81. Xie, Y., et al., *Ubiquitination regulation of aerobic glycolysis in cancer.* Life Sciences, 2022. **292**: p. 120322.
82. Lin, S., et al., *Fascin promotes lung cancer growth and metastasis by enhancing glycolysis and PFKFB3 expression.* Cancer Letters, 2021. **518**: p. 230–242.
83. Chang, X., et al., *Glycolysis in the progression of pancreatic cancer.* American Journal of Cancer Research, 2022. **12**(2): p. 861–872.

84. Wang, S., et al., *lncRNA Linc00173 modulates glucosemetabolism and multidrug chemoresistancein SCLC: Potential molecular panel for targeted therapy.* Molecular Therapy, 2021.
85. Gao, S.J., et al., *Targeting EGFR sensitizes 5-Fu-resistant colon cancer cells through modification of the lncRNA-FGD5-AS1-miR-330-3p-Hexokinase 2 axis.* Molecular Therapy — Oncolytics, 2021. **23**: p. 14–25.
86. Zhou, J., et al., *lncRNA XLOC013218 promotes cell proliferation and TMZ resistance by targeting the PIK3R2-mediated PI3K/AKT pathway in glioma.* Cancer Science, 2022.
87. He, S., et al., *The Role of the SOX9/lncRNA ANXA2P2/miR-361-3p/SOX9 Regulatory Loop in Cervical Cancer Cell Growth and Resistance to Cisplatin.* Frontiers in Oncology, 2021. **11**: p. 784525.
88. Sun, Y.F., et al., *SNHG15, a p53-regulated lncRNA, suppresses cisplatin-induced apoptosis and ROS accumulation through the miR-335-3p/ZNF32 axis.* American Journal of Cancer Research, 2022. **12**(2): p. 816–828.
89. Han, J., et al., *IGF2BP2 induces U251 glioblastoma cell chemoresistance by inhibiting FOXO1-mediated PID1 expression through stabilizing lncRNA DANCR.* Frontiers in Cell and Developmental Biology, 2021. **9**: p. 659228.
90. Wang, Y.Y. and C. Chen, *lncRNA-DANCR promotes taxol resistance of prostate cancer cells through modulating the miR-33b-5p-LDHA axis.* Disease Markers, 2022. **2022**: p. 9516774.
91. Wang, Z.W., et al., *SRSF3-mediated regulation of N6-methyladenosine modification-related lncRNA ANRIL splicing promotes resistance of pancreatic cancer to gemcitabine.* Cell Reports, 2022. **39**(6): p. 110813.
92. Zhou, M., et al., *Chitosan-gelatin-EGCG nanoparticle-meditated LncRNA TMEM44-AS1 silencing to activate the P53 signaling pathway for the synergistic reversal of 5-FU resistance in gastric cancer.* Advances Science (Weinh), 2022: p. e2105077.
93. Zhu, L., et al., *lncRNA NEAT1 promotes the taxol resistance of breast cancer via sponging the miR-23a-3p-FOXA1 axis.* Acta Biochimica et Biophysica Sinica (Shanghai), 2021. **53**(9): p. 1198–1206.
94. Wu, J., et al., *Formononetin relieves the facilitating effect of lncRNA AFAP1-AS1-miR-195/miR-545 axis on progression and*

chemo-resistance of triple-negative breast cancer. Aging (Albany NY), 2021. **13**(14): p. 18191–18222.

95. Gui, Z., et al., *LncRNA FEZF1-AS1 promotes multi-drug resistance of gastric cancer cells via upregulating ATG5.* Frontiers in Cell and Developmental Biology, 2021. **9**: p. 749129.
96. Yang, S., et al., *lncRNA PVT1 promotes cetuximab resistance of head and neck squamous cell carcinoma cells by inhibiting miR-124-3p.* Head & Neck, 2021. **43**(9): p. 2712–2723.
97. Sun, Y., et al., *MEG3 LncRNA from exosomes released from cancer-associated fibroblasts enhances cisplatin chemoresistance in SCLC via a MiR-15a-5p/CCNE1 axis.* Yonsei Medical Journal, 2022. **63**(3): p. 229–240.
98. Jiang, X., et al., *TFAP2C-mediated lncRNA PCAT1 inhibits ferroptosis in docetaxel-resistant prostate cancer through c-Myc/miR-25-3p/SLC7A11 signaling.* Frontiers in Oncology, 2022. **12**: p. 862015.
99. Cui, Z., et al., *LncRNA HCG11 promotes 5-FU resistance of colon cancer cells through reprogramming glucose metabolism by targeting the miR-144-3p-PDK4 axis.* Cancer Biomarkers, 2022. **34**(1): p. 41–53.
100. Zhang, X., et al., *Cancer-associated fibroblast-induced lncRNA UPK1A-AS1 confers platinum resistance in pancreatic cancer via efficient double-strand break repair.* Oncogene, 2022. **41**(16): p. 2372–2389.
101. Lin, C., et al., *Knockdown of lncRNA ACTA2-AS1 reverses cisplatin resistance of ovarian cancer cells via inhibition of miR-378a-3p-regulated Wnt5a.* Bioengineered, 2022. **13**(4): p. 9829–9838.
102. Smith, J., et al., *The ATM–Chk2 and ATR–Chk1 pathways in DNA damage signaling and cancer.* Advances in Cancer Research, 2010. **108**: p. 73–112.
103. Paull, T.T., *Mechanisms of ATM activation.* Annual Review of Biochemistry, 2015. **84**: p. 711–738.
104. Bakkenist, C.J. and M.B.J.N. Kastan, *DNA damage activates ATM through intermolecular autophosphorylation and dimer dissociation.* Nature, 2003. **421**(6922): p. 499–506.
105. Guo, Z., et al., *LncRNA linc00312 suppresses radiotherapy resistance by targeting DNA-PKcs and impairing DNA damage repair in nasopharyngeal carcinoma.* Cell Death and Disease, 2021. **12**(1): p. 69.

106. Ma, Y., et al., *lncRNA GAS5 sensitizes breast cancer cells to ionizing radiation by inhibiting DNA repair.* BioMed Research International, 2022. **2022**: p. 1987519.
107. Huang, Q.J.B.i.M., *Predictive relevance of ncRNAs in non-small-cell lung cancer patients with radiotherapy: a review of the published data.* Biomarkers in Medicine, 2018. **12**(10): p. 1149–1159.
108. Bhan, A., M. Soleimani, and S.S.J.C.r. Mandal, *Long noncoding RNA and cancer: A new paradigm.* Cancer Research, 2017. 77(15): p. 3965–3981.
109. Yu, H. and S.-B. Li, *Role of LINC00152 in non-small cell lung cancer.* Journal of Zhejiang University Science B, 2020. **21**(3): p. 179–191.
110. Yue, B., et al., *A positive feed-forward loop between LncRNA-CYTOR and Wnt/β-catenin signaling promotes metastasis of colon cancer.* Molecular Therapy, 2018. **26**(5): p. 1287–1298.
111. Moradi, M.-T., et al., *Circulating CYTOR as a potential biomarker in breast cancer.* International Journal of Molecular and Cellular Medicine, 2020. **9**(1): p. 83.
112. Jiang, G., et al., *lncRNA cytoskeleton regulator reduces non-small cell lung cancer radiosensitivity by downregulating miRNA-206 and activating prothymosin α.* International Journal of Oncology, 2021. **59**(5).
113. Cheng, W., et al., *LncRNA MAGI2-AS3 overexpression sensitizes esophageal cancer cells to irradiation through down-regulation of HOXB7 via EZH2.* Frontiers in Cell and Developmental Biology, 2020. **8**: p. 552822.
114. Nguyen, H.S., et al., *Molecular markers of therapy-resistant glioblastoma and potential strategy to combat resistance.* International Journal of Molecular Sciences, 2018. **19**(6): p. 1765.
115. Kazerooni, A.F., et al., *Imaging signatures of glioblastoma molecular characteristics: A radiogenomics review.* Journal of Magnetic Resonance Imaging, 2020. **52**(1): p. 54.
116. Li, W., et al., *LncRNA RBPMS-AS1 promotes NRGN transcription to enhance the radiosensitivity of glioblastoma through the microRNA-301a-3p/CAMTA1 axis.* Translational Oncology, 2022. **15**(1): p. 101282.
117. Balça-Silva, J., et al. *Cellular and molecular mechanisms of glioblastoma malignancy: Implications in resistance and therapeutic strategies.* Seminars in Cancer Biology, 2019. 58: p. 130–141. Elsevier.

118. Visvanathan, A., et al., *Essential role of METTL3-mediated m6A modification in glioma stem-like cells maintenance and radioresistance.* Oncogene, 2018. **37**(4): p. 522–533.
119. Lin, X., et al., *HBX-induced miR-5188 impairs FOXO1 to stimulate β-catenin nuclear translocation and promotes tumor stemness in hepatocellular carcinoma.* Theranostics, 2019. **9**(25): p. 7583.
120. Zou, Y., et al., *Timeless-stimulated miR-5188-FOXO1/β-catenin-c-Jun feedback loop promotes stemness via ubiquitination of β-catenin in breast cancer.* Molecular Therapy, 2020. **28**(1): p. 313–327.
121. Tang, T., et al., *lncRNA TPTEP1 inhibits stemness and radioresistance of glioma through miR-106a-5p-mediated P38 MAPK signaling.* Molecular Medicine Reports, 2020. **22**(6): p. 4857–4867.
122. Zhang, N., et al., *LncRNA LINC00963 promotes tumorigenesis and radioresistance in breast cancer by sponging miR-324-3p and inducing ACK1 expression.* Molecular Therpy Nucleic Acids, 2019. **18**: p. 871–881.
123. Wang, M., et al., *lncRNA CCAT2 promotes radiotherapy resistance for human esophageal carcinoma cells via the miR-145/p70S6K1 and p53 pathway.* International Journal of Oncology, 2020. **56**(1): p. 327–336.
124. Gou, C., et al., *Knockdown of lncRNA BLACAT1 enhances radiosensitivity of head and neck squamous cell carcinoma cells by regulating PSEN1.* The British Journal of Radiology, 2020. **93**(1108): p. 20190154.
125. Yu, Z., et al., *LncRNA SBF2-AS1 affects the radiosensitivity of non-small cell lung cancer via modulating microRNA-302a/MBNL3 axis.* Cell Cycle, 2020. **19**(3): p. 300–316.
126. Hu, M. and J. Yang, *Down-regulation of lncRNA UCA1 enhances radiosensitivity in prostate cancer by suppressing EIF4G1 expression via sponging miR-331-3p.* Cancer Cell International, 2020. **20**: p. 449.
127. Du, R., et al., *Knockdown of lncRNA X inactive specific transcript (XIST) radiosensitizes non-small cell lung cancer (NSCLC) cells through regulation of miR-16-5p/WEE1 G2 checkpoint kinase (WEE1) axis.* International Journal of Immunopathology and Pharmacology, 2021. **35**: p. 2058738420966087.
128. Liang, X., et al., *Inhibition of lncRNA RET enhances radio-sensitivity of tumor cells via miR-3179/Slug/PTEN axis.* Toxicology Research (Camb), 2022. **11**(2): p. 348–360.

129. Zuo, Z., et al., *LncRNA TTN-AS1/miR-134-5p/PAK3 axis regulates the radiosensitivity of human large intestine cancer cells through the P21 pathway and AKT/GSK-3β/β-catenin pathway.* Cell Biology International, 2020. **44**(11): p. 2284–2292.
130. Zhang, H., et al., *Cancer-associated fibroblast-promoted LncRNA DNM3OS confers radioresistance by regulating DNA damage response in esophageal squamous cell carcinoma.* Clinical Cancer Research, 2019. **25**(6): p. 1989–2000.
131. Dou, Q., et al., *LncRNA FAM83H-AS1 contributes to the radioresistance, proliferation, and metastasis in ovarian cancer through stabilizing HuR protein.* European Journal of Pharmacology, 2019. **852**: p. 134–141.
132. Liu, J., X. Liu, and R. Li, *LncRNA SNHG6 enhances the radioresistance and promotes the growth of cervical cancer cells by sponging miR-485-3p.* Cancer Cell International, 2020. **20**: p. 424.
133. Liu, H., et al., *lncRNA CASC19 contributes to radioresistance of nasopharyngeal carcinoma by promoting autophagy via AMPK-mTOR pathway.* International Journal of Molecular Sciences, 2021. **22**(3).
134. He, P., et al., *LncRNA LINC00210 regulated radiosensitivity of osteosarcoma cells via miR-342-3p/GFRA1 axis.* Journal of Clinical Laboratory Analysis, 2020. **34**(12): p. e23540.
135. Han, P.B., et al., *Upregulation of lncRNA LINC00473 promotes radioresistance of HNSCC cells through activating Wnt/β-catenin signaling pathway.* European Review for Medical and Pharmacological Sciences, 2018. **22**(21): p. 7305–7313.
136. Zou, Y., et al., *LncRNA OIP5-AS1 regulates radioresistance by targeting DYRK1A through miR-369-3p in colorectal cancer cells.* European Journal of Cell Biology, 2018. **97**(5): p. 369–378.
137. Han, D., J. Wang, and G. Cheng, *LncRNA NEAT1 enhances the radioresistance of cervical cancer via miR-193b-3p/CCND1 axis.* Oncotarget, 2018. **9**(2): p. 2395–2409.
138. Yang, H., et al., *Downregulation of lncRNA XIST represses tumor growth and boosts radiosensitivity of neuroblastoma via modulation of the miR-375/L1CAM axis.* Neurochemical Research, 2020. **45**(11): p. 2679–2690.

139. Li, C., et al., *LncRNA EGOT/miR-211-5p affected radiosensitivity of rectal cancer by competitively regulating ErbB4.* OncoTargets and Therapy, 2021. **14**: p. 2867–2878.
140. Han, Q., et al., *Downregulation of lncRNA X inactive specific transcript (XIST) suppresses cell proliferation and enhances radiosensitivity by upregulating mir-29c in nasopharyngeal carcinoma cells.* Medical Science Monitor, 2017. **23**: p. 4798–4807.
141. Wang, Z., *LncRNA CCAT1 downregulation increases the radiosensitivity of non-small cell lung cancer cells.* The Kaohsiung Journal of Medical Sciences, 2021. **37**(8): p. 654–663.
142. Ge, X., et al., *Knockdown of lncRNA PCAT1 enhances radiosensitivity of cervical cancer by regulating miR-128/GOLM1 axis.* OncoTargets and Therapy, 2020. **13**: p. 10373–10385.
143. Qin, H., et al., *LncRNA OGFRP1 promotes cell proliferation and suppresses cell radiosensitivity in gastric cancer by targeting the miR-149-5p/MAP3K3 axis.* Journal of Molecular Histology, 2022. **53**(2): p. 257–271.
144. Sun, C., et al., *LncRNA ANRIL negatively regulated chitooligosaccharide-induced radiosensitivity in colon cancer cells by sponging miR-181a-5p.* Advances in Clinical Experimental Medicine, 2021. **30**(1): p. 55–65.
145. Shi, R., et al., *Knockdown of lncRNA PCAT6 enhances radiosensitivity in triple-negative breast cancer cells by regulating miR-185-5p/TPD52 axis.* OncoTargets and Therapy, 2020. **13**: p. 3025–3037.
146. Lai, Y., et al., *Down-regulation of LncRNA CCAT1 enhances radiosensitivity via regulating miR-148b in breast cancer.* Cell Biology International, 2018. **42**(2): p. 227–236.
147. Ma, X., et al., *LncRNA ANCR promotes proliferation and radiation resistance of nasopharyngeal carcinoma by inhibiting PTEN expression.* OncoTargets and Therapy, 2018. **11**: p. 8399–8408.

https://doi.org/10.1142/9789811267390_0008

Chapter 8

Exosomal long non-coding RNAs (lncRNAs) in cancer progression and diagnosis

Mohammad Arad Zandieh[1], Nazanin Ranjbar Naeini[2], Romina Rajabi[2], Shokooh Salimimoghadam[3], Kiavash Hushmandi[1]*, Huiyan Eng[4,5] and Alan Prem Kumar[4,5]

[1]*Department of Food Hygiene and Quality Control, Division of Epidemiology & Zoonoses, Faculty of Veterinary Medicine, University of Tehran, Tehran, Iran*

[2]*Faculty of Veterinary Medicine, Islamic Azad University, Science and Research Branch, Tehran, Iran*

[3]*Department of Biochemistry and Molecular Biology, Faculty of Veterinary Medicine, Shahid Chamran University of Ahvaz, Ahvaz, Iran*

[4]*Department of Pharmacology, Yong Loo Lin School of Medicine, National University of Singapore, 117600, Singapore*

[5]*NUS Centre for Cancer Research (N2CR), Yong Loo Lin School of Medicine, National University of Singapore, Singapore 119228, Singapore*

*Corresponding author: Kiavash Hushmandi, Department of Food Hygiene and Quality Control, Division of Epidemiology & Zoonoses, Faculty of Veterinary Medicine, University of Tehran, Tehran, Iran, Email: houshmandi.kia7@ut.ac.ir

Abstract

Both treatment and early diagnosis of cancer are challenging for physicians around the world. The treatment of cancer has shown difficulties due to the resistance and inability in increasing the dose of chemotherapy agents and radiotherapy because of side effects. Besides, malignant behavior and abnormal growth and metastasis of tumor cells have resulted in therapy resistance in cancer. Besides, it is a troublesome problem to diagnose cancer patients at early stages. This chapter focuses on long non-coding RNAs (lncRNAs) present in exosomes, known as exosomal lncRNAs in cancer diagnosis and treatment. The transfer of lncRNAs by exosomes can influence proliferation, invasion, and therapy resistance in tumor cells. Furthermore, exosomal lncRNAs can be found in body fluids such as serum for use as a biomarker to diagnose cancer patients. Furthermore, exosomal lncRNAs are valuable prognostic factors in cancer patients that are discussed in this chapter.

1. Introduction

For a long time, treatment of cancer has been a dream for researchers around the world and the reason for reaching to no effective treatment for cancer is the multifactorial nature of cancer. Although cardiovascular diseases are the leading cause of death worldwide, the majority of studies have been focused on cancer, since most of the factors responsible for cardiovascular pathogenesis have been recognized; while there are a wide variety of factors involved in cancer initiation and development, many of them have not been identified yet [1–3]. About 18.1 million new cases were diagnosed with cancer in 2018 with 9.6 million cancer deaths [4]. This devastating disease is responsible for reducing the quality of life of many patients around the world, and among different factors involved in its progression, genome mutations and signaling networks have been considered as the major factors that need to be highlighted appropriately in the effective treatment of cancer and suppression of tumor cells [5–7]. Each cancer type has its own histopathological and molecular profile making it distinct from others. However, tumors share some similarities in hallmarks including sustained proliferation, abnormal migration ability, angiogenesis, and instability in genomes [8, 9]. The treatment modalities for cancer can be divided into two parts including conventional and modern therapeutics. Conventional treatments include surgery, radiotherapy, and chemotherapy, while modern therapies include immunotherapy and targeted therapy. Due to some challenges related to conventional therapies such as resistance and their side effects, it is highly suggested to combine them with new therapies. Furthermore, a number of new anti-tumor agents such as plant-derived natural products have been introduced for the treatment of cancer patients, but their clinical application is under discussion due to their poor bioavailability, rapid metabolism in body, and low therapeutic impact in cancer patients [10, 11]. Regardless of therapeutics for cancer, the changes in genes and epigenetics can lead to tumor development. The coordination among cellular and molecular mechanisms leads to tumor progression. For instance, activation of oncogenic signaling pathways such as PI3K/Akt signaling can prevent apoptosis in tumor cells and enhance their proliferation and metastasis [12, 13]. The aim of this chapter is to understand the role of long non-coding RNAs (lncRNAs) present in exosomes in regulating tumor progression and therapy response.

2. Exosomes and their importance in oncology

All cells in the human body are capable of secreting cell membrane–surrounded vesicles, known as exosomes with 30–200 nm size that can encapsulate biofunctional molecules such as genes and enzymes, lipids, and proteins [14]. After secretion by cells, exosomes flow in human body fluids and they are absorbed by cells to influence the function of cells and provide homeostasis [15–17]. The disease progression, especially cancer is mainly affected by exosomes due to cell-to-cell communication. Hence, recognition of exosomes is important for human disease diagnosis and progression and they are widely used as biomarkers for cancer diagnosis on liquid biopsy [18]. Under electron microscopy, exosomes demonstrate a cup-shaped morphology [19]. Although all cells in the human body secrete exosomes, tumor cells have more ability in exosome secretion compared to other cells [20]. In spite of significant efforts in understanding the factors involved in modulating exosome secretion by cells, there are still some unknown mechanisms that should be highlighted in further studies. A recent study has revealed the role of iron in exosome secretion by cells [21]. IRE-IRP complex can regulate CD63, a member of tetraspanin superfamily for regulating exosome secretion from cells [21]. Recently, exosomes have obtained much attention in the field of oncology due to their capacity in regulating drug resistance, immune evasion, and invasion of cancer cells [22–25].

For secretion of exosomes, three main phases are followed [26]: in the first step, an endocytic vesicle should be formed; in the second step, multivesicular bodies (MVBs) are generated that comprise intraluminal vesicles (ILVs); and in the final step, MVBs are fused with the cell membrane to secrete exosomes. The secretion of exosomes occurs in both healthy and disease states, and different arrays of cell kinds secret them [27–30]. On biogenesis of exosomes, endocytic vesicle is derived from the cell membrane and it transforms into an early endosome and then into a late endosome. Membranes of the late endosome undergo invagination to generate ILVs within the lumen of organelles [31]. The generation of MVBs is performed on assembly of ILVs into late endosomes. The proteins belonging to Rab family are involved in regulating the formation of endocyclic vesicles. Endosomal sorting complexes required for the transport (ESCRT)-dependent pathway and ESCRT-independent pathway contribute to the formation of endosomal vesicles. In addition to Rab proteins, TSG101 and ALIX participate in the generation of exosomes [32–34]. Figure 1 provides a schematic representation of exosome biogenesis and related mechanisms.

Recent experiments have evaluated the role of exosomes in cancer progression. The exosomes derived from cancer cells induce nuclear factor-κB (NF-kB) signaling to enhance the expression level of programmed death ligand 1 for mediating changes in the metabolism of tumor cells and triggering glycolysis to induce polarization of macrophages to an immuno-suppressive phenotype [35]. The macrophage-tumor chimeric exosomes have been used for immunotherapy in

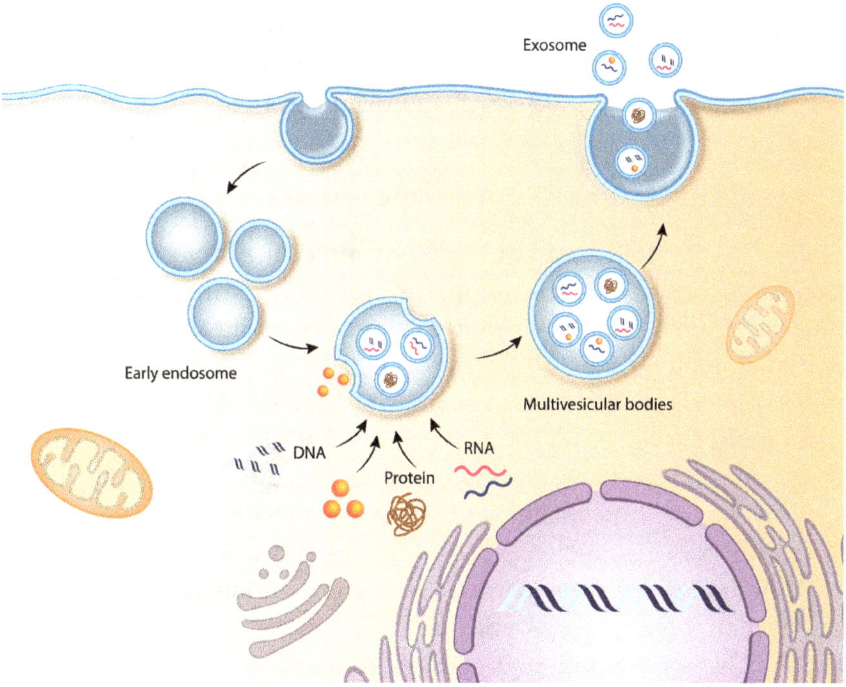

Figure 1. Exosome biogenesis in cells.

cancer. Such exosomes have the ability to accumulate in tumor lymph nodes and stimulate the immune system (T-cell activation) to boost immunotherapy against tumor cells [36]. The presence of hypoxia in the tumor microenvironment (TME) of colorectal tumor cells results in the secretion of exosomes that have high levels of miR-135a-3p for increasing progression and association with unfavorable prognosis [37]. Lin28B has been considered as a vital factor for the metastasis of breast tumor cells to lung tissue. Notably, the release of exosomes with low levels of let-7s is necessary for lin28B to suppress the immune response and to promote breast tumor progression [38]. In type II diabetic patients, exosomes derived from adipocytes can involve in enhancing breast cancer progression [39]. Furthermore, exosomes can be engineered in a way to induce M1 polarization of macrophages and to suppress cancer invasion [40, 41]. Engineered exosomes are also promising candidates for reversing drug resistance and improving immune system action [42, 43]. Therefore, exosomes are the ideal candidate for cancer progression and diagnosis [44–47].

3. lncRNAs and their importance in oncology

In mammalian cells, most of the RNA molecules are not transcribed to proteins and since their number is more than protein-coding RNA molecules, there have been much debate regarding their role in cells and pathological events. In terms of size, non-coding RNA (ncRNA) molecules are divided into small RNAs (microRNAs) and lncRNAs [48]. lncRNAs are a well-known group of ncRNAs and a member of epigenetic factors that comprised more than 200 nucleotides, while small RNA molecules such as miRNAs have less than 25 nucleotides in length [49–51]. lncRNA-coding genes and mRNA-coding genes have unique differences in terms of histone modification signature, but both of them are transcribed by RNA polymerase II. Furthermore, the lncRNA processing after formation is similar to mRNA, so that lncRNAs undergo 5′-end capping, intron splicing, 3-′end polyadenylation, and intracellular transportation that also occur in mRNAs. An interesting point regarding lncRNAs is the presence of small open reading frames, but their inability in coding proteins. A number of RNA-sequencing analysis has demonstrated that lncRNAs can interact with ribosomes and they demonstrate protein-coding regulatory capacity that shows cytoplasmic role of these ncRNAs in regulating the metabolism of mRNAs [52].

Based on high-throughput sequencing technology, it has been shown that more than 98% of the human genome undergoes transcription to RNA molecules lacking the ability in protein coding [53, 54]. According to recent lncRNA annotations, the number of lncRNAs is suggested to be between 30000 and 60000 [55, 56]. Important biological functions are mediated by lncRNAs in cells including translation regulation, splicing, post-translation modifications, chromatin remodeling, gene expression, differentiation, proliferation, development, migration, autophagy, and cell death mechanisms [57]. Inhibition translation of mRNAs and their destabilization are performed by decoy lncRNAs. The scaffold lncRNAs are involved in the assembly of high-molecular-weight protein complexes [58]. Guide lncRNAs increase direct translocation of RNPs to target genes [59]. Enhancer lncRNAs affect chromatin structure to regulate gene expression [60].

The interesting point regarding lncRNAs is their function in disease pathogenesis, especially cancer identified by their dysregulation [3, 61–66]. The overexpression of lncRNA GHET1 is observed in thyroid cancer, and it is responsible for increasing growth and migration rate of tumor cells as well as for preventing apoptosis and cell cycle arrest at G0/G1 phase [67]. The induction of epithelial–mesenchymal transition (EMT) is correlated with an increase in the invasion of lung cancer cells. lncRNA HHIP-AS1 increases PCDHGA9 expression via miR-153-3p absorbing to suppress EMT and reduce stemness of lung cancer cells [68]. lncRNA PCAT6 undergoes overexpression in bladder cancer and increases proliferation and metastasis of tumor cells. By reducing miR-143-3p expression, PCAT6 enhances PDIA6 expression in promoting bladder tumor progression [69]. By the activation of RAB14 expression, lncRNA CCAT2 functions as an oncogenic factor, and it increases growth and metastasis of cancer cells [70]. lncRNA ZFAS1 sponges miR-497-5p to upregulate HMGA2 expression in increasing growth and metastasis of pancreatic cancer cells [71]. Therefore, silencing oncogenic lncRNAs impairs tumor progression. Silencing LINC00997 promotes the expression level of miR-512-3p which is important in suppressing growth, invasion, and EMT in colorectal tumor cells [72]. Based on these studies, lncRNAs are important regulators in the field of oncology and they can regulate cancer hallmarks in different tumors in affecting progression [73–77].

4. Exosomal lncRNAs in cancer proliferation

The most obvious feature or hallmark of tumor cells is their proliferation rate which is higher compared to normal cells. Changes in metabolism, glycolysis induction, apoptosis inhibition, and cell cycle progression are the factors responsible for high growth rate of cancer cells. Activation of STAT3 signaling in esophageal cancer is in favor of tumor progression. miR-124 suppresses STAT3 signaling to impair the proliferation of esophageal cancer cells. It has been reported that exosomal lncRNA ZFAS1 stimulates STAT3 signaling via miR-124 downregulation in increasing cancer proliferation [78]. Similar to STAT3 signaling, Wnt/β-catenin signaling participates in tumor progression and drug resistance. Activation of Wnt signaling in thyroid cancer enhances growth and stemness of tumor cells. Exosomal lncRNA DOCK9-AS2 is secreted by stem cell–like cells, and it stimulates Wnt/β-catenin signaling for promoting tumor proliferation [79].

The most abundant infiltrating immune cells in TME are tumor-associated macrophages (TAMs), and they are involved in the progression of various cancers such as osteosarcoma [80–82]. TAMs demonstrate oncogenic and onco-suppressor functions based on their polarization as M2 or M1, respectively [83]. TAMs have been involved in osteosarcoma progression via inducing STAT3 signaling [84]. TAMs secrete exosomes containing lncRNA LIFR-AS1 that increases NFIA expression via miR-29a sponging in enhancing osteosarcoma growth [85].

One of the important aspects is the emphasis of studies on the role of exosomal lncRNAs in regulating miRNAs and then affecting the progression and growth of tumor cells. In fact, most well-known downstream target of exosomal lncRNAs in regulating cancer proliferation has been considered to be miRNAs [86]. Exosomal lncRNA LINC00659 can be secreted by cancer-associated fibroblasts, and by sponging miR-342-3p, it enhances ANXA2 expression to accelerate colorectal cancer proliferation [87]. In glioma and lung cancer cells, exosomal lncRNAs also regulate miRNAs in affecting their proliferation rate [88, 89]. Based on these studies, exosomal lncRNAs affect the growth and cell cycle progression of tumor cells. Silencing exosomal lncRNAs with oncogenic function impairs proliferation and stimulates cell cycle arrest in tumor cells.

5. Exosomal lncRNAs in cancer migration

After the development of cancer cells, many tumor cells prefer to disseminate to other locations that are different from their primary site and are followed by entering into bloodstream circulation and reaching to a new site for colony formation and establishing new cancer populations, which is known as metastasis [8, 90, 91]. A wide variety of molecular pathways regulate metastasis of tumor cells. Metastasis is a critical factor for poor prognosis and low survival rate of cancer patients. Therefore, it is important to reveal molecular pathways affecting tumor invasion. The current section focuses on the role of exosomal lncRNAs in regulating the invasion of cancer cells.

M2-polarized macrophages can secrete exosomes containing lncRNA AFAP1-AS1 to regulate the migration rate of esophageal cancer cells. By increasing AFAP1-AS1 expression, exosomes lead to downregulation of miR-26a and subsequent overexpression of ATF2 which is important for increasing the invasion of esophageal cancer cells to lung tissue [92]. One of the critical factors that significantly decreases the prognosis of bladder cancer patients is lymph node metastasis which is responsible for the decrease in 5-year survival from 77.6% to 18.6% [93]. Exosomal lncRNA LNMAT2 interacts with hnRNPA2B1 to be internalized in HLECs, and by recruitment of hnRNPA2B1, it enhances the expression level of PROX1 to induce lymph node metastasis of bladder tumor cells [94].

In cancer patients, bone metastasis is one of the leading causes of mortality and disease recurrence that is frequently observed in different tumors such as breast and lung cancers [95]. The incidence rate of bone metastasis in lung cancer is suggested to be as much as 66.7% [96, 97]. Exosomal lncRNA SOX2OT derived from tumor cells increase bone metastasis of lung cancer cells in vitro and in vivo. Exosomal lncRNA SOX2OT promotes RAC1 expression via miR-194-5p sponging to enhance bone metastasis [98]. lncRNAs and exosomal types have shown capacity in reducing expression level of miRNAs via acting as competing endogenous (ceRNA) or sponge. miR-152-3p suppresses invasion of colorectal tumor cells by Vascular endothelial growth factor A (VEGFA) downregulation. Exosomal lncRNA PVT1 is associated with metastasis and stemness in colorectal cancer via miR-152-3p downregulation to overexpress VEGFA [99]. Cancer-associated fibroblasts are important partners in increasing metastasis of osteosarcoma cells. Cancer-associated fibroblasts secrete exosomal lncRNA SNHG17 that promotes matrix metalloproteinase 2 (MMP-2) expression via miR-2861 sponging in enhancing the invasion of osteosarcoma [100]. In addition to MMPs that can increase tumor invasion via degrading extracellular matrix and destroying basement membrane, it has been shown that exosomal lncRNA SOX2OT derived from cancer cells acts as a sponge for miR-200 family to induce EMT mechanism for pancreatic cancer progression [101]. Based on these studies, exosomal lncRNAs are key players in regulating the metastasis of tumor cells by affecting signaling networks and regulating factors such as MMPs and EMT.

6. Exosomal lncRNAs in cancer angiogenesis

The formation of new vessels from pre-existing ones is known as angiogenesis which is an irreplaceable stage in cancer progression. Induction of angiogenesis not only is vital for energy and oxygen for cancer cells but also mediates their migration to different parts of the body for establishing new colonies [102]. lncRNAs are potential regulators of angiogenesis in cancer. In hypoxic conditions, pancreatic tumor cells secrete exosomes containing lncRNA UCA1 for acting as the sponge for miR-96-5p in upregulating AMOTL2 to induce ERK1/2 signaling, resulting in angiogenesis and increased growth [103]. VEGFA is the most well-known regulator of angiogenesis in cancer cells, and its downregulation has been shown to be a promising strategy. Exosomal lncRNA RAMP2-AS1 is derived from chondrosarcoma cells and by miR-2355-5p downregulation, and it promotes VEGFR2 expression to induce angiogenesis in favor of tumor progression [104]. Exosomal lncRNA FAM225A is able to decrease miR-206 expression via sponging where this process is a prerequisite for the upregulation of NETO2 and FOXP1 in inducing angiogenesis and increasing the progression of squamous cancer cells [105]. Sponging miRNAs and affecting their downstream targets are

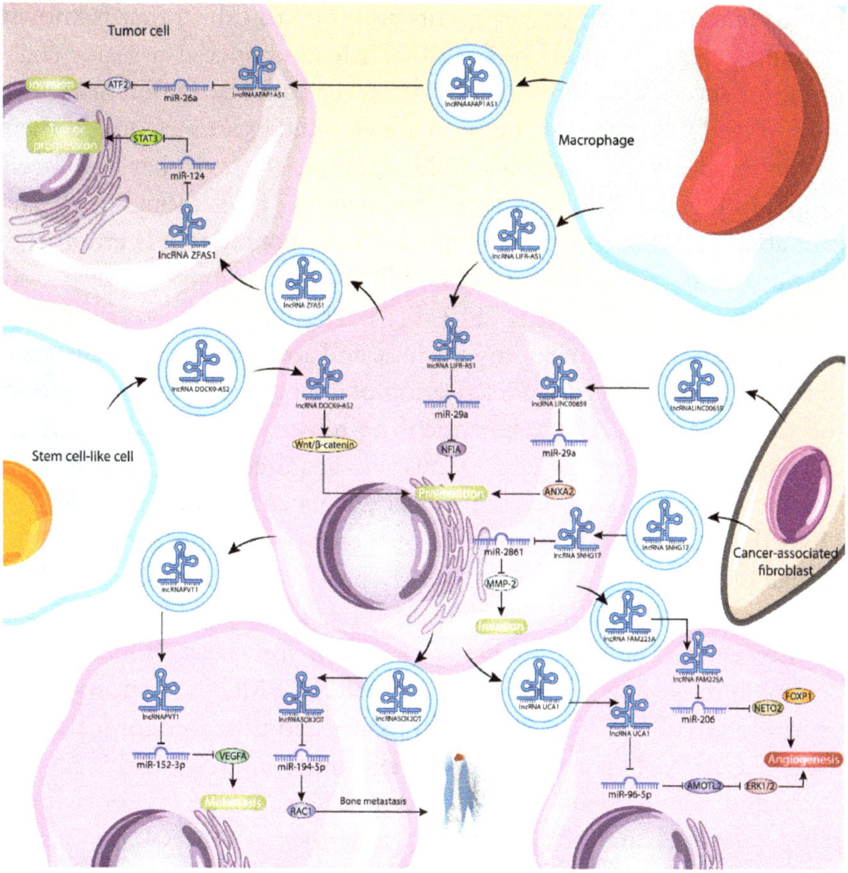

Figure 2. lncRNAs in regulating proliferation, invasion, and angiogenesis in cancers.

followed mainly by exosomal lncRNAs in regulating angiogenesis in cancer [106, 107]. Furthermore, angiogenesis induction by exosomal lncRNAs leads to a significant enhancement in the growth rate of cancer cells (Figure 2) [108].

7. Exosomal lncRNAs in cancer drug resistance

Chemotherapy is one of the gold standards in the treatment of cancer, but a majority of cancer patients develop resistance to chemotherapy, first to one of the anti-cancer agents and then to others that is known as multi-drug resistance [109, 110]. Drug resistance is a major challenge for successful chemotherapy of cancer patients. Different factors are involved in process of chemo-resistance and exosomes due to their role in the delivery of proteins, lipids, and nucleic acids that have been shown to regulate drug resistance in cancer [111]. Although a significant attempt has been made in improving the potential of chemotherapeutic agents, drug resistance is still an obstacle to survival and prognosis of cancer patients [112–115]. There are two major categories of drug resistance including intrinsic and acquired chemo-resistance [116]. Cancer stem cells and activation of oncogenic factors are among the factors that can induce intrinsic drug resistance before exposure to any chemotherapeutic agent. However, acquired drug resistance is observed after exposure to anti-cancer agents and can be provided by DNA damage repair, upregulation of tumor-promoting genes, down-regulation of tumor-suppressor genes, pro-survival autophagy induction, apoptosis inhibition, and increased drug efflux [117, 118].

Exosomal lncRNA SBF2-AS1 has been shown to induce temozolomide resistance in glioblastoma. lncRNA SBF2-AS1 shows over-expression in glioblastoma cells and tissues and is higher compared to normal cells and tissues. Silencing exosomal lncRNA SBF2-AS1 is correlated with enhanced temozolomide sensitivity of glioblastoma cells. Exosomal lncRNA SBF2-AS1 functions as ceRNA for down-regulating miR-151a-3p expression to upregulate XRCC4 in triggering drug resistance [119]. The cells present in the TME are capable of secreting exosomes containing lncRNAs in mediating tumor progression and drug resistance. Cancer-associated fibroblasts are able to secrete exosomal lncRNA H19 to increase stemness of colorectal cancer and to stimulate drug resistance. Exosomal lncRNA H19 sponges miR-141 to induce β-catenin signaling in triggering chemo-resistance [120]. Furthermore, cancer-associated fibroblasts secrete exosomal lncRNA UCA1 in triggering drug resistance in vulvar carcinoma. Exosomal UCA1 diminishes miR-103a expression to upregulate WEE1, resulting in autophagy induction, apoptosis inhibition, and increased tumor proliferation, which are important for cisplatin resistance [121].

In addition to TME components, cancer cells can secrete exosomes. Exosomal lncRNA POU3F3 is involved in cisplatin resistance of esophageal cancer. Exosomal lncRNA POU3F3 stimulates the differentiation of fibroblasts into cancer-associated fibroblasts to secrete interleukin 6 for increasing the growth rate of tumor cells and triggering cisplatin resistance in esophageal cancer [122]. Trastuzumab has been popular in the treatment of breast cancer, but up to 27%–42% of breast cancer patients exposing to trastuzumab demonstrate resistance and recurrence [123, 124]. Overexpression of exosomal lncRNA AGAP2-AS1 in breast cancer has been implicated in a decrease in cytotoxicity of trastuzumab by enhancing the survival rate of tumor cells [125].

The interesting point toward exosomal lncRNAs is their ability in affecting the expression level of miRNAs in tumors. Exosomal lncRNA HEIH shows overexpression in tongue carcinoma and is responsible for cisplatin resistance. By acting as ceRNA, lncRNA HEIH promotes the expression level of HDGF to prevent apoptosis that is in favor of cisplatin resistance [126]. Cisplatin is a well-known anti-cancer agent in tumor suppression for solid tumors, adult and pediatric cancers. This platinum compound forms adducts with DNA and also induces apoptosis and cell cycle arrest in cancer suppression [127, 128]. However, increasing evidence has shown the role of lncRNAs in cisplatin resistance of tumor cells [129–131]. Exosomal lncRNA HNF1A-AS1 shows overexpression in cervical cancer and stimulates cisplatin resistance in tumor cells. Exosomal lncRNA HNF1A-AS1 promotes TUFT1 expression via miR-34b inhibition to stimulate cisplatin resistance [132]. Based on the studies, it can be concluded that exosomes can be derived from different cells such as tumor cells and cancer-associated fibroblasts, and by transferring oncogenic lncRNAs, they induce drug resistance in cancers [133, 134]. There are two limitations that should be considered in future studies. First, studies are about oncogenic exosomal lncRNAs, and researchers should also recognize onco-suppressor lncRNAs regulating drug resistance in cancer. Second, the role of exosomal lncRNAs derived from other sources such as macrophages and mesenchymal stem cells in affecting chemoresistance in cancer should be considered.

8. Exosomal lncRNAs in cancer radio-resistance

DNA strand break occurs on exposure of tumor cells to radiation therapy that impairs the ability of cancer cells in proliferation and leads to their elimination. However, some factors including hypoxia, overexpression of oncogenic factors, DNA damage repair, and tumor size increase result in radio-resistance in cancer [135, 136]. Increasing evidence has revealed the role of lncRNAs in regulating radio-resistance/sensitivity in tumors. For instance, lncRNA TP53TG1 acts as oncogenic factor and stimulates radio-resistance in glioma via miR-524-5p downregulation and subsequent overexpression of RAB5A [137]. By stabilizing SIRT6, lncRNA RBM5-AS1 prevents apoptosis and DNA damage for inducing radio-resistance in medulloblastoma [138]. However, one experiment has examined the role of exosomal lncRNA in radio-resistance. M2-polarized macrophages can secrete exosomal lncRNA AGAP2-AS1 that induces NOTCH2 signaling via miR-296 downregulation for providing radiotherapy immunity in lung cancer [139]. The capacity of exosomal lncRNAs in regulating apoptosis and autophagy, as well as affecting DNA damage as regulators of radio-resistance should be considered in next studies (Figure 3).

9. Exosomal lncRNAs in cancer diagnosis and prognosis

Previous sections revealed the role of exosomal lncRNAs in affecting tumor progression and therapy response. Although the treatment of cancer is an important step and much effort has been put into it, another important step in cancer is its diagnosis. The interesting point related to exosomes is their presence in body fluids that can be used as a minimally invasive method for cancer diagnosis and prognosis. Exosomal lncRNA DLX6-AS1 shows high levels in the serum of cervical cancer patients and it positively correlates with lymph node metastasis, differentiation, and low survival rate of patients. Furthermore, high exosomal lncRNA DLX6-AS1 levels mediate more chance of relapse compared to its low levels. It is also a prognostic factor and high levels of exosomal lncRNA DLX6-AS1 provide poor prognosis for cervical cancer patients [140]. Notably, serum vesicles

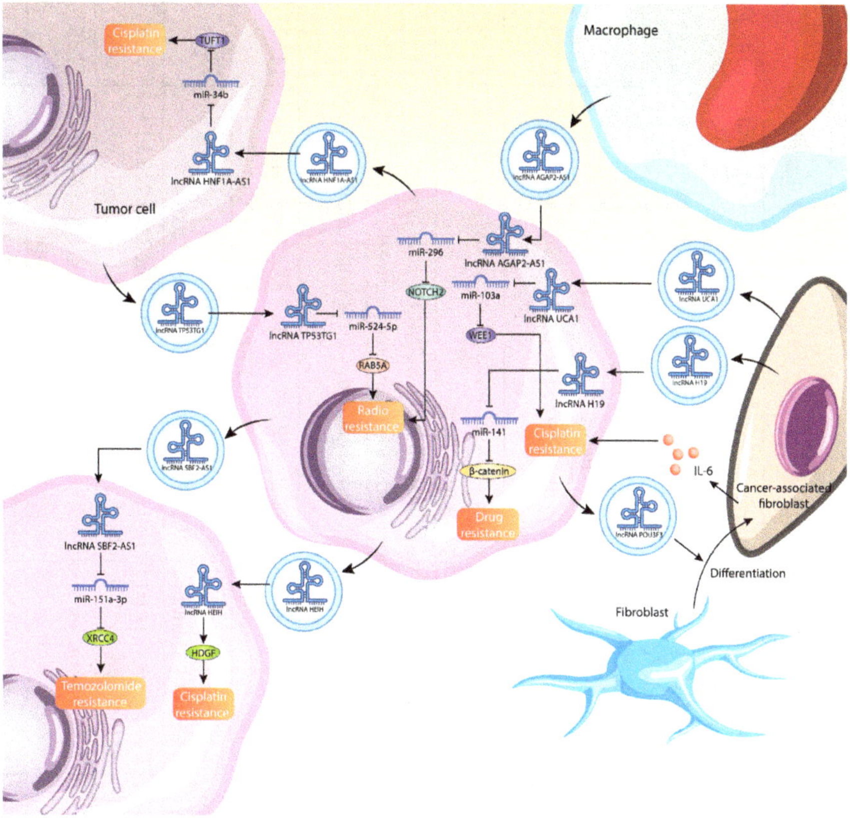

Figure 3. lncRNAs in therapy response of cancers.

and exosomes can be easily isolated [141]. To increase specificity in the diagnosis of cancer, more than one exosomal lncRNA can be used. Exosomal lncRNA TBILA and AGAP2-AS1 are stable in the serum of lung cancer patients, and they are potential diagnostic tools. However, the results of this experiment provide some controversial discussions that individual exosomal lncRNA TBILA or AGAP2-AS1 has more accuracy in lung cancer diagnosis compared to their combination [142]. The most important limitation of current works is their focus on individual exosomal lncRNAs, and it is better for future studies to develop signatures in cancer diagnosis and prognosis based

Table 1. An overview of exosomal lncRNAs in cancer progression and diagnosis.

Exosomal lncRNA	Molecular Pathway	Cancer Type	Remarks	Ref
FMR1-AS1	TLR7/ NF-κB/c-Myc	Female esophageal carcinoma	Association of exosomal lncRNA FMR1-AS1 with poor clinical outcomes. FMR1-AS1 binds to TLR7 to induce its downstream target NF-κB/c-Myc. Apoptosis inhibition. Proliferation and migration increase.	[147]
HOXD-AS1	miR-361-5p/ FOXM1	Prostate cancer	Exosomal HOXD-AS1 is internalized in tumor cells and enhances prostate cancer metastasis.	[148]
UEGC1	—	Gastric cancer	High expression level of exosomal UEGC1 in gastric cancer patients and acting as biomarker.	[149]
SUMO1P3	—	Triple-negative breast cancer	Overexpression of exosomal lncRNA SUMO1P3 in breast cancer patients and association with poor survival rate.	[150]
MALAT1	—	Ovarian cancer	MALAT1 induces angiogenesis and mediates unfavorable prognosis in patients.	[151]
SNHG15	—	Lung cancer	Overexpression of exosomal lncRNA SNHG15 in lung cancer patients and providing unfavorable prognosis.	[152]
BCYRN1	WNT5A/VEGF-C/ VEGFR3	Bladder cancer	Lymph node metastasis of bladder tumor cells. BCYRN1 stimulates WNT5A/VEGF-C/VEGFR3 axis.	[153]
NEAT1	miR-26a/b-5p/ STAT3	Endometrial cancer	Cancer-associated fibroblasts secrete exosomal lncRNA NEAT1. miR downregulation by NEAT1 to induce STAT3 signaling.	[154]
MMP2-2	MMP2	Lung cancer	TGF-β induces exosomal lncRNA MMP2-2 to increase MMP2 expression in enhancing metastasis of lung tumor cells.	[155]
HOTTIP	miR-214/KPNA3	Colorectal cancer	Exosomal lncRNA HOTTIP is involved in mitomycin resistance via miR-214 inhibition and increasing stability of KPNA3.	[156]

on exosomal lncRNAs [143, 144]. High levels of exosomal lncRNA H19 are found in the serum of gastric cancer patients and it mediates poor prognosis [145]. As a minimally invasive prognostic factor, high serum levels of exosomal lncRNA RP5-977B1 mediates poor prognosis in lung cancer patients [146]. Table 1 provides a summary of exosomal lncRNAs in cancer progression.

10. Conclusion and remarks

Exosomes are a member of extracellular vesicles with low size that can carry cargo such as proteins, lipids, and genetic materials between normal cells and cancerous cells. The cell-to-cell communication and homeostasis are provided by exosomes. These small extracellular vesicles can carry lncRNAs derived from macrophages, cancer-associated fibroblasts, mesenchymal stem cells, and tumor cells. Exosomal lncRNAs regulate apoptosis, cell cycle progression, growth, metastasis, and EMT mechanism in cancers to affect their progression. Exosomal lncRNAs can induce drug resistance and radio-resistance in cancers and due to their presence in serum, they are widely used as biomarkers in cancer patients. The limitation of current works is their focus on oncogenic exosomal lncRNAs. Furthermore, it has been reported that exosomal lncRNAs affect different molecular pathways such as STAT3 and Wnt/β-catenin signaling in regulating the progression of tumor cells.

Conflict of interest:

The authors declare no conflict of interest.

Acknowledgment

H.E. is supported by a Postdoctoral Fellowship under the NRF-NUS Resilience & Growth PDF Fellowship from the National University of Singapore.

Funding

The work was supported by a grant from the Singapore Ministry of Education Tier 2 (MOET2EP30120-0016) to A.P.K.

References

1. Aggarwal, V., et al., *Molecular mechanisms of action of hesperidin in cancer: Recent trends and advancements.* Experimental Biology and Medicine (Maywood), 2020. **245**(5): p. 486–497.
2. Paskeh, M.D.A., et al., *Emerging role of exosomes in cancer progression and tumor microenvironment remodeling.* Journal of Hematology & Oncology, 2022. **15**(1): p. 1–39.
3. Mirzaei, S., et al., *The long and short non-coding RNAs modulating EZH2 signaling in cancer.* Journal of Hematology & Oncology, 2022. **15**(1): p. 1–34.
4. Khazaei, Z., et al., *Global cancer statistics 2018: GLOBOCAN estimates of incidence and mortality worldwide stomach cancers and their relationship with the human development index (HDI).* Epidemiology, 2019. **6**(9).
5. Banik, K., et al., *Piceatannol: A natural stilbene for the prevention and treatment of cancer.* Pharmacological Research, 2020. **153**: p. 104635.
6. Patra, S., et al., *Autophagy-modulating phytochemicals in cancer therapeutics: Current evidences and future perspectives.* Seminars in Cancer Biology, 2022. **80**: p. 205–217.
7. Mohan, C.D., et al., *Targeting STAT3 signaling pathway in cancer by agents derived from mother nature.* Seminars in Cancer Biology, 2022. **80**: p. 157–182.
8. Hanahan, D. and R.A. Weinberg, *The hallmarks of cancer.* Cell, 2000. **100**(1): p. 57–70.
9. Roy, N.K., et al., *The potential role of boswellic acids in cancer prevention and treatment.* Cancer Letters, 2016. **377**(1): p. 74–86.
10. Abadi, A.J., et al., *Curcumin and its derivatives in cancer therapy: Potentiating antitumor activity of cisplatin and reducing side effects.* Phytotherapy Research, 2022. **36**(1): p. 189–213.

11. Mirzaei, S., et al., *Caffeic acid and its derivatives as potential modulators of oncogenic molecular pathways: New hope in the fight against cancer.* Pharmacological Research, 2021. **171**: p. 105759.
12. Xue, C., et al., *Crosstalk between circRNAs and the PI3K/AKT signaling pathway in cancer progression.* Signal Transduction and Targeted Therapy, 2021. **6**(1): p. 400.
13. He, Y., et al., *Targeting PI3K/Akt signal transduction for cancer therapy.* Signal Transduction and Targeted Therapy, 2021. **6**(1): p. 425.
14. Nakase, I., T. Takatani-Nakase, *Exosomes: Breast cancer-derived extracellular vesicles; recent key findings and technologies in disease progression, diagnostics, and cancer targeting.* Drug Metabolism and Pharmacokinetics, 2021. **42**: p. 100435.
15. Tan, A., J. Rajadas, and A. Seifalian, *Exosomes as nano-theranostic delivery platforms for gene therapy.* Advanced Drug Delivery Reviews, 2013. **65**(3): p. 357–367.
16. Yamamoto, T., et al., *Latest advances in extracellular vesicles: From bench to bedside.* Science and Technology of Advanced Materials, 2019. **20**(1): p. 746–757.
17. Nakase, I.J.P., *Biofunctional peptide-modified extracellular vesicles enable effective intracellular delivery via the induction of macropinocytosis.* Processes, 2021. **9**(2): p. 224.
18. Jiang, L., et al., *Exosomes: Diagnostic biomarkers and therapeutic delivery vehicles for cancer.* Molecular Pharmaceutics, 2019. **16**(8): p. 3333–3349.
19. Channon, L.M., et al., *Small extracellular vesicles (exosomes) and their cargo in pancreatic cancer: Key roles in the hallmarks of cancer.* Biochimica et Biophysica Acta. Reviews on Cancer, 2022. **1877**(3): p. 188728.
20. Kalluri, R., *The biology and function of exosomes in cancer.* The Journal of Clinical Investigation, 2016. **126**(4): p. 1208–1215.
21. Yanatori, I., et al., *CD63 is regulated by iron via the IRE-IRP system and is important for ferritin secretion by extracellular vesicles.* Blood, 2021. **138**(16): p. 1490–1503.
22. Fang, Y., et al., *Exosomal miRNA-106b from cancer-associated fibroblast promotes gemcitabine resistance in pancreatic cancer.* Experimental Cell Research, 2019. **383**(1): p. 111543.

23. Shen, T., et al., *Pancreatic cancer derived exosomes induce apoptosis of T lymphocytes through the p38 MAPK mediated endoplasmic reticulum stress.* FASEB Journal, 2020. **34**(6): p. 8442–8458.
24. Yu, Z., et al., *Pancreatic cancer-derived exosomes promote tumor metastasis and liver pre-metastatic niche formation.* Oncotarget, 2017. **8**(38): p. 63461.
25. Hoshino, A., et al., *Tumour exosome integrins determine organotropic metastasis.* Nature, 2015. **527**(7578): p. 329–335.
26. Kumar, D.N., et al., *Exosomes as emerging drug delivery and diagnostic modality for breast cancer: Recent advances in isolation and application.* Cancers (Basel), 2022. **14**(6).
27. Sliwińska-Mossoń, M., I. Zieleń, and H. Milnerowicz, *New trends in the treatment of nicotine addiction.* Acta Poloniae Pharmaceutica, 2014. **71**(4): p. 525–530.
28. Trajkovic, K., et al., *Ceramide triggers budding of exosome vesicles into multivesicular endosomes.* Science, 2008. **319**(5867): p. 1244–1247.
29. Batista, B.S., et al., *Identification of a conserved glycan signature for microvesicles.* Journal of Proteome Research, 2011. **10**(10): p. 4624–4633.
30. Beach, A., et al., *Exosomes: An overview of biogenesis, composition and role in ovarian cancer.* Journal of Ovarian Research, 2014. **7**(1): p. 1–11.
31. Hessvik, N.P. and A. Llorente, *Current knowledge on exosome biogenesis and release.* Cellular and Molecular Life Sciences, 2018. **75**(2): p. 193–208.
32. Schmidt, O. and D. Teis, *The ESCRT machinery.* Current Biology, 2012. **22**(4): p. R116–R120.
33. Mercier, V., et al., *ALG-2 interacting protein-X (Alix) is essential for clathrin-independent endocytosis and signaling.* Scientific Reports, 2016. **6**(1): p. 1–15.
34. Słomka, A., et al., *EVs as potential new therapeutic tool/target in gastrointestinal cancer and HCC.* Cancers (Basel), 2020. **12**(10): p. 3019.
35. Morrissey, S.M., et al., *Tumor-derived exosomes drive immunosuppressive macrophages in a pre-metastatic niche through glycolytic dominant metabolic reprogramming.* Cell Metabolism, 2021. **33**(10): p. 2040–2058.e10.

36. Wang, S., et al., *Macrophage-tumor chimeric exosomes accumulate in lymph node and tumor to activate the immune response and the tumor microenvironment.* Science Translational Medicine, 2021. **13**(615): p. eabb6981.
37. Sun, H., et al., *Hypoxia-inducible exosomes facilitate liver-tropic pre-metastatic niche in colorectal cancer.* Hepatology, 2021. **74**(5): p. 2633–2651.
38. Qi, M., et al., *Lin28B-high breast cancer cells promote immune suppression in the lung pre-metastatic niche via exosomes and support cancer progression.* Nature Communications, 2022. **13**(1): p. 897.
39. Jafari, N., et al., *Adipocyte-derived exosomes may promote breast cancer progression in type 2 diabetes.* Science Signaling, 2021. **14**(710): p. eabj2807.
40. Patwardhan, S., et al., *ECM stiffness-tuned exosomes drive breast cancer motility through thrombospondin-1.* Biomaterials, 2021. **279**: p. 121185.
41. Gunassekaran, G.R., et al., *M1 macrophage exosomes engineered to foster M1 polarization and target the IL-4 receptor inhibit tumor growth by reprogramming tumor-associated macrophages into M1-like macrophages.* Biomaterials, 2021. **278**: p. 121137.
42. Zhao, Y., et al., *M1 Macrophage-derived exosomes loaded with gemcitabine and deferasirox against chemoresistant pancreatic cancer.* Pharmaceutics, 2021. **13**(9).
43. Huang, L., et al., *Engineered exosomes as an in situ DC-primed vaccine to boost antitumor immunity in breast cancer.* Molecular Cancer, 2022. **21**(1): p. 45.
44. Jiang, Z., et al., *Cancer derived exosomes induce macrophages immunosuppressive polarization to promote bladder cancer progression.* Cell Communication and Signaling, 2021. **19**(1): p. 93.
45. Wen, H., et al., *MiR-185-5p targets RAB35 gene to regulate tumor cell-derived exosomes-mediated proliferation, migration and invasion of non-small cell lung cancer cells.* Aging (Albany NY), 2021. **13**(17): p. 21435–21450.
46. Tang, Q., et al., *Tumor-derived exosomes in the cancer immune microenvironment and cancer immunotherapy.* Cancer Letters, 2022. **548**: p. 215823.

47. Wu, J., S. Li, and P. Zhang, *Tumor-derived exosomes: Immune properties and clinical application in lung cancer.* Cancer Drug Resistance, 2022. **5**(1): p. 102–113.
48. Shabgah, A.G., et al., *Curcumin and cancer; are long non-coding RNAs missing link?* Progress in Biophysics and Molecular Biology, 2021. **164**: p. 63–71.
49. Chen, Z., et al., *miR-342-3p regulates the proliferation and apoptosis of NSCLC cells by targeting BCL-2.* Technology in Cancer Research & Treatment, 2021. **20**: p. 15330338211041193.
50. Gong, Y., et al., *Bioinformatics analysis of long non-coding RNA and related diseases: An overview.* Frontiers in Genetics, 2021. **12**.
51. Janaththani, P., S.L. Srinivasan, and J. Batra, *Long non-coding RNAs at the chromosomal risk loci identified by prostate and breast cancer GWAS.* Genes (Basel), 2021. **12**(12): p. 2028.
52. Yoon, J.-H., K. Abdelmohsen, and M. Gorospe, *Posttranscriptional gene regulation by long noncoding RNA.* Journal of Molecular Biology, 2013. **425**(19): p. 3723–3730.
53. Kopp, F. and J.T. Mendell, *Functional classification and experimental dissection of long noncoding RNAs.* Cell, 2018. **172**(3): p. 393–407.
54. Zamaraev, A.V., et al., *Long non-coding RNAs: A view to kill ovarian cancer.* Biochimica et Biophysica Acta. Reviews on Cancer, 2021. **1876**(1): p. 188584.
55. Hon, C.-C., et al., *An atlas of human long non-coding RNAs with accurate 5′ ends.* Nature, 2017. **543**(7644): p. 199–204.
56. Iyer, M.K., et al., *The landscape of long noncoding RNAs in the human transcriptome.* Nature Genetics, 2015. **47**(3): p. 199–208.
57. Schmitz, S.U., et al., *Mechanisms of long noncoding RNA function in development and disease.* Cellular and Molecular Life Sciences, 2016. **73**(13): p. 2491–2509.
58. Fang, Y. and M.J. Fullwood, *Roles, functions, and mechanisms of long non-coding RNAs in cancer.* Genomics Proteomics Bioinformatics, 2016. **14**(1): p. 42–54.
59. Grote, P., et al., *The tissue-specific lncRNA Fendrr is an essential regulator of heart and body wall development in the mouse.* Developmental Cell, 2013. **24**(2): p. 206–214.

60. Hou, Y., R. Zhang, and X.J. Sun, *Enhancer LncRNAs influence chromatin interactions in different ways.* Frontiers in Genetics, 2019. **10**: p. 936.
61. Mirzaei, S., et al., *Molecular landscape of LncRNAs in prostate cancer: A focus on pathways and therapeutic targets for intervention.* Journal of Experimental & Clinical Cancer Research, 2022. **41**(1): p. 1–26.
62. Entezari, M., et al., *Long non-coding RNAs and exosomal lncRNAs: Potential functions in lung cancer progression, drug resistance and tumor microenvironment remodeling.* Biomédecine & Pharmacothérapie, 2022. **150**: p. 112963.
63. Ashrafizadeh, M., et al., *Long noncoding RNAs (lncRNAs) in pancreatic cancer progression.* Drug Discovery Today, 2022. **27**(8): p. 2181–2198.
64. Entezari, M., et al., *Non-coding RNAs and macrophage interaction in tumor progression.* Critical Reviews in Oncology/Hematology, 2022. **173**: p. 103680.
65. Iranmanesh, H., et al., *The association of clinicopathological characterizations of colorectal cancer with membrane-bound mucins genes and LncRNAs.* Pathology — Research and Practice, 2022. **233**: p. 153883.
66. Liu, T., et al., *MicroRNA-216b targets HK2 to potentiate autophagy and apoptosis of breast cancer cells via the mTOR signaling pathway.* International Journal of Biological Sciences, 2021. **17**(11): p. 2970.
67. Liu, Y., et al., *Long non-coding RNA GHET1 promotes thyroid cancer cell proliferation and invasion.* Translational Cancer Research, 2021. **10**(9): p. 4148–4157.
68. Zhou, Z., et al., *Long non-coding RNA HHIP-AS1 inhibits lung cancer epithelial-mesenchymal transition and stemness by regulating PCDHGA9.* Molecuar Medicine Reports, 2021. **24**(6).
69. Zhang, Y., L. Chen, and G. Luo, *Long non-coding RNA PCAT6 regulates bladder cancer progression via the microRNA-143-3p/PDIA6 axis.* Experimental and Therapeutic Medicine, 2021. **22**(3): p. 947.
70. Wang, D., Z. Li, and H. Yin, *Long non-coding RNA CCAT2 activates RAB14 and acts as an oncogene in colorectal cancer.* Frontiers Oncology, 2021. **11**: p. 751903.

71. Rao, M., et al., *Long non-coding RNA ZFAS1 promotes pancreatic cancer proliferation and metastasis by sponging miR-497-5p to regulate HMGA2 expression.* Cell Death & Disease, 2021. **12**(10): p. 859.
72. Shi, Z., et al., *Long non-coding RNA LINC00997 silencing inhibits the progression and metastasis of colorectal cancer by sponging miR-512-3p.* Bioengineered, 2021. **12**(1): p. 627–639.
73. Xiao, H., et al., *Targeting long non-coding RNA TTN-AS1 suppresses bladder cancer progression.* Frontiers in Genetics, 2021. **12**: p. 704712.
74. Ye, G.Y., et al., *Long non-coding RNA LINC01569 promotes proliferation and metastasis in colorectal cancer by miR-381-3p/RAP2A axis.* Frontiers in Oncology, 2021. **11**: p. 727698.
75. Zhang, M., et al., *Long non-coding RNA TRG-AS1 promoted proliferation and invasion of lung cancer cells through the miR-224-5p/SMAD4 axis.* OncoTargets and Therapy, 2021. **14**: p. 4415–4426.
76. Zhou, Q., et al., *Long non-coding RNA GRIK1-AS1 inhibits the proliferation and invasion of gastric cancer cells by regulating the miR-375/IFIT2 axis.* Frontiers in Oncology, 2021. **11**: p. 754834.
77. Liang, H., et al., *Long non-coding RNA Duxap8 facilitates cell proliferation and induces apoptosis in colorectal cancer via miR-519b/ZNF277 axis.* OncoTargets and Therapy, 2021. **14**: p. 4693–4703.
78. Li, Z., et al., *Exosomal lncRNA ZFAS1 regulates esophageal squamous cell carcinoma cell proliferation, invasion, migration and apoptosis via microRNA-124/STAT3 axis.* Journal of Experimental & Clinical Cancer Research, 2019. **38**(1): p. 477.
79. Dai, W., et al., *Exosomal lncRNA DOCK9-AS2 derived from cancer stem cell-like cells activated Wnt/β-catenin pathway to aggravate stemness, proliferation, migration, and invasion in papillary thyroid carcinoma.* Cell Death & Disease, 2020. **11**(9): p. 743.
80. Wang, M., et al., *Role of tumor microenvironment in tumorigenesis.* Journal of Cancer, 2017. **8**(5): p. 761.
81. Zhu, J., et al., *The role of tumor associated macrophages in the tumor microenvironment: mechanism and functions.* Anti-cancer Agents in Medicinal Chemistry, 2016. **16**(9): p. 1133–1141.
82. Liang, X., et al., *Macrophages reduce the sensitivity of osteosarcoma to neoadjuvant chemotherapy drugs by secreting Interleukin-1 beta.* Cancer Letters, 2020. **480**: p. 4–14.

83. Martinez, F.O. and S. Gordon, *The M1 and M2 paradigm of macrophage activation: Time for reassessment.* F1000 Prime Reports, 2014. **6**.
84. Han, Y., et al., *Tumor-associated macrophages promote lung metastasis and induce epithelial-mesenchymal transition in osteosarcoma by activating the COX-2/STAT3 axis.* Cancer Letters, 2019. **440**: p. 116–125.
85. Zhang, H., et al., *Macrophages-derived exosomal lncRNA LIFR-AS1 promotes osteosarcoma cell progression via miR-29a/NFIA axis.* Cancer Cell International, 2021. **21**(1): p. 192.
86. Jia, J., et al., *Exosomal-lncRNA DLEU1 accelerates the proliferation, migration, and invasion of endometrial carcinoma cells by regulating microRNA-E2F3.* OncoTargets and Therapy, 2020. **13**: p. 8651–8663.
87. Zhou, L., et al., *Exosomal LncRNA LINC00659 transferred from cancer-associated fibroblasts promotes colorectal cancer cell progression via miR-342-3p/ANXA2 axis.* Journal of Translatonal Medicine, 2021. **19**(1): p. 8.
88. Chai, Y., et al., *Exosomal lncRNA ROR1-AS1 derived from tumor cells promotes glioma progression via regulating miR-4686.* International Journal of Nanomedicine, 2020. **15**: p. 8863–8872.
89. Lv, X., et al., *Exosomal long non-coding RNA LINC00662 promotes non-small cell lung cancer progression by miR-320d/E2F1 axis.* Aging (Albany NY), 2021. **13**(4): p. 6010–6024.
90. Lambert, A.W., D.R. Pattabiraman, and R.A. Weinberg, *Emerging biological principles of metastasis.* Cell, 2017. **168**(4): p. 670–691.
91. Hanahan, D. and R.A. Weinberg, *Hallmarks of cancer: The next generation.* Cell, 2011. **144**(5): p. 646–674.
92. Mi, X., et al., *M2 macrophage-derived exosomal lncRNA AFAP1-AS1 and MicroRNA-26a affect cell migration and metastasis in esophageal cancer.* Molecular Therapy Nucleic Acids, 2020. **22**: p. 779–790.
93. Hautmann, R.E., et al., *Radical cystectomy for urothelial carcinoma of the bladder without neoadjuvant or adjuvant therapy: Long-term results in 1100 patients.* European Urology, 2012. **61**(5): p. 1039–1047.
94. Chen, C., et al., *Exosomal long noncoding RNA LNMAT2 promotes lymphatic metastasis in bladder cancer.* Journal of Clinical Investigation, 2020. **130**(1): p. 404–421.
95. Roodman, G.D., *Mechanisms of bone metastasis.* The New England Journal of Medicine, 2004. **350**(16): p. 1655–1664.

96. Suva, L.J., et al., *Bone metastasis: Mechanisms and therapeutic opportunities.* Nature Reviews. Endocrinology, 2011. 7(4): p. 208–218.
97. Mundy, G.R., *Metastasis to bone: Causes, consequences and therapeutic opportunities.* Nature Reviews. Cancer, 2002. **2**(8): p. 584–593.
98. Ni, J., et al., *Tumour-derived exosomal lncRNA-SOX2OT promotes bone metastasis of non-small cell lung cancer by targeting the miRNA-194-5p/RAC1 signalling axis in osteoclasts.* Cell Death & Disease, 2021. **12**(7): p. 662.
99. Lai, S.W., et al., *Exosomal lncRNA PVT1/VEGFA axis promotes colon cancer metastasis and stemness by downregulation of tumor suppressor miR-152-3p.* Oxidative Medicine and Cell Longevity, 2021. **2021**: p. 9959807.
100. Zhao, A., et al., *Carcinoma-associated fibroblasts promote the proliferation and metastasis of osteosarcoma by transferring exosomal LncRNA SNHG17.* American Journal of Translational Research, 2021. **13**(9): p. 10094–10111.
101. Li, Z., et al., *Tumor-derived exosomal lnc-Sox2ot promotes EMT and stemness by acting as a ceRNA in pancreatic ductal adenocarcinoma.* Oncogene, 2018. **37**(28): p. 3822–3838.
102. Maiborodin, I., et al., *Cancer angiogenesis and opportunity of influence on tumor by changing vascularization.* Journal of Personalized Medicine, 2022. **12**(3).
103. Guo, Z., et al., *Hypoxic tumor-derived exosomal long noncoding RNA UCA1 promotes angiogenesis via miR-96-5p/AMOTL2 in pancreatic cancer.* Molecular Therapy — Nucleic Acids, 2020. **22**: p. 179–195.
104. Cheng, C., et al., *Exosomal lncRNA RAMP2-AS1 derived from chondrosarcoma cells promotes angiogenesis through miR-2355-5p/VEGFR2 axis.* OncoTargets and Therapy, 2020. **13**: p. 3291–3301.
105. Zhang, C., et al., *Exosomal lncRNA FAM225A accelerates esophageal squamous cell carcinoma progression and angiogenesis via sponging miR-206 to upregulate NETO2 and FOXP1 expression.* Cancer Medicine, 2020. **9**(22): p. 8600–8611.
106. Yuan, D., et al., *Exosomal lncRNA ATB derived from ovarian cancer cells promotes angiogenesis via regulating miR-204-3p/TGFβR2 axis.* Cancer Management and Research, 2022. **14**: p. 327–337.

107. Li, Y., et al., *Highly enriched exosomal lncRNA OIP5-AS1 regulates osteosarcoma tumor angiogenesis and autophagy through miR-153 and ATG5.* American Journal of Translational Research, 2021. **13**(5): p. 4211–4223.
108. Lei, L. and Q. Mou, *Exosomal taurine up-regulated 1 promotes angiogenesis and endothelial cell proliferation in cervical cancer.* Cancer Biology & Therapy, 2020. **21**(8): p. 717–725.
109. Li, J., et al., *The emerging role of exosomes in cancer chemoresistance.* Frontiers in Cell and Developmental Biology, 2021. **9**: p. 737962.
110. Gottesman, M.M., *Mechanisms of cancer drug resistance.* Annual Review of Medicine, 2002. **53**(1): p. 615–627.
111. Mc Namee, N. and L. O'Driscoll, *Extracellular vesicles and anti-cancer drug resistance.* Biochimica et Biophysica Acta. Reviews on Cancer. 2018. **1870**(2): p. 123–136.
112. Console, L. and M. Scalise, *extracellular vesicles and cell pathways involved in cancer chemoresistance.* Life (Basel), 2022. **12**(5).
113. Mostafazadeh, M., et al., *Potential roles and prognostic significance of exosomes in cancer drug resistance.* Cell and Bioscience, 2021. **11**(1): p. 1–15.
114. Vasan, N., J. Baselga, and D.M. Hyman, *A view on drug resistance in cancer.* Nature, 2019. **575**(7782): p. 299–309.
115. Shomar, A., O. Barak, and N. Brenner, *Cancer progression as a learning process.* iScience, 2022. **25**(3): p. 103924.
116. Kelderman, S., T.N. Schumacher, and J.B. Haanen, *Acquired and intrinsic resistance in cancer immunotherapy.* Molecular Oncology, 2014. **8**(6): p. 1132–1139.
117. Li, J., et al., *The emerging role of exosomes in cancer chemoresistance.* Frontiers in Cell and Developmental Biology, 2021. **9**: p. 2985.
118. Bukowski, K., M. Kciuk, and R. Kontek, *Mechanisms of multidrug resistance in cancer chemotherapy.* International Journal of Molecular Sciences, 2020. **21**(9): p. 3233.
119. Zhang, Z., et al., *Exosomal transfer of long non-coding RNA SBF2-AS1 enhances chemoresistance to temozolomide in glioblastoma.* Journal of Experimental & Clinical Cancer Research, 2019. **38**(1): p. 166.

120. Ren, J., et al., *Carcinoma-associated fibroblasts promote the stemness and chemoresistance of colorectal cancer by transferring exosomal lncRNA H19.* Theranostics, 2018. **8**(14): p. 3932–3948.
121. Gao, Q., et al., *Exosomal lncRNA UCA1 from cancer-associated fibroblasts enhances chemoresistance in vulvar squamous cell carcinoma cells.* Journal of Obstetrics and Gynaecology Research, 2021. **47**(1): p. 73–87.
122. Tong, Y., et al., *Tumor-secreted exosomal lncRNA POU3F3 promotes cisplatin resistance in ESCC by inducing fibroblast differentiation into CAFs.* Molecular Therapy — Oncolytics, 2020. **18**: p. 1–13.
123. Doss, S., J. Robertson, and J. Adam, *Lapatinib or trastuzumab in combination with an aromatase inhibitor for first-line treatment of metastatic hormone-receptor-positive breast cancer that overexpresses HER2.* Health Technology Assessment, 2012. **13**(8): p. 766–767.
124. Molina, M.A., et al., *Trastuzumab (herceptin), a humanized anti-Her2 receptor monoclonal antibody, inhibits basal and activated Her2 ectodomain cleavage in breast cancer cells.* Cancer Research, 2001. **61**(12): p. 4744–4749.
125. Zheng, Z., et al., *Increased expression of exosomal AGAP2-AS1 (AGAP2 antisense RNA 1) in breast cancer cells inhibits trastuzumab-induced cell cytotoxicity.* Medical Science Monitor, 2019. **25**: p. 2211–2220.
126. Wang, X., et al., *Exosomal lncRNA HEIH promotes cisplatin resistance in tongue squamous cell carcinoma via targeting miR-3619-5p/HDGF axis.* Acta Histochemica, 2020. **122**(8): p. 151647.
127. Dasari, S. and P.B. Tchounwou, *Cisplatin in cancer therapy: Molecular mechanisms of action.* European Journal of Pharmacology, 2014. **740**: p. 364–378.
128. Ghosh, S., *Cisplatin: The first metal based anticancer drug.* Bio-organic Chemistry, 2019. **88**: p. 102925.
129. Fang, Z., et al., *LncRNA UCA1 promotes proliferation and cisplatin resistance of oral squamous cell carcinoma by sunppressing miR-184 expression.* Cancer Medicine, 2017. **6**(12): p. 2897–2908.
130. Ge, P., et al., *LncRNA SNHG1 contributes to the cisplatin resistance and progression of NSCLC via miR-330-5p/DCLK1 axis.* Experimental and Molecular Pathology, 2021. **120**: p. 104633.

131. Wu, Y., et al., *LncRNA WDFY3-AS2 promotes cisplatin resistance and the cancer stem cell in ovarian cancer by regulating hsa-miR-139-5p/SDC4 axis.* Cancer Cell International, 2021. **21**(1): p. 284.
132. Luo, X., et al., *Exosomal lncRNA HNF1A-AS1 affects cisplatin resistance in cervical cancer cells through regulating microRNA-34b/TUFT1 axis.* Cancer Cell International, 2019. **19**: p. 323.
133. Domvri, K., et al., *Exosomal lncRNA PCAT-1 promotes Kras-associated chemoresistance via immunosuppressive miR-182/miR-217 signaling and p27/CDK6 regulation.* Oncotarget, 2020. **11**(29): p. 2847–2862.
134. Wang, Z., et al., *Induction of m(6)A methylation in adipocyte exosomal LncRNAs mediates myeloma drug resistance.* Journal of Experimental & Clinical Cancer Research, 2022. **41**(1): p. 4.
135. Tian, Y., et al., *MiRNAs in radiotherapy resistance of nasopharyngeal carcinoma.* Journal of Cancer, 2020. **11**(13): p. 3976.
136. Xiao, J. and X. He, *Involvement of non-coding RNAs in chemo- and radioresistance of nasopharyngeal carcinoma.* Cancer Management and Research, 2021. **13**: p. 8781–8794.
137. Gao, W., M. Qiao, and K. Luo, *Long noncoding RNA TP53TG1 contributes to radioresistance of glioma cells via miR-524-5p/RAB5A axis.* Cancer Biother Radiopharm, 2021. **36**(7): p. 600–612.
138. Zhu, C., et al., *RBM5-AS1 promotes radioresistance in medulloblastoma through stabilization of SIRT6 protein.* Acta Neuropathologica Communications, 2021. **9**(1): p. 123.
139. Zhang, F., et al., *M2 macrophage-derived exosomal long non-coding RNA AGAP2-AS1 enhances radiotherapy immunity in lung cancer by reducing microRNA-296 and elevating NOTCH2.* Cell Death & Disease, 2021. **12**(5): p. 467.
140. Ding, X.Z., et al., *Serum exosomal lncRNA DLX6-AS1 is a promising biomarker for prognosis prediction of cervical cancer.* Technology in Cancer Research & Treatment, 2021. **20**: p. 1533033821990060.
141. Guo, Y., et al., *Appraising the value of serum and serum-derived exosomal LncRNA-EXOC7 as a promising biomarker in cervical cancer.* Clinical Laboratory, 2020. **66**(7).
142. Tao, Y., et al., *Exploration of serum exosomal LncRNA TBILA and AGAP2-AS1 as promising biomarkers for diagnosis of non-small cell lung*

cancer. International Journal of Biological Sciences, 2020. **16**(3): p. 471–482.

143. Li, C., et al., *Tumor-derived exosomal lncRNA GAS5 as a biomarker for early-stage non-small-cell lung cancer diagnosis.* Journal of Cellular Physiology, 2019. **234**(11): p. 20721–20727.
144. Liu, T., et al., *Exosomal long noncoding RNA CRNDE-h as a novel serum-based biomarker for diagnosis and prognosis of colorectal cancer.* Oncotarget, 2016. 7(51): p. 85551–85563.
145. Zhou, H., et al., *Circulating exosomal long non-coding RNA H19 as a potential novel diagnostic and prognostic biomarker for gastric cancer.* Journal of International Medical Research, 2020. **48**(7): p. 300060520934297.
146. Min, L., et al., *Exosomal LncRNA RP5-977B1 as a novel minimally invasive biomarker for diagnosis and prognosis in non-small cell lung cancer.* International Journal of Clinical Oncology, 2022. **27**(6): p. 1013–1024.
147. Li, W., et al., *Exosomal FMR1-AS1 facilitates maintaining cancer stem-like cell dynamic equilibrium via TLR7/NFκB/c-Myc signaling in female esophageal carcinoma.* Molecular Cancer, 2019. **18**(1): p. 22.
148. Jiang, Y., et al., *Exosomal long noncoding RNA HOXD-AS1 promotes prostate cancer metastasis via miR-361-5p/FOXM1 axis.* Cell Death & Disease, 2021. **12**(12): p. 1129.
149. Lin, L.Y., et al., *Tumor-originated exosomal lncUEGC1 as a circulating biomarker for early-stage gastric cancer.* Molecular Cancer, 2018. **17**(1): p. 84.
150. Na-Er, A., et al., *Upregulation of serum exosomal SUMO1P3 predicts unfavorable prognosis in triple negative breast cancer.* European Review of Medical and Pharmacological Sciences, 2021. **25**(1): p. 154–160.
151. Qiu, J.J., et al., *Exosomal metastasis-associated lung adenocarcinoma transcript 1 promotes angiogenesis and predicts poor prognosis in epithelial ovarian cancer.* International Journal of Biological Sciences, 2018. **14**(14): p. 1960–1973.
152. Han, P., J. Zhao, and L. Gao, *Increased serum exosomal long non-coding RNA SNHG15 expression predicts poor prognosis in non-small cell lung cancer.* Journal of Clinical Laboratory Analysis, 2021. **35**(11): p. e23979.

https://doi.org/10.1142/9789811267390_0009

Chapter 9

Circular RNAs (circRNAs) in cancer proliferation: Molecular interactions and possible therapeutic targets

Sepideh Mirzaei[1], Maryam Majidinia[2], Sima Orouei[3], Vihan Moodi[4], Shokooh Salimimoghadam[5], Maliheh Entezari[6,7], Kiavash Hushmandi[8]*, Zhaowu Ma[9] and Lingzhi Wang[10,11]

[1]*Department of Biology, Faculty of Science, Islamic Azad University, Science and Research Branch, Tehran, Iran*
[2]*Solid Tumor Research Center, Urmia University of Medical Sciences, Urmia, Iran*
[3]*Department of Biology, Science and Research Branch, Islamic Azad University, Tehran, Iran*
[4]*School of Medicine, Tehran University of Medical Sciences, Tehran, Iran*
[5]*Department of Biochemistry and Molecular Biology, Faculty of Veterinary Medicine, Shahid Chamran University of Ahvaz, Ahvaz, Iran*
[6]*Farhikhtegan Medical Convergence Sciences Research Center, Farhikhtegan Hospital Tehran Medical Sciences, Islamic Azad University, Tehran, Iran*
[7]*Department of Genetics, Faculty of Advanced Science and Technology, Tehran Medical Sciences, Islamic Azad University, Tehran, Iran*
[8]*Department of Food Hygiene and Quality Control, Division of Epidemiology & Zoonoses, Faculty of Veterinary Medicine, University of Tehran, Tehran, Iran*

*Corresponding author: Kiavash Hushmandi, Department of Food Hygiene and Quality Control, Division of Epidemiology & Zoonoses, Faculty of Veterinary Medicine, University of Tehran, Tehran, Iran, Email: houshmandi.kia7@ut.ac.ir

[9]*School of Basic Medicine, Health Science Center, Yangtze University, Hubei, China*
[10]*Department of Pharmacology, Yong Loo Lin School of Medicine, National University of Singapore, Singapore*
[11]*Cancer Science Institute of Singapore, National University of Singapore, Singapore*

Abstract

Circular RNAs (circRNAs) are a member of non-coding RNA transcripts that do not encode proteins, but they exert important biological functions in cells such as regulation of proliferation, migration, differentiation, cell cycle progression, cell death mechanisms, and autophagy. circRNAs have high stability and are reliable biomarkers due to their structure and resistance to degradation by RNase enzymes. circRNA dysregulation has been implicated in disease pathogenesis, especially in cancer. circRNAs affect molecular pathways to regulate the progression of tumor cells and their targeting is important in the treatment of cancer patients. This chapter emphasizes the role of circRNAs in affecting proliferation of tumor cells via regulating apoptosis mechanism, autophagy machinery, and glucose metabolism with a focus on related molecular pathways to pave the way for the development of novel therapeutics for cancer patients.

1. Introduction

A serious public health problem that is a major reason of death in recent years is cancer [1]. This complicated and multifactorial disease is caused by a variety of factors including genetic and epigenetic alterations [2–4]. Changes in genes and related signaling networks not only provide insights toward cancer therapy but also pave the way for cancer diagnosis [5–7]. One of the hot topics in recent years has been epigenetic changes in cancer. Based on the data from human genome sequencing, up to 98% of the genome is formed by non-coding genes [8]. The transcripts of such genes do not have the ability in protein coding and they are known as non-coding RNA (ncRNA) molecules [9, 10]. Although ncRNAs are one of the hot topics in the recent decade, they were first considered as transcriptional by-products [11]. The development and emergence of high-throughput sequencing technology have been beneficial in identifying many ncRNAs, and this family includes microRNAs (miRNAs), long non-coding RNAs (lncRNAs), and circular RNAs (circRNAs) [12–14]. circRNA is considered as a single-stranded RNA molecule that has been covalently closed lacking 5′-end caps or 3′-end poly (A) tails [15]. Non-canonical splicing is involved in the generation of circRNAs from its precursor mRNA [16]. The first identification of circRNAs occurred in 1976, and it was discovered in the virus [17]. However, it was first considered as a by-product of splicing error with no function in cells [18, 19]. With respect to the unique structure of circRNAs that are covalently closed loops, their expression level appears to be higher compared to linear mRNA and miRNAs and other RNA molecules in blood, plasma, and platelets. The half-life of circRNAs is suggested to be higher and due to their resistance to degradation by RNase enzymes, they are more detectable compared to other linear RNA molecules. Therefore, they can be used as ideal candidates for disease diagnosis [20, 21]. Gene expression level regulation and protein activity are also regulated by circRNAs in physiological and pathological conditions [22]. Growing evidence has shown an association of circRNAs with various diseases including lupus erythematosus [23], diabetes mellitus [24], neurological diseases [25], liver diseases [26], and cancer [27].

There are three major kinds of circRNAs including exonic circRNAs, intronic circRNAs, and exon-intron circRNAs, and most of the circRNAs are exonic circRNAs [28]. circRNAs have four important features that make them different from others including multiplicity, abundant expression, stability, and conservation. Multiplicity is defined as the fact that different genes can encode various circRNAs with different exons and introns; due to the unique structures of circRNAs, their stability is high and for instance, they make up 14% of transcribed genes in fibroblasts; Finally, in mammals, circRNAs demonstrate higher sequence conservation compared to others [29–33]. circRNAs demonstrate great biological activities and they are important players in the clinical course. circRNAs can directly regulate the expression level of genes or they can interact with micromolecules to affect biological mechanisms. miRNA sponging, protein interaction, gene expression regulation, and translation template are among the mechanisms regulated by circRNAs [34] (Figure 1).

In recent years, circRNAs have obtained much attention in the treatment of cancer and their interaction with other signaling

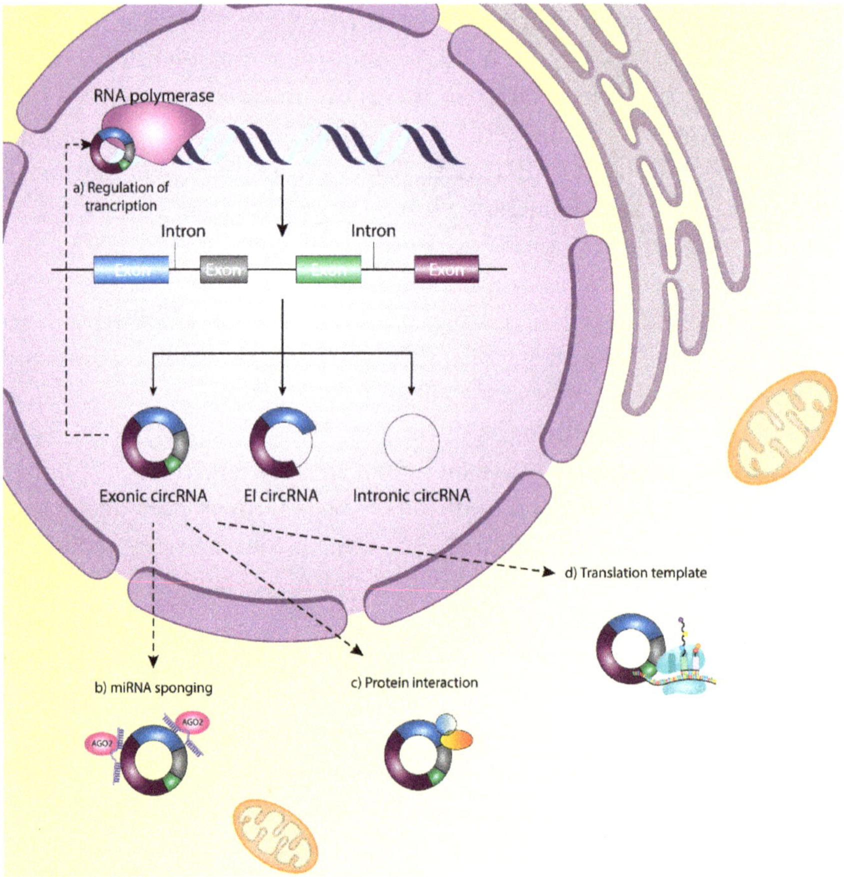

Figure 1. The process of circRNA biogenesis and a summary of their action in cells.

networks has been highlighted. These RNA molecules can affect both oncogenic and onco-suppressor factors in cancer cells. Furthermore, they can have both tumor suppressor and tumor-promoting functions in tumors and that is context-dependent. Even in a certain type of cancer, a circRNA may demonstrate dual functions, complicating the process of cancer treatment. Both molecular pathways and mechanisms are tightly regulated by circRNAs and in following sections of this chapter, it is highlighted how circRNAs affect apoptosis, autophagy, and other factors related to the proliferation of cancer cells.

2. circRNAs in apoptosis regulation

Tissue formation and structuring, embryogenesis, immune system function, and damaged cell destruction are regulated by programmed cell death in physiological conditions [35]. Although a number of programmed cell death mechanisms have been identified, apoptosis is the most well-known and best-studied one that is based on the activation of caspase cascade in the elimination of cells [36]. The pathogen-invaded cells can be eliminated by apoptosis, and this mechanism is also involved in suppressing malignant cells and affecting immune cells. Two distinct pathways including intrinsic and extrinsic pathways of apoptosis can induce activation of the caspase cascade [37, 38]. Apoptosis is regulated and controlled by cellular proteins and signal transduction cascades. There are two kinds of apoptotic proteins including pro- and anti-apoptotic proteins. Caspases are pro-apoptotic proteins, while Bcl-2 family is anti-apoptotic protein [39]. Caspases are members of the cysteine protease family with 14 proteins that include inflammatory, effector, and initiator caspases. Bcl-2 family proteins are localized in outer membrane of mitochondria, and they include a large number of proteins, such as Bax, Bak, Bad, Bid, Bcl-2, and Bcl-xL [40–42]. The extrinsic pathway of apoptosis is based on attachment of apoptosis-inducing ligands to death receptors on surface of cells, while intrinsic pathway of apoptosis occurs by a number of signals such as DNA damage, and other stimuli such as exposure to chemical agents [43–45]. Figure 2 schematically depicts apoptosis mechanism in cells.

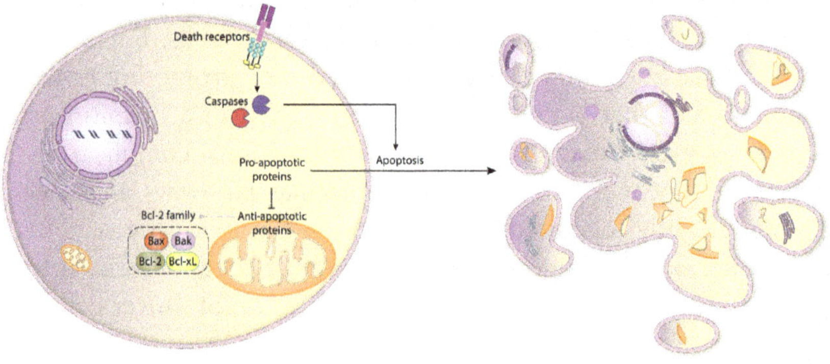

Figure 2. A schematic representation of apoptosis mechanism. Based on this figure, apoptosis can occur due to two pathways including mitochondrial pathway and death receptors that activate caspase cascade.

circRNAs regulate the progression of tumor cells by affecting apoptosis. circSEPT9 shows overexpression in triple-negative breast cancer and shows a positive association with unfavorable prognosis and advanced clinical stage. circSEPT9 promotes LIF expression via miR-637 sponging to induce STAT3 signaling in enhancing cancer progression. Notably, the expression level and biogenesis of circSETP9 enhance by E2F1 and EIF4A3 in breast tumor cells, Silencing circSEPT9 stimulates apoptosis and impairs proliferation of breast cancer cells [46]. The strategy of circRNAs in preventing apoptosis and increasing tumor progression is based on the activation of oncogenic signaling networks. Wnt/β-catenin signaling activation prevents apoptosis and increases hepatocellular carcinoma progression. It has been demonstrated that hsa-circRNA-104348 is able to promote progression of hepatocellular carcinoma and for this purpose, it stimulates Wnt/β-catenin signaling to increase tumor proliferation and to mediate resistance to apoptosis [47]. The nuclear translocation of β-catenin is vital for oncogenesis. On nuclear translocation, β-catenin stimulates the expression of oncogenic factors and interacts with TCF3, TCF4, and LEF1. circ-102171 negatively interacts with CTNNBIP1 to activate β-catenin signaling in enhancing thyroid cancer progression. Silencing circ-102171 stimulates apoptosis in cancer cells via inactivation of Wnt signaling [48].

The proliferation of cancer cells and apoptosis have a close association. Preventing apoptosis paves the way for the increase in proliferation rate of tumor cells. circ-UBAP2 has been implicated in increasing the progression of ovarian cancer cells. circ-UBAP2 upregulates PRPF8 expression via miR-382-5p inhibition to increase the proliferation rate of ovarian cancer cells via apoptosis inhibition [49]. Downregulation of such oncogenic factors stimulates apoptosis in tumor cells and significantly reduces their survival rate. For instance, the expression level of circFNDC3B enhances in esophageal cancer tissues and its silencing is associated with apoptosis induction and a decrease in the proliferation of tumor cells [50]. The impact of circRNAs in apoptosis in cancers is attributed to their capacity in regulating miRNA expression. circ-000166 has been implicated in increasing colorectal cancer progression. By sponging miR-326, circ-000166 increases LASP1 expression to prevent apoptosis and increase abnormal growth of colorectal tumor cells [51]. A similar strategy also occurs in esophageal cancer. circ-0004370 shows overexpression in esophageal cancer cells and tissues, and it is vital for aberrant growth and apoptosis inhibition in tumor cells. circ-0004370 promotes COL1A1 expression via miR-1301-3p inhibition to enhance esophageal cancer proliferation and to prevent apoptosis in tumor cells [52]. Although a majority of studies have focused on oncogenic circRNAs, it appears that restoring the expression level of onco-suppressor circRNAs can pave the way for apoptosis induction in tumor cells. Expression level of circ-0001776 and its downstream target LRIG2 decreases in endometrial cancer, while miR-182 as oncogenic factor shows overexpression. Overexpression of circ-0001776 stimulates apoptosis and impairs proliferation of tumor cells via miR-182 inhibition to increase the expression level of LRIG2 [53]. Therefore, circRNA/apoptosis axis is an important and promising target in cancer therapy.

3. circRNAs in autophagy regulation

Autophagy is defined as a conserved homeostasis mechanism vital for the degradation of various cargo, including proteins, organelles, and pathogens [54]. The survival of cells enhances by autophagy during environmental stresses, but it may result in cell death [55]. Targeting autophagy has been a promising approach in the treatment of cancer, inducing cell death, impairing proliferation and invasion of tumor cells, and enhancing therapy sensitivity of cancer cells [56]. A wide variety of molecular pathways are involved in the regulation of autophagy, such as STAT3, Wnt/β-catenin, and miRNAs [57], but the most well-known regulators of autophagy are ATGs, beclin-1, AMPK, and mTOR pathways [56, 58, 59]. Figure 3 schematically represents the autophagy mechanism in cells.

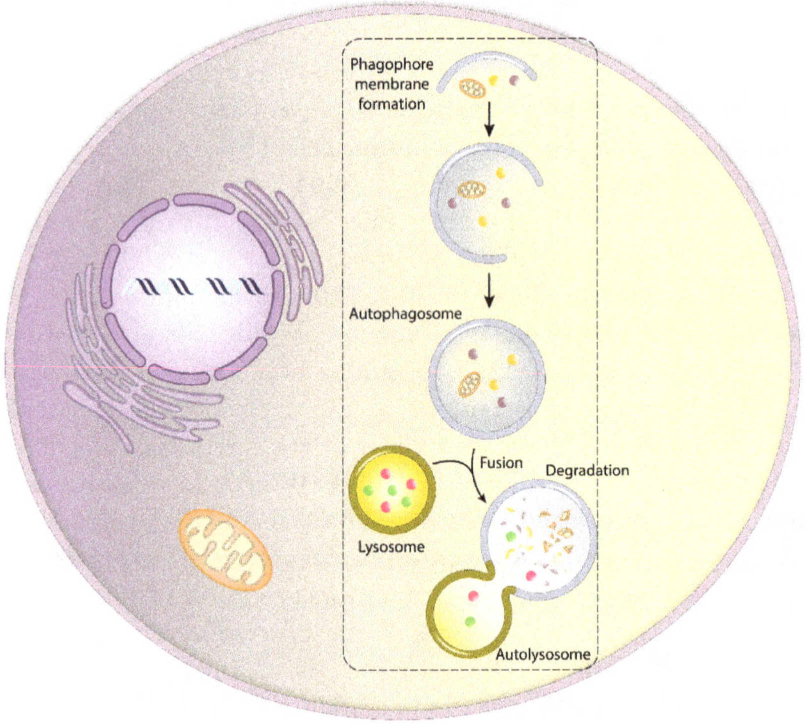

Figure 3. A schematic representation of autophagy mechanism in cells.

The regulation of autophagy by circRNAs affects the progression of tumor cells. The expression level of circ-LRP6 demonstrates an increase in oral cancer and silencing circ-LRP6 impairs autophagy in tumor cells. circ-LRP6 increases LCB levels and decreases p62 expression in inducing autophagy and increasing progression of oral tumor cells [60]. The induction of pro-survival autophagy occurs by oncogenic circRNAs in increasing tumor progression, and it has been shown that circ-EEF2 impedes miR-6881-3p expression to increase expression levels of ATG5 and ATG7 in triggering autophagy to promote growth and metastasis of ovarian tumor cells [61]. In addition to the association with proliferation and invasion of cancer cells, circRNA/autophagy axis can affect therapy response. hsa-circ-0092276 is involved in increasing the proliferation rate of breast tumor cells and mediating doxorubicin resistance. circ-0092276 promotes the expression level of ATG7 via miR-348 sponging to stimulate autophagy for purpose of doxorubicin resistance in breast cancer [62].

Gastric cancer is at the fifth place in causing cancer-related death in patients [63, 64]. The survival rate and prognosis of gastric cancer patients have been improved using chemotherapy, radiotherapy, endoscopy, and serology [65, 66]. One of the most well-known anticancer agents in the treatment of gastric tumors is cisplatin [67]. However, when tumor cells are exposed to cisplatin, they obtain acquired drug resistance due to the activation of oncogenic pathways and resistance to apoptosis [68, 69]. circ-PVT1 has been implicated in cisplatin resistance in gastric cancer. circ-PVT1 promotes YAP1 expression via miR-30a-5p downregulation to induce pro-survival autophagy in preventing apoptosis and mediating cisplatin resistance in gastric cancer [70].

For in vivo, it has been shown that circRNA-mediated pro-survival autophagy induction participates in enhancing tumor growth in xenografts. Furthermore, circRNAs inducing autophagy can prevent senescence in cancer cells and provide a condition for growth [71]. One of the urological cancers responsible for high death among men is prostate cancer, and radiation therapy has been considered as one of the therapeutic modalities for this disease. circ-CCNB2 shows overexpression in irradiation-resistant prostate tumor cells and by miR-30b-5p inhibition, it increases the expression level of KIF18A to induce autophagy in triggering radio-resistance [72]. It appears that the capacity of autophagy in triggering drug resistance is due to preventing apoptosis in cancer cells. hsa-circ-0085131 functions as competing endogenous RNA (ceRNA) for miR-654-5p inhibition to upregulate ATG7 in triggering autophagy and subsequent cisplatin resistance in lung cancer [73]. Based on these studies, circRNA/autophagy axis is vital for the progression of tumor cells [74–76]. However, future studies should also focus on pro-death autophagy and its regulation by circRNAs in cancer.

4. circRNAs in cancer cell glycolysis

Otto Warburg made a vital discovery in the field of tumor metabolism, and it was shown that in spite of the presence of oxygen, tumor cells prefer to use glucose and generate lactate for providing their energy [77]. Warburg suggested a cancer cell–centric model in which carcinogenesis is based on disruption and interference of mitochondrial electron transport chain, and it is shared among various tumor types [78]. However, one of the challenges was that tumor microenvironment comprised both normal and cancer cells, and it failed to identify duality of metabolic demands. It has been shown that metabolic reprogramming is vital for immune cell fates. Metabolic networks have been shown to be associated with immune cell–mediated tumor removal [79]. Cancer cells show high proliferation rate and this rapid dividing requires high amount of energy. Therefore, cancer cells increase their glucose metabolism to meet their biosynthetic demands [80]. Although the volume of ATP production during glycolysis is suggested to be low, these changes in metabolism are vital for pathways of de novo lipid, nucleotide, and amino acid synthesis. This is vital for the proliferation of cancer cells, dysregulation of cell cycle, and activation of immune cells [77]. The final aim of glycolysis is to change metabolism from oxidative phosphorylation to glucose metabolism in increasing tumor progression and malignancy [81]. The glucose membrane transporters and enzymes including hexokinase 2, phosphofructokinase 1, and pyruvate kinase 2 are involved in regulating glycolysis in cells [82]. Increasing evidence has shown the

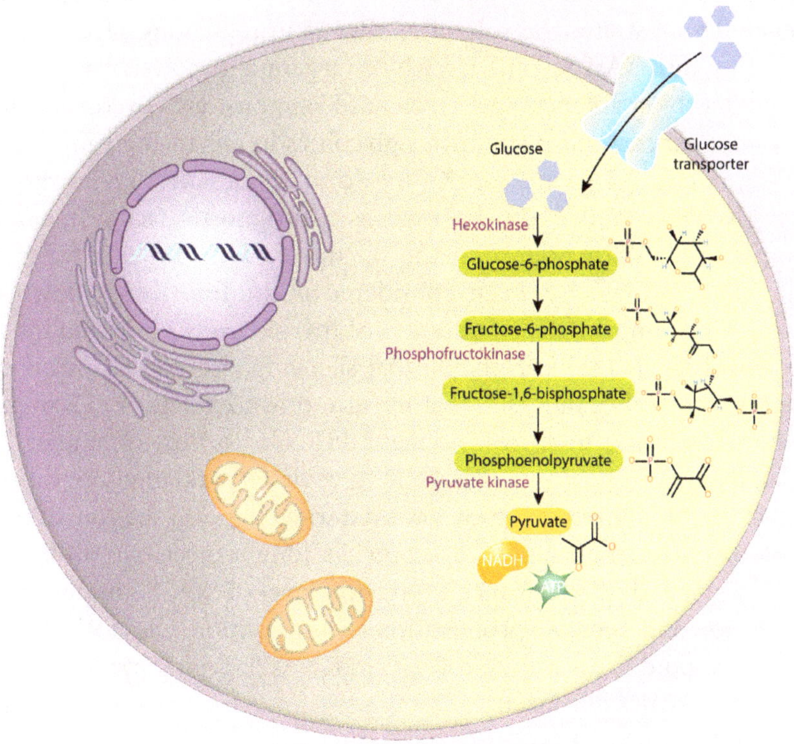

Figure 4. Glycolysis and related mechanisms in cells.

role of glycolysis in enhancing the progression of tumor cells [83, 84]. Figure 4 provides a schematic representation of glycolysis.

circ-ENO1 shows overexpression in lung cancer, and it is vital for the induction of glycolysis. It has been shown that circ-ENO1 functions as ceRNA to reduce miR-22-3p expression in upregulating ENO1 to stimulate glycolysis and enhance lung cancer proliferation [85]. The activation of aerobic glycolysis has been implicated in increasing the progression of triple-negative breast cancer cells. circ-PDCD11 mediates poor prognosis in breast cancer patients, and it increases glucose uptake, lactate production, ATP formation, and extracellular acidification rate. circ-PDCD11 promotes LDHA expression via miR-432-5p inhibition in increasing breast cancer progression by glycolysis induction [86]. First of all, increasing evidence demonstrates the role of circRNAs in regulating glycolysis by affecting miRNAs. Second, circRNAs targeting glycolysis can be considered as biomarkers in cancer. circYY1 demonstrates overexpression in breast cancer, and it stimulates glycolysis in enhancing tumor progression. circYY1 sponges miR-769-3p to upregulate YY1 in triggering glycolysis, and it can be used as a prognostic factor in breast cancer [87]. With respect to the oncogenic function of circRNAs, their knock-down has been considered in studies. Knock-down of circ-PRKCI impairs the progression of thyroid cancer cells and inhibits glycolysis. It has been shown that silencing circ-PRKCI promotes expression level of miR-335 that in turn, downregulates E2F3 in glycolysis inhibition in thyroid cancer [88]. Up to 90% of studies are related to oncogenic circRNAs in glycolysis regulation in cancer. However, an interesting study has shed some light on the role of circ-0006677 as onco-suppressor factor in lung cancer. circ-0006677 sponges miR-578 to enhance expression level of SOCS2 in glycolysis inhibition and decrease proliferation of lung tumor cells [89]. Future studies should focus on the role of circRNAs in regulating glycolysis-related enzymes in cancers.

5. circRNAs with oncogenic function

Previous sections demonstrated the role of circRNAs in regulating tumor proliferation via affecting related mechanisms such as apoptosis, autophagy, and glycolysis. This section briefly discusses some of the newly recognized circRNAs that can enhance the proliferation of tumor cells. circ-ACACA drives progression of cervical cancer cells by affecting miR-582-5p/ERO1A axis. It has been shown that circ-ACACA overexpression is in favor of proliferation, metastasis, and glycolysis in cervical tumor cells. circ-ACACA promotes ERO1A expression by miR-582-5p downregulation [90]. The ability of circRNAs in affecting the promoter of miRNAs has been associated with regulating the progression of tumor cells. circ-POLA2 mediates methylation of miR-31 promoter to enhance the proliferation rate of endometrial tumor cells [91]. One of the features of tumor cells is their stemness that can be considered as a supporter for their progression and also provide therapy resistance. It has been reported that hsa-circ-0003222 elevates PHF21B expression via miR-527 sponging to increase the stemness and progression of lung tumor cells. Silencing circ-0003222 increases sensitivity of lung tumor cells to anti-programmed death-ligand 1-based immunotherapy in vivo [92]. Based on the studies, three major arms are vital for the abnormal progression of tumors, including growth, metastasis, and angiogenesis. It has been shown that circ-0000467 sponges miR-4766-5p to increase the expression level of KLF12 in promoting proliferation and invasion of colorectal tumor cells as well as triggering angiogenesis in improving tumor malignancy [93]. Since a high number of oncogenic circRNAs involved in tumor progression have been identified, studies have focused on reducing their expression for cancer therapy. For instance, silencing circ-BIRC6 [94] or circ-0000517 [95] is associated with a significant diminution in the growth, invasion, and glucose metabolism of tumor cells.

6. circRNAs with onco-suppressor function

Although growing evidence has focused on the role of oncogenic circRNAs in cancer, there are also attempts in the identification of onco-suppressor circRNAs. Radiation mainly stimulates DNA damage in mediating cell death and impairing the progression of tumor cells. In some cases, chemotherapy agents can also induce DNA damage. Therefore, conventional therapies stimulate DNA damage in decreasing survival and progression of cancer cells; however, DNA damage repair mechanisms can prevent cytotoxicity of these therapies and mediate resistance. circSMARCA5 has been involved in impairing DNA damage repair via interacting with host gene. Restoring the expression level of circSMARCA5 promotes chemosensitivity of breast tumor cells in vitro and in vivo. circSMARCA5 is capable of generating an R-loop to induce transcriptional pause at exon 15 of SMARCA5 for preventing DNA damage repair and increasing the cytotoxicity of drugs against breast tumor cells [96]. The onco-suppressor circRNAs are capable of decreasing proliferation and metastasis of tumor cells. This capacity is obtained via interacting with complicated signaling networks that are core regulators of tumor progression. circ-cRAPGEF5 decreases the growth and migration of renal cancer cells. For this purpose, circ-cRAPGEF5 sponges miR-27a-3p to upregulate TXNIP in restraining renal cancer progression [97].

Colorectal cancer is one of the invasive and malignant diseases of gastrointestinal tumors, and autophagy has been shown to play a significant role in its progression. Autophagy induction during hypoxia is in favor of increasing the progression of colorectal tumor cells [98]. Furthermore, autophagy inhibition is beneficial in enhancing apoptosis during hypoxia in colorectal cancer [99]. The ability of SOX2 in triggering epithelial–mesenchymal transition (EMT), drug resistance, and promoting stemness in colorectal cancer is attributed to the induction of beclin-1/autophagy axis [100]. An interesting experiment has shown that circ-103948 promotes the expression level of TPT1 via miR-1236-3p sponging to suppress autophagy in impairing the progression of colorectal tumor cells [101]. On the other hand, stimulation of PI3K/Akt signaling significantly increases the progression of gastric tumor cells. hsa-circ-100269 inhibits PI3K/Akt signaling to induce apoptosis, G0/G1 cell cycle arrest and to impair proliferation and metastasis of gastric cancer cells [102]. Table 1 provides a summary of circRNAs involved in regulating the progression of tumor cells.

7. Conclusion and remarks

The abnormal proliferation of cancer cells depends on different factors, and the best strategy is to target the main factor responsible for tumor growth instead of affecting a certain type of mechanism or molecular pathway. For instance, it is true that activation of pro-survival autophagy can increase the growth of cancer cells, but only targeting autophagy is not effective in the complete eradication of tumors. The purpose of this chapter was to show that circRNAs are among the main regulators of cancer proliferation and they can be targeted for effective cancer therapy. The overexpression of oncogenic

Table 1. circRNAs and related molecular pathways in regulating tumor progression.

Cancer Type	circRNA	Molecular Pathway	Remark(s)	Ref
Ovarian cancer	circ-100395	miR-1228/ p53/EMT	circ-100395 reduces miR-12228 expression to inhibit EMT and increase p53 expression in impairing tumor progression.	[103]
Glioma	circ-ITCH	miR-106a-5p/ SASH1	circ-ITCH promotes SASH1 expression by miR-106a-5p sponging to reduce the growth and invasion of tumor cells.	[104]
Lung adenocarcinoma	circ-0018414	miR-6807-3p/ DKK1	Decrease in proliferation and stemness. Apoptosis induction. circ-0018414 promotes DKK1 expression via miR-6807-3p sponging.	[105]
Prostate cancer	circ-UCK2	miR-767-5p/ TET1	circ-UCK2 sponges miR-767-5p to enhance TET1 expression in decreasing metastasis and growth of tumor cells.	[106]
Cervical cancer	circ-0000730	miR-942-3p/ PTEN	Limiting growth and invasion of tumor cells. circ-0000730 induces PTEN signaling via miR-942-3p sponging.	[107]
Colorectal cancer	circ-RNF121	miR-1224-5p/ FOXM1	Overexpression of circ-RNF121 and FOXM1, and downregulation of miR-1224-5p in cancer. Increasing progression and glucose metabolism in tumor cells.	[108]
Gastric cancer	circ-000423	miR-582-3p/ DIXDC1	Increase in proliferation and metastasis of tumor cells. circ-000423 promotes DIXDC1 expression via miR-582-3p sponging.	[109]

(*Continued*)

Table 1. (*Continued*)

Cancer Type	circRNA	Molecular Pathway	Remark(s)	Ref
Colorectal cancer	circ-0087862	miR-142-3p/ BACH1	Increase in the progression of colorectal tumor cells by circ-0087862 via miR-142-3p sponging and subsequent overexpression of BACH1.	[110]
Colorectal cancer	circ-0006174	miR-142-3p	Preventing apoptosis and increasing growth and invasion of tumor cells by circ-0006174 via miR-142-3p sponging.	[111]
Breast cancer	circ-0103552	miR-515-5p/ CYR61	Enhanced growth and invasion of tumor cells by circ-0103552 via miR-515-5p sponging and upregulating CYR61 expression.	[112]
Colorectal cancer	circ-0062682	miR-940/ PHGDH	Increased serine metabolism and cancer proliferation. circ-0062682 promotes PHGDH expression via miR-940 sponging.	[113]
Non-small cell lung cancer	circ-100565	miR-337-3p/ ADAM28	Apoptosis inhibition and cisplatin resistance. circ-100565 promotes ADAM28 expression via miR-337-3p sponging.	[114]
Cervical cancer	hsa-circ-0001400	miR-326	Silencing circ-0001400 promotes apoptosis in tumor cells preventing sponging of miR-326.	[115]

circRNAs prevents apoptosis and induce pro-survival autophagy in enhancing the survival of tumor cells and growth rate. Glucose metabolism, lactate production, and glycolysis enhance by circRNAs in promoting proliferation of tumor cells. Silencing oncogenic circRNAs or restoring the expression level of onco-suppressor circRNAs can be used in cancer therapy.

Conflict of interest:

The authors declare no conflict of interest.

References

1. Xue, C., et al., *The functional roles of the circRNA/Wnt axis in cancer.* Molecular Cancer, 2022. **21**(1): p. 108.
2. Zhou, S., A.E. Treloar, and M. Lupien, *Emergence of the noncoding cancer genome: A target of genetic and epigenetic alterations.* The Noncoding Cancer Genome, 2016. **6**(11): p. 1215–1229.
3. Morel, D., et al., *Combining epigenetic drugs with other therapies for solid tumours — past lessons and future promise.* Nature Reviews. Clinical Oncology, 2020. **17**(2): p. 91–107.
4. Van Der Pol, Y. and F. Mouliere, *Toward the early detection of cancer by decoding the epigenetic and environmental fingerprints of cell-free DNA.* Cancer Cell, 2019. **36**(4): p. 350–368.
5. Calses, P.C., et al., *Hippo pathway in cancer: aberrant regulation and therapeutic opportunities.* Trends in Cancer, 2019. **5**(5): p. 297–307.
6. Pópulo, H., J.M. Lopes, and P. Soares, *The mTOR signalling pathway in human cancer.* International Journal of Molecular Sciences, 2012. **13**(2): p. 1886–1918.
7. Dhillon, A.S., et al., *MAP kinase signalling pathways in cancer.* Oncogene, 2007. **26**(22): p. 3279–3290.
8. Engreitz, J.M., et al., *Local regulation of gene expression by lncRNA promoters, transcription and splicing.* Nature, 2016. **539**(7629): p. 452–455.
9. Matsui, M. and D.R. Corey, *Non-coding RNAs as drug targets.* Nature Reviews. Drug Discovery, 2017. **16**(3): p. 167–179.

10. Li, G., et al., *Long noncoding RNA GAS8-AS1: A novel biomarker in human diseases.* Biomedicine & Pharmacotherapy, 2021. **139**: p. 111572.
11. Anastasiadou, E., L.S. Jacob, and F.J. Slack, *Non-coding RNA networks in cancer.* Nature Reviews. Cancer. 2018. **18**(1): p. 5–18.
12. Beermann, J., et al., *Non-coding RNAs in development and disease: Background, mechanisms, and therapeutic approaches.* Physiological Reviews, 2016. **96**(4): p. 1297–1325.
13. Zhu, K.-P., et al., *Analyzing the interactions of mRNAs and ncRNAs to predict competing endogenous RNA networks in osteosarcoma chemo-resistance.* Molecular Therapy, 2019. **27**(3): p. 518–530.
14. Chan, J.J. and Y. Tay, *Noncoding RNA:RNA regulatory networks in cancer.* International Journal of Molecular Sciences, 2018. **19**(5).
15. Meng, S., et al., *CircRNA: Functions and properties of a novel potential biomarker for cancer.* Molecular Cancer, 2017. **16**(1): p. 1–8.
16. Chen, X., et al., *Circular RNAs in immune responses and immune diseases.* Theranostics, 2019. **9**(2): p. 588.
17. Wang, P., et al., *The function and regulation network mechanism of circRNA in liver diseases.* Cancer Cell International, 2022. **22**(1): p. 141.
18. Danan, M., et al., *Transcriptome-wide discovery of circular RNAs in Archaea.* Nucleic Acids Research, 2012. **40**(7): p. 3131–3142.
19. Cocquerelle, C., et al., *Mis-splicing yields circular RNA molecules.* FASEB Journal, 1993. 7(1): p. 155–160.
20. Patop, I.L., S. Kadener, *circRNAs in cancer.* Current Opinion in Genetics & Development, 2018. **48**: p. 121–127.
21. Memczak, S., et al., *Identification and characterization of circular RNAs as a new class of putative biomarkers in human blood.* PLoS One, 2015. **10**(10): p. e0141214.
22. Chen, L.-L., *The expanding regulatory mechanisms and cellular functions of circular RNAs.* Nature Reviews. Molecular Cell Biology, 2020. **21**(8): p. 475–490.
23. Li, H., et al., *Comprehensive circular RNA profiles in plasma reveals that circular RNAs can be used as novel biomarkers for systemic lupus erythematosus.* Clinica Chimica Acta, 2018. **480**: p. 17–25.
24. Sakshi, S., et al., *Role of circRNA-miRNA-mRNA interaction network in diabetes and its associated complications.* Molecular Therapy. Nucleic Acids, 2021. **26**: p. 1291–1302.

25. Zhang, Y., et al., *CircRNA-ceRNA network revealing the potential regulatory roles of CircRNA in alzheimer's disease involved the cGMP-PKG signal pathway.* Frontiers in Molecular Neuroscience, 2021. **14**: p. 665788.
26. Chien, Y., et al., *CircularRNA as novel biomarkers in liver diseases.* Journal of the Chinese Medical Association, 2020. **83**(1): p. 15–17.
27. Tang, X., et al., *Review on circular RNAs and new insights into their roles in cancer.* Computational and Structural Biotechnology Journal, 2021. **19**: p. 910–928.
28. Guo, J.U., et al., *Expanded identification and characterization of mammalian circular RNAs.* Genome Biology, 2014. **15**(7): p. 1–14.
29. Lasda, E. and R. Parker, *Circular RNAs: diversity of form and function.* RNA, 2014. **20**(12): p. 1829–1842.
30. Jeck, W.R., et al., *Circular RNAs are abundant, conserved, and associated with ALU repeats.* RNA, 2013. **19**(2): p. 141–157.
31. Suzuki, H., et al., *Characterization of RNase R-digested cellular RNA source that consists of lariat and circular RNAs from pre-mRNA splicing.* Nucleic Acids Research, 2006. **34**(8): p. e63–e63.
32. Enuka, Y., et al., *Circular RNAs are long-lived and display only minimal early alterations in response to a growth factor.* Nucleic Acids Research, 2016. **44**(3): p. 1370–1383.
33. Rybak-Wolf, A., et al., *Circular RNAs in the mammalian brain are highly abundant, conserved, and dynamically expressed.* Molecular Cell, 2015. **58**(5): p. 870–885.
34. Zhu, G., et al., *CircRNA: A novel potential strategy to treat thyroid cancer (Review).* International Journal of Molecular Medicine, 2021. **48**(5).
35. Castillo Ferrer, C., K. Berthenet, and G. Ichim, *Apoptosis — Fueling the oncogenic fire.* FEBS Journal, 2021. **288**(15): p. 4445–4463.
36. Fuchs, Y. and H. Steller, *Live to die another way: Modes of programmed cell death and the signals emanating from dying cells.* Nature Reviews. Molecular Cell Biology, 2015. **16**(6): p. 329–344.
37. Wu, X.-y., et al., *Mechanisms of cancer cell killing by metformin: A review on different cell death pathways.* Molecular and Cellular Biochemistry, 2022: p. 1–18.
38. Huang, J., et al., *Nobiletin as an inducer of programmed cell death in cancer: A review.* Apoptosis, 2022. **27**(5–6): p. 1–14.

63. Bray, F., et al., *Global cancer statistics 2018: GLOBOCAN estimates of incidence and mortality worldwide for 36 cancers in 185 countries.* CA: A Cancer Journal for Clinicians, 2018. **68**(6): p. 394–424.
64. Ferlay, J., et al., *Estimating the global cancer incidence and mortality in 2018: GLOBOCAN sources and methods.* International Journal of Cancer, 2019. **144**(8): p. 1941–1953.
65. Li, S., D.C. Chung, and J.T. Mullen, *Screening high-risk populations for esophageal and gastric cancer.* Journal of Surgical Oncology, 2019. **120**(5): p. 831–846.
66. Venerito, M., et al., *Gastric cancer: Epidemiology, prevention, and therapy.* Helicobacter, 2018. **23**: p. e12518.
67. Tokunaga, M., et al., *Perioperative chemotherapy for locally advanced gastric cancer in Japan: current and future perspectives.* Surgery Today, 2020. **50**(1): p. 30–37.
68. Ashrafizadeh, M., et al., *Association of the epithelial–mesenchymal transition (EMT) with cisplatin resistance.* International Journal of Molecular Sciences, 2020. **21**(11): p. 4002.
69. Mirzaei, S., et al., *Nrf2 signaling pathway in cisplatin chemotherapy: Potential involvement in organ protection and chemoresistance.* Pharmacological Research, 2021. **167**: p. 105575.
70. Yao, W., et al., *Exosome-derived Circ-PVT1 contributes to cisplatin resistance by regulating autophagy, invasion, and apoptosis via miR-30a-5p/YAP1 axis in gastric cancer cells.* Cancer Biotherapy and Radiopharmaceuticals, 2021. **36**(4): p. 347–359.
71. Du, W.W., et al., *A circular RNA circ-DNMT1 enhances breast cancer progression by activating autophagy.* Oncogene, 2018. **37**(44): p. 5829–5842.
72. Cai, F., et al., *Knockdown of Circ_CCNB2 sensitizes prostate cancer to radiation through repressing autophagy by the miR-30b-5p/KIF18A axis.* Cancer Biotherapy and Radiopharmaceuticals, 2020.
73. Kong, R., *Circular RNA hsa_circ_0085131 is involved in cisplatin-resistance of non-small-cell lung cancer cells by regulating autophagy.* Cell Biology International, 2020. **44**(9): p. 1945–1956.
74. Guo, J., et al., *Hsa_circ_0023404 enhances cervical cancer metastasis and chemoresistance through VEGFA and autophagy signaling by*

sponging miR-5047. Biomedicine & Pharmacotherapy, 2019. **115**: p. 108957.

75. Duan, X., X. Yu, and Z. Li, *Circular RNA hsa_circ_0001658 regulates apoptosis and autophagy in gastric cancer through microRNA-182/Ras-related protein Rab-10 signaling axis.* Bioengineered, 2022. **13**(2): p. 2387–2397.
76. Yang, X.P., et al., *Circ_0020123 regulates autophagy, glycolysis, and malignancy by upregulating IRF4 through eliminating miR-193a-3p-mediated suppression of IRF4 in non-small cell lung cancer.* Neoplasma, 2022. **69**(2): p. 392–403.
77. Reinfeld, B.I., et al., *The therapeutic implications of immunosuppressive tumor aerobic glycolysis.* Cellular & Molecular Immunology, 2022. **19**(1): p. 46–58.
78. Warburg, O., *On the origin of cancer cells.* Science, 1956. **123**(3191): p. 309–314.
79. Andrejeva, G. and J.C. Rathmell, *Similarities and distinctions of cancer and immune metabolism in inflammation and tumors.* Cell Metabolism, 2017. **26**(1): p. 49–70.
80. Vander Heiden, M.G., L.C. Cantley, and C.B. Thompson, *Understanding the Warburg effect: The metabolic requirements of cell proliferation.* Science, 2009. **324**(5930): p. 1029–1033.
81. Lin, X., et al., *Glucose metabolism on tumor plasticity, diagnosis, and treatment.* Frontiers in Oncology, 2020. **10**: p. 317.
82. Pralea, I.-E., et al., *Phytochemicals as regulators of tumor glycolysis and hypoxia signaling pathways: Evidence from In vitro studies.* Pharmaceuticals, 2022. **15**(7): p. 808.
83. Yang, J., et al., *Circular RNA UBE2Q2 promotes malignant progression of gastric cancer by regulating signal transducer and activator of transcription 3-mediated autophagy and glycolysis.* Cell Death & Disease, 2021. **12**(10): p. 910.
84. Xu, F., et al., *LncRNA HIF1A-AS1 promotes gemcitabine resistance of pancreatic cancer by enhancing glycolysis through modulating the AKT/YB1/HIF1α pathway.* Cancer Research, 2021. **81**(22): p. 5678–5691.
85. Zhou, J., et al., *CircRNA-ENO1 promoted glycolysis and tumor progression in lung adenocarcinoma through upregulating its host gene ENO1.* Cell Death & Disease, 2019. **10**(12): p. 885.

86. Xing, Z., et al., *CircRNA circ-PDCD11 promotes triple-negative breast cancer progression via enhancing aerobic glycolysis.* Cell Death Discovery, 2021. 7(1): p. 218.
87. Zhang, X., J. Li, and Q. Feng, *CircRNA circYY1 (hsa_circ_0101187) modulates cell glycolysis and malignancy through regulating YY1 expression by sponging miR-769-3p in breast cancer.* Cancer Management and Research, 2021. **13**: p. 1145–1158.
88. Liu, Y., et al., *Silencing circRNA protein kinase C iota (circ-PRKCI) suppresses cell progression and glycolysis of human papillary thyroid cancer through circ-PRKCI/miR-335/E2F3 ceRNA axis.* Endocrine Journal, 2021. **68**(6): p. 713–727.
89. Yang, B., et al., *CircRNA circ_0006677 inhibits the progression and glycolysis in non-small-cell lung cancer by sponging miR-578 and regulating SOCS2 expression.* Frontiers in Pharmacology, 2021. **12**: p. 657053.
90. Huang, D. and C. Li, *circ-ACACA promotes proliferation, invasion, migration and glycolysis of cervical cancer cells by targeting the miR-582-5p/ERO1A signaling axis.* Oncology Letters, 2021. **22**(5): p. 795.
91. Fang, X., et al., *circRNA circ_POLA2 increases microRNA-31 methylation to promote endometrial cancer cell proliferation.* Oncology Letters, 2021. **22**(5): p. 762.
92. Li, C., et al., *hsa_circ_0003222 accelerates stemness and progression of non-small cell lung cancer by sponging miR-527.* Cell Death & Disease, 2021. **12**(9): p. 807.
93. Chen, H., et al., *circ_0000467 promotes the proliferation, metastasis, and angiogenesis in colorectal cancer cells through regulating KLF12 expression by sponging miR-4766-5p.* Open Medicine (Warsaw), 2021. **16**(1): p. 1415–1427.
94. Zhou, L., et al., *Silencing circ-BIRC6 inhibits the proliferation, invasion, migration and epithelial-mesenchymal transition of bladder cancer cells by targeting the miR-495-3p/XBP1 signaling axis.* Molecular Medicine Reports, 2021. **24**(5).
95. Bing, Z.X., et al., *Silencing of circ_0000517 suppresses proliferation, glycolysis, and glutamine decomposition of non-small cell lung cancer by modulating miR-330-5p/YY1 signal pathway.* The Kaohsiung Journal of Medical Sciences, 2021. **37**(12): p. 1027–1037.

96. Xu, X., et al., *CircRNA inhibits DNA damage repair by interacting with host gene.* Molecular Cancer, 2020. **19**(1): p. 128.
97. Chen, Q., et al., *CircRNA cRAPGEF5 inhibits the growth and metastasis of renal cell carcinoma via the miR-27a-3p/TXNIP pathway.* Cancer Letters, 2020. **469**: p. 68–77.
98. Qureshi-Baig, K., et al., *Hypoxia-induced autophagy drives colorectal cancer initiation and progression by activating the PRKC/PKC-EZR (ezrin) pathway.* Autophagy, 2020. **16**(8): p. 1436–1452.
99. Dong, Y., et al., *Inhibition of autophagy by 3-MA promotes hypoxia-induced apoptosis in human colorectal cancer cells.* Europen Review for Medical and Pharmacological Sciences, 2019. **23**(3): p. 1047–1054.
100. Zhu, Y., et al., *SOX2 promotes chemoresistance, cancer stem cells properties, and epithelial-mesenchymal transition by β-catenin and Beclin1/autophagy signaling in colorectal cancer.* Cell Death & Disease, 2021. **12**(5): p. 449.
101. Zhang, N., et al., *CircRNA_103948 inhibits autophagy in colorectal cancer in a ceRNA manner.* Annals of the New York Academy of Sciences, 2021. **1503**(1): p. 88–101.
102. Wang, Z. and C. Liu, *Upregulated hsa_circRNA_100269 inhibits the growth and metastasis of gastric cancer through inactivating PI3K/Akt axis.* PLoS One, 2021. **16**(4): p. e0250603.
103. Li, X., et al., *CircRNA_100395 inhibits cell proliferation and metastasis in ovarian cancer via regulating miR-1228/p53/epithelial-mesenchymal transition (EMT) axis.* Journal of Cancer, 2020. **11**(3): p. 599–609.
104. Chen, W., et al., *CircRNA Circ-ITCH inhibits the proliferation and invasion of glioma cells through targeting the miR-106a-5p/SASH1 axis.* Cell Transplantation, 2021. **30**: p. 963689720983785.
105. Yao, Y., Y. Zhou, and Q. Hua, *circRNA hsa_circ_0018414 inhibits the progression of LUAD by sponging miR-6807-3p and upregulating DKK1.* Molecular Therapy Nucleic Acids, 2021. **23**: p. 783–796.
106. Xiang, Z., et al., *CircRNA-UCK2 increased TET1 inhibits proliferation and invasion of prostate cancer cells via sponge MiRNA-767-5p.* Open Medicine (Warsaw), 2019. **14**: p. 833–842.
107. Yuan, D.D., et al., *Circular RNA hsa_circ_0000730 restrains cell proliferation, migration, and invasion in cervical cancer through*

miR-942-5p/PTEN axis. The Kaohsiung Journal of Medical Sciences, 2021. **37**(11): p. 964–972.

108. Jiang, Z., et al., *Circ-RNF121 regulates tumor progression and glucose metabolism by miR-1224-5p/FOXM1 axis in colorectal cancer.* Cancer Cell International, 2021. **21**(1): p. 596.
109. Huang, C.Q., et al., *Circular RNA circ_0000423 promotes gastric cancer cell proliferation, migration and invasion via the microR-582-3p/disheveled-axin domain containing 1 axis.* Bioengineered, 2021. **12**(2): p. 12755–12766.
110. Huang, B., et al., *Circ_0087862 promotes the progression of colorectal cancer by sponging miR-142-3p and up-regulating BACH1 expression.* The Kaohsiung Journal of Medical Sciences, 2021. **37**(12): p. 1048–1057.
111. Huang, B., et al., *Circ_0006174 promotes colorectal cancer progression by sponging microRNA-142-3p and regulating X-linked inhibitor of apoptosis expression.* The International Journal of Biological Markers, 2021. **36**(3): p. 3–13.
112. Huang, Q., et al., *Circular RNA hsa_circ_0103552 promotes proliferation, migration, and invasion of breast cancer cells through upregulating cysteine-rich angiogenic inducer 61 (CYR61) expression via sponging microRNA-515-5p.* The Tohoku Journal of Experimental Medicine, 2021. **255**(2): p. 171–181.
113. Sun, S., et al., *Hsa_circ_0062682 promotes serine metabolism and tumor growth in colorectal cancer by regulating the miR-940/PHGDH axis.* Frontiers in Cell and Developmental Biology, 2021. **9**: p. 770006.
114. Zhong, Y., et al., *CircRNA_100565 contributes to cisplatin resistance of NSCLC cells by regulating proliferation, apoptosis and autophagy via miR-337-3p/ADAM28 axis.* Cancer Biomarkers, 2021. **30**(2): p. 261–273.
115. Cai, Y., et al., *Downregulation of hsa_circRNA_0001400 helps to promote cell apoptosis through disruption of the circRNA_0001400-miR-326 sponge in cervical cancer cells.* Frontiers in Genetics, 2021. **12**: p. 779195.

https://doi.org/10.1142/9789811267390_0010

Chapter 10

Circular RNAs (circRNAs) in cancer metastasis: Molecular interactions and possible therapeutic targets

Rasoul Raesi[1,2], Amirhossein Zabolian[3], Farzaneh Hasani Sadi[4], Salar Javanshir[5], Shokooh Salimimoghadam[6], Young Yun Jung[7], Kwang Seok Ahn[7] and Sepideh Mirzaei[8]*

[1]*Department of Health Services Management, Mashhad University of Medical Sciences, Mashhad, Iran*
[2]*Department of Medical-Surgical Nursing, Mashhad University of Medical Sciences, Mashhad, Iran*
[3]*Resident of Orthopedics, Department of Orthopedics, School of Medicine, 5th Azar Hospital, Golestan University of Medical Sciences, Golestan, Iran*
[4]*General Practitioner, Kerman University of Medical Sciences, Kerman, Iran*
[5]*Young Researchers and Elite Club, Tehran Medical Sciences, Islamic Azad University, Tehran, Iran*
[6]*Department of Biochemistry and Molecular Biology, Faculty of Veterinary Medicine, Shahid Chamran University of Ahvaz, Ahvaz, Iran*
[7]*Department of Science in Korean Medicine, Kyung Hee University, Seoul, Republic of Korea*
[8]*Department of Biology, Faculty of Science, Islamic Azad University, Science and Research Branch, Tehran, Iran*

*Corresponding author: Sepideh Mirzaei, Department of Biology, Faculty of Science, Islamic Azad University, Science and Research Branch, Tehran, Iran, Email: sepideh mirzaei.smv@gmail.com

Abstract

Metastasis is defined as a complicated process in which tumor cells migrate from their primary site to a secondary site for establishing new colonies and ensuring their progression. During this process, cancer cells invade surrounding tissue and enter into bloodstream, which is known as intravasation, and then on reaching to an appropriate site, they exit blood vessels, which is called extravasation. Up to 90% of cancer-related mortality is due to metastasis, and it can reduce the survival rate of patients. Although genetic alterations play a significant role in metastasis of tumor cells, epigenetic changes have been shown to be involved in the process of cancer metastasis. Circular RNAs (circRNAs) are RNA transcripts with no capacity in encoding proteins that exert regulatory effects in cells during physiological functions and their dysregulation is observed in diseases such as diabetes mellitus, neurological diseases, and cancers. circRNAs regulate epithelial–mesenchymal transition (EMT), matrix metalloproteinases (MMPs), and angiogenesis in regulating the invasion of cancer cells. Knock-down of oncogenic circRNAs is important in impairing metastasis in tumors. circRNA-miRNA axis plays a remarkable role in the invasion of tumor cells. Targeting circRNAs regulating tumor invasion is beneficial in impairing cancer malignancy and improving the prognosis and survival rate of patients.

1. Introduction

Circular RNAs (circRNAs) are a kind of RNA transcripts with covalently closed loop structures that result from back-splicing in mammals [1]. About 40 years ago, the first circRNA was identified in plant viroids that were shown to be covalently closed circRNA molecules [2]. The investigation by electron microscopy in 1979 showed that RNA molecules with circular structures are present in viruses under specific denaturing conditions and for the first time, circRNA was detected in the hepatitis delta virus in 1986 [3, 4]. circRNAs are endogenous RNA molecules partly originate from protein-coding genes, and they can be represented by one exon or a combination of multiple exons [5]. The interesting feature of circRNAs is the lack of

3′-poly(A) tails and 5′-end caps. Since there is no available end at circRNAs, they show resistance to degradation by RNase enzymes and are more stable compared to linear RNA molecules [6, 7]. Although it is not a rule, it has been shown that circRNAs demonstrate lower expression levels compared to their host genes [8–10]. There are different kinds of circRNAs, and among them exonic circRNAs are the most abundant ones; however, there are other kinds of circRNAs including intronic, anti-sense, 5′- or 3′-untranslated and intergenic genomic regions that participate in biogenesis of circRNAs [9]. The process of back-splicing is involved in the biogenesis of exonic circRNAs in which a downstream 5′-splice site of an exon is joined to an upstream 3′-splice site of another exon that can involve one exon or more than one exon [5]. As it was mentioned, most of the circRNAs are originated from protein-coding genes and RNA polymerase II participates in their transcription, and their biogenesis occurs by spliceosomes [5]. Figure 1 demonstrates the biogenesis of circRNAs in cells.

circRNAs have demonstrated various functions, and microRNA (miRNA) sponge is one of them. miRNAs bind to 3′-untranslated region (UTR) region for affecting the stability of mRNAs and are capable of modulating gene expression at the nucleus by binding to the promoter of genes [11]. circRNAs can function as competing endogenous RNA and by absorbing miRNAs, decrease their expression [12]. circ-ZNF609 can regulate the expression level of AKT3 by miR-150-5p sponging [13]. circRNAs are also involved in the regulation of alternative splicing in cells. The competition of back-splicing of circRNA with linear splicing of pre-mRNA for splicing sites occurs. It has been shown that circMbl is formed by the second exon of MBL and has MBL-binding sites in flanking introns [14, 15].

Regardless of the important functions of circRNAs in cells, they have demonstrated a close association with disease pathogenesis. For instance, in diabetes mellitus (DM), circRNA-010383 sponges miR-135a to increase renal fibrosis during diabetic nephropathy. Silencing circRNA-010383 is associated with enhanced accumulation of extracellular matrix and low expression of TRPC1 in ameliorating diabetic nephropathy [16]. Furthermore, low expression level of circRNA

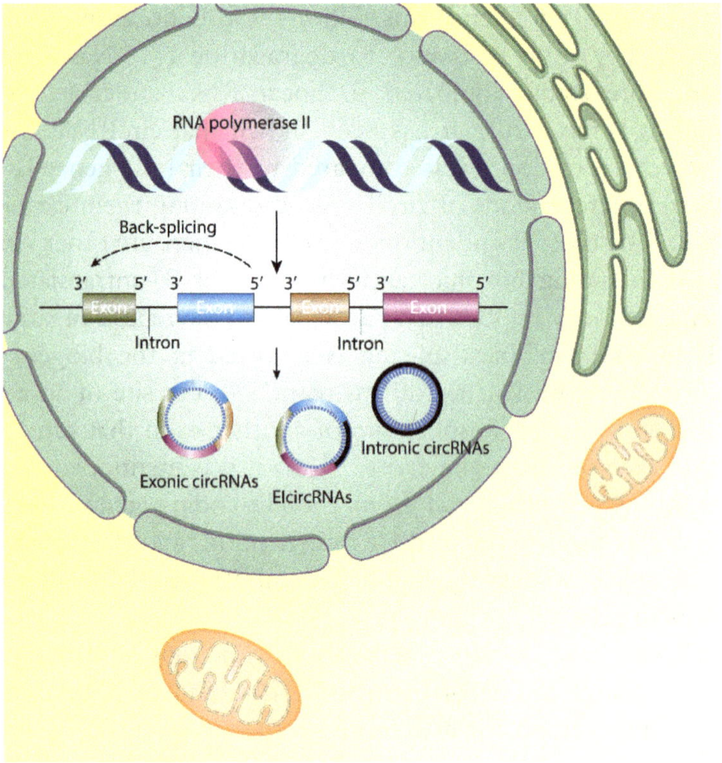

Figure 1. A schematic representation of circRNA biogenesis in cells.

DMNT3B is correlated with diabetic retinal vascular dysfunction [17]. circ-0000950 sponges miR-103 to increase neuronal apoptosis and to prevent neurite outgrowth in Alzheimer's disease [18]. circ-0005835 sponges miR-576-3p to increase proliferation of neuronal stem cells and to prevent inflammatory cytokines in Alzheimer's disease [19]. Although circRNAs have been considered as important players in disease pathogenesis and progression, the role of these RNA transcripts and their dysregulation in cancer have been of importance in recent years. Cancer hallmarks and their response to therapy are regulated by circRNAs, and these RNA transcripts can be used as biomarkers for the diagnosis and prognosis of cancer patients [20–24].

2. An overview of cancer metastasis and related pathways

It has been reported that 90% of cancer-related deaths can be attributed to a process, known as metastasis. However, it is still one of the poorly understood mechanisms in the process of cancer pathogenesis. After the establishment of colony and proliferation at their primary site, tumor cells tend to invade other organs and tissues of the body to increase their malignancy and set up new colonies there. The metastasis is a multi-step process, and at the first stage, tumor cells should invade the surrounding tissues to enter the microvasculature of the lymph and blood system which is known as intravasation (Figure 2). Then, cancer cells should survive at the stage and by

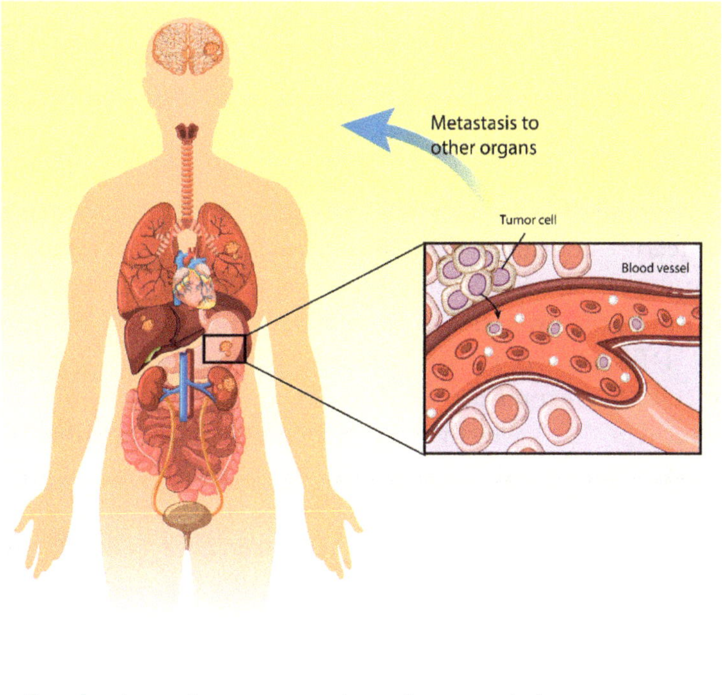

Figure 2. A schematic representation of metastasis in tumor progression. After the proliferation of cancer cells at their primary site, they enter into blood circulation known as intravasation and then they diffuse into the body to reach their intended site. Then, they exit blood vessels known as extravasation and establish new colonies.

transferring into bloodstream circulation, they can reach microvessels of distant tissues. Then, they exit from the bloodstream which is known as extravasation. Then, tumor cells survive in the new tumor microenvironment (TME) and by adapting to new conditions, they can increase their proliferation and establish new colonies [25]. Although different phases are followed for metastasis, this mechanism can be summarized into two main phases including physical transfer of cancer cells and second colonization [26].

By the time of diagnosis of cancer patients, 60–70 of these individuals demonstrate metastasis of tumor cells [27]. The experiments have shown that a single molecular pathway is not responsible for cancer metastasis and complicated signaling networks interact with each other in providing tumor migration and invasion. Phosphoglycerate dehydrogenase (PHGDH) is involved in increasing the metastasis of tumor cells. PHGDH heterogeneity has been associated with cancer invasion [28]. Slit2 has been considered as an inhibitor of metastasis in breast cancer. Slit2 stimulates M1-like phagocytic and anti-fibrotic macrophages to significantly enhance the invasion of breast tumor cells [29]. Hypoxia is one of the well-known features of tumor cells, and it reduces the expression level of FTO to upregulate MTA1 in increasing colorectal cancer metastasis [30]. During the progression of colorectal tumor cells, downregulation of DEM1C occurs to increase invasion [31]. In pancreatic tumor cells, overexpression of HMGB1 leads to the downregulation of E-cadherin that paves the way for metastasis of tumor cells [32]. Some anti-cancer agents with anti-metastatic activity have been introduced. Ginsenoside Rh2 promotes the expression level of miR-491 to suppress metastasis of colon cancer cells [33]. Metformin induces AMPK signaling to suppress mTOR expression for preventing invasion and metastasis of colorectal tumor cells [34]. These studies demonstrate that the regulation of metastasis in tumor cells is completely complex and interactions among molecular pathways are involved [35–37]. The following sections focus on the role of circRNAs in regulating tumor metastasis.

3. circRNAs in EMT regulation

Epithelial–mesenchymal transition (EMT) is a dynamic and reversible mechanism that cells lose their epithelial features, such as apico-basal polarity, epithelial markers, intercellular junctions, reorganization of cytoskeletal structure, immobility, and differentiation. On the other hand, they obtain mesenchymal marker phenotype and features such as high invasion and migration [38–40]. There are three types of EMTs and of which type III EMT occurs in human cancers for increasing their migration and metastasis. EMT induction has been shown to promote the invasion of tumor cells. LINC00355 promotes HMGA2 expression via miR-424-54p sponging via EMT induction and enhancing cancer metastasis [41]. miR-149-3p reduces the expression level of TIMP2 and CDKN1A to trigger EMT and cisplatin resistance in ovarian cancer [42]. LINC01410 promotes Snail1 expression via miR-4319 sponging in EMT induction and promoting bladder cancer metastasis [43]. LINC00922 promotes ARK5 expression via miR-424-5p sponging in EMT induction and promotes liver cancer progression [44]. These studies demonstrate that a variety of molecular pathways are involved in EMT regulation and affect cancer metastasis [45–47].

The induction of EMT in non-small cell lung tumor cells mainly depends on transforming growth factor beta (TGF-β) signaling. Although circPTK2 has poor expression in lung cancer, its overexpression can suppress EMT and migration ability of tumor cells. On circPTK2 upregulation, it inhibits TGF-β signaling to increase the expression level of TIF1γ in impairing EMT and metastasis of lung tumor cells [48]. In addition to lung tumors, TGF-β signaling has been implicated in triggering EMT and promoting metastasis of gastric tumor cells. Low expression level of circ-OXCT1 is observed in gastric cancer, and this poor expression mediates lymph node metastasis, pathological stage, and low survival rate in patients. circ-OXCT1 inhibits TGF-β signaling and SMAD4 expression in suppressing EMT and interfering with metastasis in gastric cancer [49].

miR-25-3p has been considered as an oncogenic factor in different tumors and it is the driver of progression of retinoblastoma, glioma, and liver tumor [50–52]. Overexpression of miR-25-3p is observed in lung cancer and increases the growth and invasion of tumor cells [53–55]. hsa-circ-0043265 is an inhibitor of EMT in lung cancer and impairs the progression of tumor cells. circ-0043265 sponges miR-25-3p to increase FOXP2 expression in EMT inhibition and interfere with lung cancer progression [56].

Gastric cancer is among one of the leading causes of death around the world and due to some procedures such as diagnosis and early screening, the mortality and morbidity of gastric cancer in patients have demonstrated a decrease [57–60]. However, when gastric cancer patients are diagnosed at advanced stages, their prognosis is poor and less than 30% can be attributed to the malignant behavior of tumor cells and recurrence [61, 62]. circRNAs mainly regulate miRNAs in affecting EMT in gastric cancer. circ-0021087 sponges miR-184 to increase the expression level of FOSB in EMT inhibition and reduces the invasion of gastric tumor cells [63]. Besides, circ-0049447 sponges miR-324-5p in impairing EMT-mediated metastasis in gastric cancer [64].

These studies focused on onco-suppressor circRNAs in inhibiting EMT in cancers. Notably, most of the studies have shown the role of circRNAs in triggering EMT and enhancing cancer metastasis. The invasion of gastric tumor cells significantly enhances by hsa-circ-101882 by N-cadherin and vimentin upregulation and E-cadherin downregulation to induce EMT [65]. Silencing such oncogenic circRNAs interferes with the progression of tumor cells. Knock-down of circ-0001666 promotes the expression level of miR-1251 to downregulate SOX4 in suppressing pancreatic cancer progression and preventing EMT in decreasing tumor metastasis [66].

HMGA2 is a member of HMG protein family that shows overexpression in undifferentiated mesenchymal cells [67–69]. HMGA2 can function as a transcriptional co-regulator and is involved in gene transcriptional activation [70]. Overexpression of HMGA2 has been observed in various tumors such as colorectal cancer and lung cancer [68, 71, 72]. Overexpression of HMGA2 promotes metastasis of gastric tumor cells via EMT induction. circ-0000267 sponges miR-503-5p to upregulate HMGA2 by triggering EMT and increasing metastasis of gastric tumor cells [73]. During hypoxia, EMT commonly occurs in gastric cancer to promote tumor progression. miR-497-5p overexpression suppresses EMT in hypoxia to interfere with the migration of gastric tumor cells. circ-0081143 promotes EGFR expression via miR-497-5p sponging to inhibit EMT in impairing gastric cancer progression in hypoxia [74]. Based on these studies, affecting circRNAs is a promising approach to regulating EMT and metastasis of cancer cells (Figure 3).

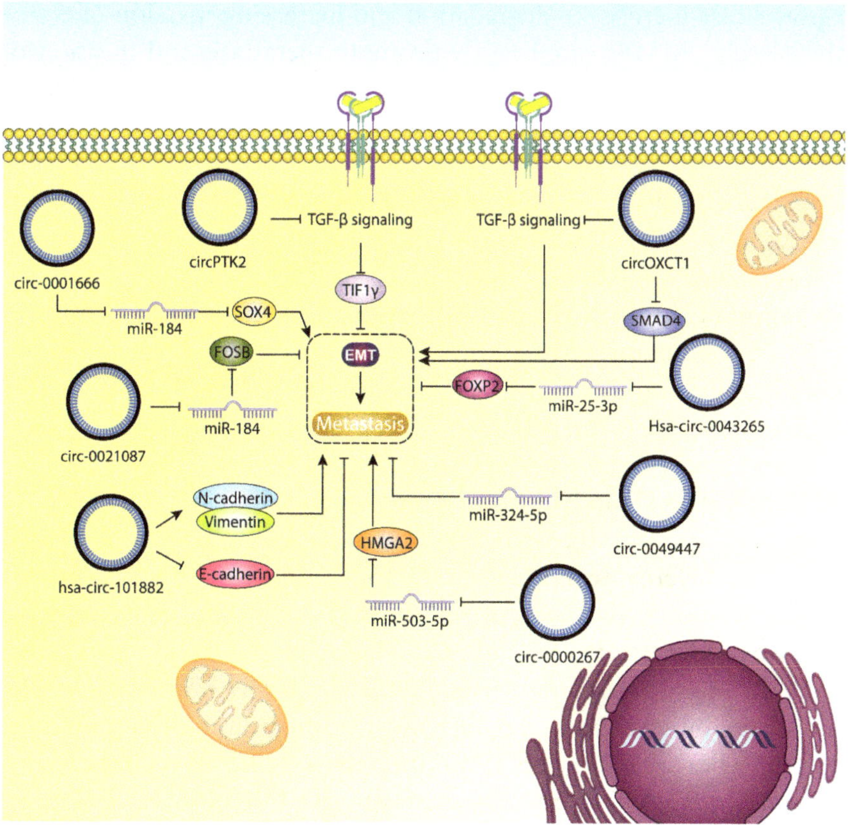

Figure 3. The ability of circRNAs in EMT regulation and affecting tumor progression. The most well-known mechanism in regulating metastasis and invasion of cancer cells is EMT mechanism, which is modulated by circRNAs via affecting molecular pathways, such as SOX4, SMAD4, HMGA2, and FOSB. circRNAs can affect molecular imprints of EMT mechanisms, such as vimentin, N-cadherin, and E-cadherin.

4. circRNAs in MMP regulation

Matrix metalloproteinases (MMPs) are a family of proteins that have related and homologous structures, and these zinc-dependent endopeptidases are capable of degrading extracellular matrix and basement membrane [75]. Several physiological and pathological mechanisms are regulated by MMPs such as wound healing, tissue remodeling, embryonic development, and bone resorption [76, 77]. The role of MMPs in cancer has been of interest and because of their ability in extracellular membrane degradation and increasing invasion of endothelial cells, MMPs significantly promote metastasis and invasion of cancer cells [78–81]. Neterin-like domain of sFRP4 is capable of inhibiting MMP-2 to impair the progression and metastasis of glioma cells [82]. As an anti-cancer agent, λ-carrageenan reduces MMP-2 expression in decreasing brain cancer invasion [83]. The migration and invasion of oral cancer cells enhance oral submucous fibrosis via the activation of MMP-2 [84]. Furthermore, heteronemin and fluoroquinolones downregulate MMP-9 in impairing cancer metastasis [85, 86]. Bisdemethoxycurcumin has been involved in impairing glioblastoma suppression via downregulation of MMP-2 [87]. This section focuses on the role of circRNAs in regulating MMP expression and affecting cancer metastasis.

circ-0016347 and its downstream target KCNH1 demonstrate overexpression in osteosarcoma, while miR-1225-3p expression level decreases. Overexpression of circ-0016347 and KCNH1 in osteosarcoma promotes invasion of tumor cells. circ-0016347 increases KCNH1 expression via miR-12225-3p sponging to upregulate MMP-9 in osteosarcoma metastasis [88]. It was shown that EMT induction by circRNAs can increase the metastasis of tumor cells. Notably, both MMPs and EMT mechanism can be regulated by a certain circRNA for cancer metastasis. circ-0006948 is capable of increasing lymph node metastasis and progression of bladder tumor cells. circ-0006948 promotes MMP-9 expression and induces EMT via vimentin and N-cadherin upregulation, and E-cadherin downregulation in enhancing bladder cancer metastasis [89]. Although most of the studies demonstrate that circRNAs reduce the expression level of miRNAs in affecting cancer progression, it appears that circRNAs can also positively regulate miRNA expression. circ-KATNAL1 suppresses the progression and migration of prostate tumor cells. circ-KATNAL1 promotes the expression level of miR-145-3p to downregulate WISP1, resulting in the inhibition of MMP-2 and MMP-9 in impairing prostate cancer metastasis [90]. Therefore, the interaction between circRNAs and miRNAs is important in regulating MMP expression in tumor progression [91–93]. Based on these studies, MMP-2 and MMP-9 are the most well-known downstream targets of circRNAs in process of cancer metastasis (Figure 4).

5. circRNAs in angiogenesis regulation

In 1971, the process of angiogenesis was coined and a scientist called Folkman suggested that angiogenesis is vital for metastasis and proliferation of tumor cells [94]. It is a highly dynamic and complicated event in which new vessels are formed from pre-existing ones [95]. Although angiogenesis is an important process for physiological mechanisms, its induction can significantly promote the progression of tumor cells. HBXIP has been implicated in triggering angiogenesis and increasing bladder cancer proliferation via induction of Akt/mTOR signaling [96]. FAK is able to increase the expression level of VEGFR2 in triggering angiogenesis and enhancing breast cancer progression [97]. SERPINE2 has been involved in triggering angiogenesis and promoting lymphangiogenesis in increasing oral cancer progression [98]. CELKF2 as an RNA-binding protein decreases NFATc1 expression to prevent angiogenesis and suppress the invasion of breast tumor cells [99]. LINC00261 suppresses angiogenesis in pancreatic cancer via overexpressing SCP2 [100]. Cancer-associated fibroblasts secrete exosomes containing miR-135b-5p that downregulate TXNIP for angiogenesis induction and enhancing colorectal cancer progression [101]. Anti-cancer agents targeting angiogenesis have been also used. Crocetin is able to inhibit angiogenesis and migration of gastric tumor cells via downregulation of Sonic hedgehog signaling [102]. The current section focuses on the role of circRNAs in regulating angiogenesis in cancers.

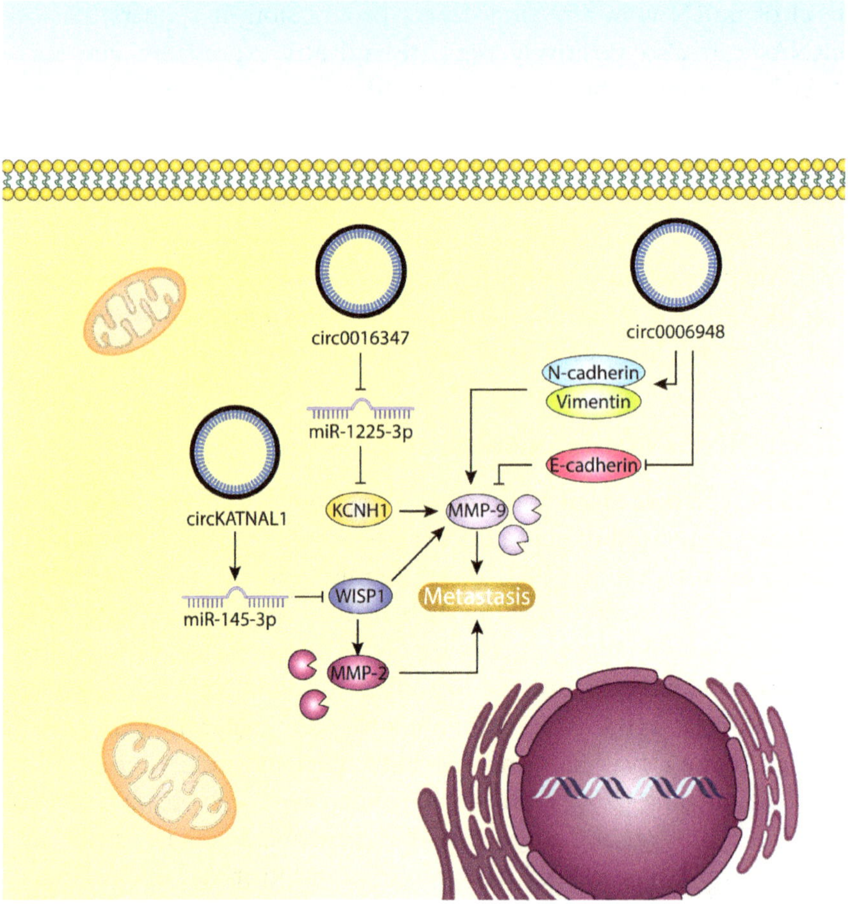

Figure 4. circRNAs in the regulation of MMPs in cancer metastasis. circRNAs can induce/inhibit miRNA expression in affecting tumor progression via decreasing/increasing MMP levels. Notably, molecular imprints of the EMT mechanism, including N-cadherin, vimentin, and E-cadherin, can regulate MMP expression.

The metastasis of cancer cells has a close association with angiogenesis. Angiogenesis induction significantly increases the migration ability of hepatocellular carcinoma cells. It has been reported that circRNA-100338 shows overexpression in hepatocellular carcinoma and enhances invasive features of tumor cells. circRNA-100338 overexpression in patients who underwent hepatectomy is considered as a risk factor for lung metastasis due to its capacity for angiogenesis induction [103]. In addition to metastasis, the process of angiogenesis appears to be vital for increasing the growth of cancer cells, since microvessels can provide a high amount of energy and oxygen for tumor cells. circ-0006988 overexpression in lung cancer is in favor of the progression of tumor cells. circ-0006988 promotes MAP3K3 expression via miR-491-5p sponging to induce angiogenesis and to promote the growth and invasion of lung tumor cells [104].

Papillary thyroid cancer (PTC) is considered as an endocrine tumor that is the most common subtype of thyroid cancer [105, 106]. Although the growth rate of PTC is slow and patients overall demonstrate a good survival rate and prognosis [107], some of them demonstrate signs of metastasis and recurrence that are challenging for physicians [108, 109]. Five-year survival of PTC patients is suggested to be 97%, and this number drops to 59% for patients at advanced stages [110]. Overexpression of circ-0000144 occurs in PTC and is a positive factor for enhancing the progression of tumor cells. circ-0000144 promotes YWHAH expression via miR-1178-3p sponging to induce angiogenesis in enhancing the progression and malignancy of PTC cells [111].

Vascular endothelial growth factor-A (VEGFA) is the most well-known factor responsible for angiogenesis induction in cancers that is tightly modulated by circRNAs. It has been shown that circ-AFAP1 shows high expression in renal cell carcinoma and its knock-down impairs the growth rate of tumor cells. circ-AFAP1 promotes VEGFA expression via miR-374b-3p downregulation in angiogenesis induction in renal cell carcinoma [112]. Another experiment also reveals the role of circ-0056618 in increasing the progression of colorectal tumor cells. circ-0056618 sponges miR-206 to promote the expression level of VEGFA in angiogenesis induction and enhance the progression of colorectal cancer cells [113]. Therefore, related molecular pathways of angiogenesis are affected by circRNAs in regulating cancer progression.

The interesting point is the interaction of TME components with circRNAs in regulating tumor progression. Macrophages are among the most abundant components of TME and they are observed in two phenotypes including M1 and M2. Although M1-polarized macrophages demonstrate tumor-suppressor function, M2-polarized macrophages are vital for the process of tumor progression [114–116]. Non-coding RNAs tightly regulate the polarization of macrophages in affecting tumor progression [117]. Although it is obvious that non-coding RNA transcripts can regulate macrophage phenotype, macrophages can also regulate the expression level of RNA molecules. It has been reported that M2-polarized macrophages increase the progression of cutaneous squamous cell carcinoma and induce angiogenesis via circ-TNFRSF21 overexpression to promote ROCK2 expression via miR-3619-5p sponging [118].

Although a huge amount of experiments has revealed the role of oncogenic circRNAs in triggering angiogenesis and promoting tumor progression, there are studies showing that onco-suppressor circRNAs can inhibit angiogenesis in the process of tumor treatment. hsa-circRNA-001587 binds to miR-223 in increasing the expression level of SLC4A4 to inhibit angiogenesis in impairing the progression and proliferation of pancreatic cancer cells [119]. Taking everything together, circRNAs that majority of them are oncogenic factors, have the ability of regulating affecting various factors such as FRMD6, TGFB1, S100A14, miR-130a-3p and other downstream targets to regulate angiogenesis in cancers and affect tumor progression [120–123]. Figure 5 shows angiogenesis regulation by circRNAs in cancer.

6. circRNA/miRNA axis in regulating cancer metastasis

The fact that 98% of the human genome is not translated to protein has resulted in directing researchers toward finding the reason and also understanding the function of this high amount of RNA molecules that are produced, but they do not translate into proteins. miRNAs are such RNA molecules have no ability in protein coding, and these endogenous RNA molecules regulate the expression level of more than 30% of genes [124]. miRNAs mainly reduce the expression level of their targets by binding to 3′-UTR [125]. Increasing evidence has revealed the role of miRNAs in human cancers, their mutations and dysregulation, regulation of cancer hallmarks, and affecting therapy response [126–128].

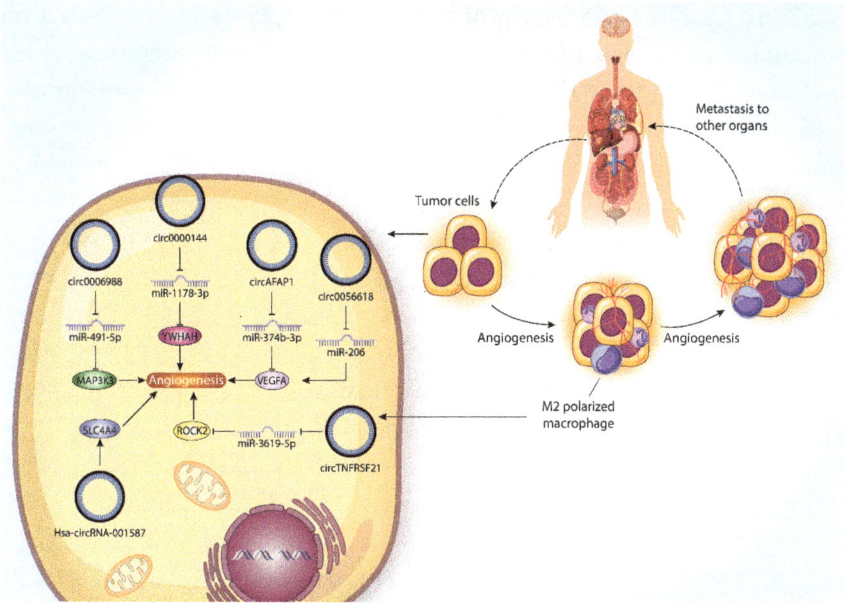

Figure 5. The regulation of angiogenesis by circRNAs in cancer. The process of angiogenesis is different from the generation of vessels during embryogenesis. During angiogenesis, new vessels are produced from previously existing vessels and circRNAs affect the genes related to angiogenesis in cancer.

The increased metastasis of gastric tumor cells is attributed to oncogenic function of circ-0043691. It has been shown that circ-0043691 sponges miR-873-3p to increase the expression level of GART as its downstream target, which is vital for the migration and survival of gastric tumor cells [129]. One of the strategies in cancer therapy is knock-down of circRNAs with oncogenic function. Silencing circDUSP16 decreases metastasis and migration rate of colorectal tumor cells. circDUSP16 promotes the expression level of E2F6 via miR-432-5p sponging in enhancing colorectal cancer progression [130]. Colorectal cancer is one of the most common malignancies of gastrointestinal tract and ranks third among cancers worldwide [131, 132]. Although colorectal cancer treatment has witnessed great hope using chemotherapy and immunotherapy, patients with this disease demonstrate recurrence and metastasis

[133, 134]. The progression of colorectal cancer can be facilitated by mutations in genes and epigenetic changes [135]. Overexpression of circ-002178 and CREB1 occurs in colorectal cancer, while miR-542-3p shows a decrease in expression. circ-002178 increases migration and invasion of colorectal tumor cells by miR-542-3p sponging and upregulation of CREB1 [136].

One of the urological cancers affecting the life of many men around the world is prostate cancer [137]. Irradiation treatment is widely used for early prostate cancer patients and for those who are in the middle stages, a combination of irradiation and surgery is applied [138, 139]. The life quality and prognosis of prostate cancer patients at advanced stages are poor [140]. The progression of prostate cancer is accelerated by circ-PAPPA which has been implicated in increasing migration and invasion of tumor cells. circ-PAPPA sponges miR-515-5p to upregulate the expression level of FKBP1A for prostate cancer progression acceleration [141]. Another urological cancer malignancy is bladder cancer with a high incidence rate in both males and females in both developed and developing countries. Although new therapeutics have been introduced for bladder cancer such as nanotherapeutics [142], there is still much space for the treatment of this malignancy. hsa-circ-0014130 has been implicated in increasing bladder cancer progression with overexpression in tumor cells and tissues. By sponging miR-132-3p, circ-0014130 promotes the expression level of KCNJ12 to facilitate metastasis of bladder cancer cells [143]. A recent experiment has shown a close association between circ-CRIM1 and distant metastasis in bladder cancer. circRNA CRIM1 promotes Foxo3a expression via miR-182 inhibition in enhancing the progression and metastasis of bladder cancer [144].

A common type of liver cancer is hepatocellular carcinoma (HCC), and its high lethality has made it a leading cause of death worldwide [145]. The incidence rate of HCC continues to increase around the world, and 75% of HCC cases have occurred in a time ranging from 1990 to 2015 [146], which can be attributed to alterations in lifestyle and unhealthy diet [147, 148]. Furthermore, changes in the genetic background can pre-dispose to the development of liver cancer [149, 150]. It has been shown that circ-PTPRA is able to sponge miR-582-3p in MMP-9 overexpression to enhance the metastasis of HCC cells [151]. Silencing circRNA DOCK1 impairs metastasis in HCC. circRNA DOCK1 promotes expression level of SMAD2 via miR-654-5p sponging to increase progression and metastasis of HCC cells [152]. In addition to MMP-9 that was mentioned in previous experiments for increasing metastasis of HCC, it has been shown that MMP-16 is also involved in HCC invasion. Hsa-circ-0001806 decreases miR-193a-5p expression for MMP-16 upregulation to elevate metastasis of HCC cells (Table 1) [153]. These studies clearly demonstrate the role of circRNA/miR axis in regulating invasion in different cancers and how they can affect various

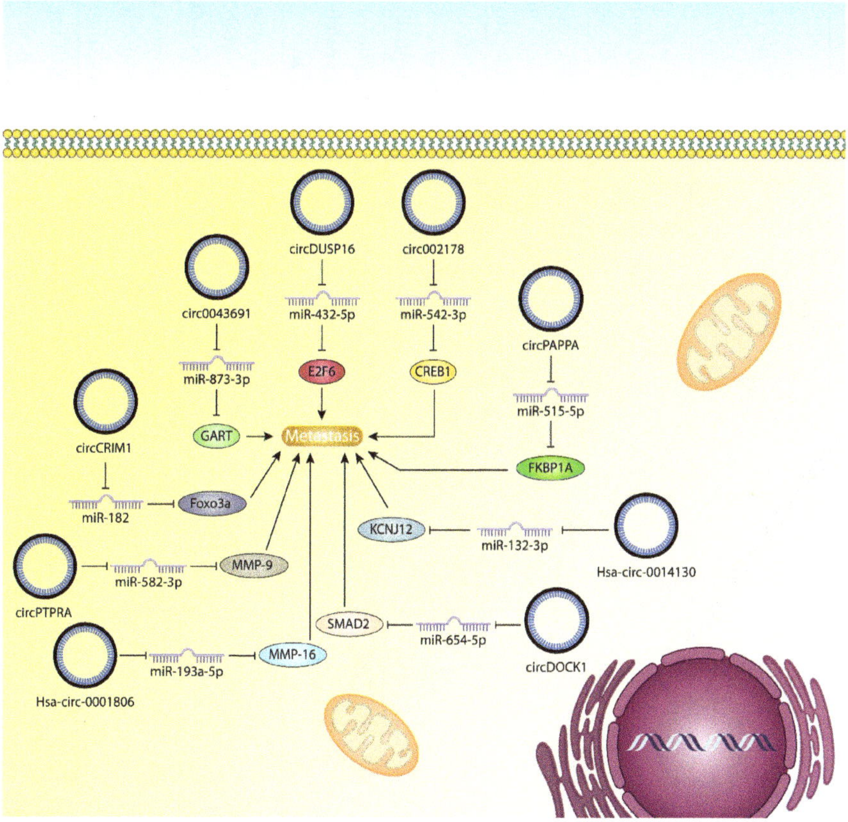

Figure 6. The role of circRNA/miRNA axis in affecting cancer metastasis.

Table 1. The role of circRNAs in regulating metastasis of cancer cells.

circRNA	Molecular Pathway	Cancer Type	Remark	Ref
hsa-circ-0043280	miR-203a-3p/ PAQR3	Cervical cancer	circ-0043280 promotes PAQR3 expression via miR-203a-3p sponging in suppressing cancer metastasis.	[155]
circ-0000517	miR-326/ miR-330-5p	Non-small cell lung cancer	circ-00000517 promotes MMP-2 expression via miR-326/miR-330-4p sponging in accelerating tumor metastasis.	[156]
circ-ERBB2	miR-136-5p miR-198	Breast cancer	circ-ERBB2 increases TFAP2C expression via miR-136-5p and miR-198 sponging in enhancing breast cancer invasion.	[157]
circ-0016760	miR-646/AKT3	Non-small cell lung cancer	circ-0016760 increases migration and invasion of tumor cells via miR-646 sponging and inducing AKT3 signaling.	[158]
hsa-circ-0004296	EIF4A3/ETS1	Prostate cancer	circ-0004296 promotes nuclear retention of EIF4A3 to avoid nuclear translocation of ETS1 in metastasis inhibition.	[159]
circ-EIF6	EIF6-224aa/MYH9	Triple-negative breast cancer	circ-EIF6 promotes the expression level of EIF6-224aa to stabilize MYH9 and to induce Wnt/β-catenin signaling in increasing cancer progression.	[160]
hsa_circ_0000497 hsa_circ_0000918	—	Ovarian cancer	Overexpression of hsa_circ_0000497 and hsa_circ_0000918 leads to peritoneal metastasis of ovarian tumor cells.	[161]
circ-TNPO3	IGF2BP3/MYC	Gastric cancer	circ-TNPO3 inhibits IGF2BP3/MYC axis in impairing metastasis of tumor cells.	[162]

(Continued)

Table 1. (*Continued*)

hsa-circ-0067514	miR-654-3p/ LATS2	Gastric cancer	circ-0067514 promotes the expression level of LATS2 via miR-654-3p sponging in suppressing tumor progression.	[163]
circ-0008797	miR-301a-3p/ SOCS2	Non-small cell lung cancer	circ-0008797 promotes SOCS2 expression via miR-301a-3p sponging in suppressing tumor metastasis.	[164]
circ-0010235	miR-338-3p/ KIF2A	Non-small cell lung cancer	circ-0010235 increases the expression level of KIF2A via miR-338-3p sponging in enhancing cancer metastasis.	[165]
circ-0082182	miR-411/ miR-1205-Wnt/ β-catenin	Colorectal cancer	circ-0082182 induces Wnt signaling via sponging miR-411 and miR-1205 in increasing cancer metastasis in vitro and in vivo.	[166]
circ-0019435	DKK1 PTEN	Cervical cancer	circ-0019435 epigenetically silences DKK1 and PTEN in increasing invasion of tumor cells and EMT induction.	[167]
hsa-circ-0006948	miR-490-3p/ HMGA2	Esophageal cancer	circ-0006948 promotes HMGA2 expression via miR-490-3p inhibition in EMT induction and enhancing cancer metastasis.	[168]
circ-0058106	miR-185-3p/ Wnt2b/β-catenin/c-Myc	Hypopharyngeal squamous cell carcinoma	miR-185-3p inhibition by circ-0058106 to induce Wnt signaling in increasing cancer metastasis and EMT induction.	[169]
circ-CSPP1	miR-1236-3p	Ovarian cancer	circ-CSPP1 sponges miR-1236-3p to increase cancer metastasis via upregulation of VEGFA and MMP-2.	[170]
circ-0000554	miR-567	Ovarian cancer	circ-0000554 increases ovarian cancer metastasis via miR-567 sponging.	[171]

downstream targets in the process of cancer metastasis (Figure 6) [11, 125, 154].

7. Conclusion and remarks

Although proliferation is a well-known hallmark of cancers, metastasis is also another challenge for physicians and those aiming to effectively treat cancer patients. The alleviation of metastasis can significantly increase the overall survival of cancer patients and is advantageous in improving prognosis. Among the different signaling networks that interact with each other in regulating cancer metastasis, circRNAs have gained much attention due to their ability in cell signaling regulation. EMT induction is commonly observed in cancer and is responsible for increase in the invasion of tumor cells. Most of the circRNAs increase cancer metastasis via EMT induction to change the phenotype of tumor cells to mesenchymal ones and increase their motility. Furthermore, circRNAs promote/decrease the expression levels of MMPs in regulating the degradation of extracellular matrix and basement membrane in affecting tumor metastasis. Angiogenesis is a vital mechanism for increasing the progression of tumor cells, their entrance into the bloodstream, and promoting metastasis of cancer cells, and this important mechanism is regulated by circRNAs in affecting tumor progression. Although a wide variety of downstream targets have been identified for circRNAs, such as Wnt/β-catenin and STAT3 signaling, miRNAs have been considered as the most well-known ones and circRNA/miRNA axis mainly affects tumor progression.

Conflict of interest:

The authors declare no conflict of interest.

References

1. Chen, L. and G. Shan, *CircRNA in cancer: Fundamental mechanism and clinical potential.* Cancer Letters, 2021. **505**: p. 49–57.

2. Sanger, H.L., et al., *Viroids are single-stranded covalently closed circular RNA molecules existing as highly base-paired rod-like structures.* Proceedings of the National Academy of Sciences of the United States of America, 1976. **73**(11): p. 3852–3856.
3. Hsu, M.-T. and M. Coca-Prados, *Electron microscopic evidence for the circular form of RNA in the cytoplasm of eukaryotic cells.* Nature, 1979. **280**(5720): p. 339–340.
4. Kos, A., et al., *The hepatitis delta (δ) virus possesses a circular RNA.* Nature, 1986. **323**(6088): p. 558–560.
5. Verduci, L., et al., *The circRNA-microRNA code: Emerging implications for cancer diagnosis and treatment.* Molecular Oncology, 2019. **13**(4): p. 669–680.
6. Jeck, W.R. and N.E. Sharpless, *Detecting and characterizing circular RNAs.* Nature Biotechnology, 2014. **32**(5): p. 453–461.
7. Memczak, S., et al., *Circular RNAs are a large class of animal RNAs with regulatory potency.* Nature, 2013. **495**(7441): p. 333–338.
8. Enuka, Y., et al., *Circular RNAs are long-lived and display only minimal early alterations in response to a growth factor.* Nucleic Acids Research, 2016. **44**(3): p. 1370–1383.
9. Salzman, J., et al., *Circular RNAs are the predominant transcript isoform from hundreds of human genes in diverse cell types.* PLoS One, 2012. 7(2): p. e30733.
10. Salzman, J., et al., *Cell-type specific features of circular RNA expression.* PLoS Genetics, 2013. **9**(9): p. e1003777.
11. Paskeh, M.D.A., et al., *Revealing the role of miRNA-489 as a new onco-suppressor factor in different cancers based on pre-clinical and clinical evidence.* International Journal of Biological Macromolecules, 2021. **191**: p. 727–737.
12. Li, J., et al., *The biological functions and regulations of competing endogenous RNA.* Yi Chuan, 2015. **37**(8): p. 756–764.
13. Peng, L., et al., *Circular RNA ZNF609 functions as a competitive endogenous RNA to regulate AKT3 expression by sponging miR-150-5p in Hirschsprung's disease.* Oncotarget, 2017. **8**(1): p. 808.
14. Li, R., et al., *CircRNA: A rising star in gastric cancer.* Cellular and Molecular Life Sciences, 2020. 77(9): p. 1661–1680.

15. Ashwal-Fluss, R., et al., *circRNA biogenesis competes with pre-mRNA splicing*. Molecular Cell, 2014. **56**(1): p. 55–66.
16. Peng, F., et al., *circRNA_010383 acts as a sponge for miR-135a, and its downregulated expression contributes to renal fibrosis in diabetic nephropathy*. Diabetes, 2021. **70**(2): p. 603–615.
17. Zhu, K., et al., *Downregulation of circRNA DMNT3B contributes to diabetic retinal vascular dysfunction through targeting miR-20b-5p and BAMBI*. EBioMedicine, 2019. **49**: p. 341–353.
18. Yang, H., et al., *Circular RNA circ_0000950 promotes neuron apoptosis, suppresses neurite outgrowth and elevates inflammatory cytokines levels via directly sponging miR-103 in Alzheimer's disease*. Cell Cycle, 2019. **18**(18): p. 2197–2214.
19. Xu, X., et al., *Circular RNA circ_0005835 promotes promoted neural stem cells proliferation and differentiate to neuron and inhibits inflammatory cytokines levels through miR-576-3p in Alzheimer's disease*. Environmental Science and Pollution Research International, 2022. **29**(24): p. 35934–35943.
20. Yan, J.S., et al., *Hsa_circ_0065217 promotes growth and metastasis of renal cancer through regulating the miR-214-3p-ALPK2 axis*. Cell Cycle, 2021. **20**(23): p. 2519–2530.
21. Wang, Y.W., et al., *Elevated circRNAs circ_0000745, circ_0001531 and circ_0001640 in human whole blood: Potential novel diagnostic biomarkers for breast cancer*. Experimental and Molecular Pathology, 2021. **121**: p. 104661.
22. Zhang, X., N. Wu, and J. Wang, *Hsa-circ_0058106 induces EMT and metastasis in laryngeal cancer via sponging miR-153 and inducing Twist1 nuclear translocation*. Cell Oncology (Dordrecht), 2021. **44**(6): p. 1373–1386.
23. Zhu, J., et al., *Circ_0061140 knockdown inhibits tumorigenesis and improves PTX sensitivity by regulating miR-136/CBX2 axis in ovarian cancer*. Journal of Ovarian Research, 2021. **14**(1): p. 136.
24. Zhang, B., S. Yang, and J. Wang, *Circ_0084615 is an oncogenic circular RNA in colorectal cancer and promotes DNMT3A expression via repressing miR-599*. Pathology — Research and Practice, 2021. **224**: p. 153494.

25. Fidler, I.J., *The pathogenesis of cancer metastasis: The'seed and soil'hypothesis revisited.* Nature Reviews. Cancer, 2003. **3**(6): p. 453–458.
26. Chaffer, C.L. and R.A. Weinberg, *A perspective on cancer cell metastasis.* Science, 2011. **331**(6024): p. 1559–1564.
27. Li, J., et al., *Regulation of lncRNA and its role in cancer metastasis.* Oncology Research, 2016. **23**(5): p. 205–217.
28. Rossi, M., et al., *PHGDH heterogeneity potentiates cancer cell dissemination and metastasis.* Nature, 2022. **605**(7911): p. 747–753.
29. Ahirwar, D.K., et al., *Slit2 inhibits breast cancer metastasis by activating M1-like phagocytic and antifibrotic macrophages.* Cancer Research, 2021. **81**(20): p. 5255–5267.
30. Ruan, D.Y., et al., *FTO downregulation mediated by hypoxia facilitates colorectal cancer metastasis.* Oncogene, 2021. **40**(33): p. 5168–5181.
31. Huang, R., et al., *Downregulation of FEM1C enhances metastasis and proliferation in colorectal cancer.* Annals of Translational Medicine, 2021. **9**(17): p. 1391.
32. Zhu, L., et al., *Exogenous HMGB1 promotes the proliferation and metastasis of pancreatic cancer cells.* Frontiers in Medicine (Lausanne), 2021. **8**: p. 756988.
33. Wei, W., et al., *Ginsenoside Rh2 suppresses metastasis and growth of colon cancer via miR-491.* Journal of Oncology, 2021. **2021**: p. 6815713.
34. Sugiura, K., et al., *Metformin inhibits the development and metastasis of colorectal cancer.* Medical Oncology, 2022. **39**(9): p. 136.
35. Huang, C., et al., *EZH2-triggered methylation of SMAD3 promotes its activation and tumor metastasis.* Journal of Clinical Investigation, 2022. **132**(5).
36. Bolik, J., et al., *Inhibition of ADAM17 impairs endothelial cell necroptosis and blocks metastasis.* Journal of Experimental Medicine, 2022. **219**(1).
37. Mochizuki, Y., et al., *Alternative microexon splicing by RBFOX2 and PTBP1 is associated with metastasis in colorectal cancer.* International Journal of Cancer, 2021. **149**(10): p. 1787–1800.
38. Usman, S., et al., *Vimentin is at the heart of epithelial mesenchymal transition (EMT) mediated metastasis.* Cancers (Basel), 2021. **13**(19).
39. Ashrafizadeh, M., et al., *New insight towards development of paclitaxel and docetaxel resistance in cancer cells: EMT as a novel molecular*

mechanism and therapeutic possibilities. Biomedicine & Pharmacotherapy, 2021. **141**: p. 111824.

40. Ashrafizadeh, M., et al., *Crosstalk of long non-coding RNAs and EMT: Searching the missing pieces of an incomplete puzzle for lung cancer therapy*. Current Cancer Drug Targets, 2021. **21**(8): p. 640–665.
41. Li, W.J., et al., *LncRNA LINC00355 promotes EMT and metastasis of bladder cancer cells through the miR-424-5p/HMGA2 axis*. Neoplasma, 2021. **68**(6): p. 1225–1235.
42. Wang, J. and L. Liu, *MiR-149-3p promotes the cisplatin resistance and EMT in ovarian cancer through downregulating TIMP2 and CDKN1A*. Journal of Ovarian Research, 2021. **14**(1): p. 165.
43. Guo, W., et al., *LINC01410 leads the migration, invasion and EMT of bladder cancer cells by modulating miR-4319/Snail1*. Cancer Cell International, 2021. **21**(1): p. 429.
44. Ye, Z., et al., *LINC00922 promotes the proliferation, migration, invasion and EMT process of liver cancer cells by regulating miR-424-5p/ARK5*. Molecular and Cellular Biochemistry, 2021. **476**(10): p. 3757–3769.
45. Ma, Y., et al., *Dihydroartemisinin suppresses proliferation, migration, the Wnt/β-catenin pathway and EMT via TNKS in gastric cancer*. Oncol Letters, 2021. **22**(4): p. 688.
46. Bhat, S., et al., *ZNF471 modulates EMT and functions as methylation regulated tumor suppressor with diagnostic and prognostic significance in cervical cancer*. Cell Biology and Toxicology, 2021. **37**(5): p. 731–749.
47. Guerra, E., et al., *Trop-2 induces ADAM10-mediated cleavage of E-cadherin and drives EMT-less metastasis in colon cancer*. Neoplasia, 2021. **23**(9): p. 898–911.
48. Wang, L., et al., *Circular RNA hsa_circ_0008305 (circPTK2) inhibits TGF-β-induced epithelial-mesenchymal transition and metastasis by controlling TIF1γ in non-small cell lung cancer*. Molecular Cancer, 2018. **17**(1): p. 140.
49. Liu, J., et al., *Circ-OXCT1 suppresses gastric cancer EMT and metastasis by attenuating TGF-β pathway through the Circ-OXCT1/miR-136/SMAD4 axis*. OncoTargets and Therpy, 2020. **13**: p. 3987–3998.

50. Chen, H., et al., *MiR-25-3p promotes the proliferation of triple negative breast cancer by targeting BTG2.* Molecular Cancer, 2018. **17**(1): p. 1–11.
51. Wan, W., et al., *MiR-25-3p promotes malignant phenotypes of retinoblastoma by regulating PTEN/Akt pathway.* Biomedicine & Pharmacotherapy, 2019. **118**: p. 109111.
52. Peng, G., et al., *miR-25-3p promotes glioma cell proliferation and migration by targeting FBXW7 and DKK3.* Experimental and Therapeutic Medicine, 2019. **18**(1): p. 769–778.
53. Ding, X., et al., *miR-25 enhances cell migration and invasion in non-small-cell lung cancer cells via ERK signaling pathway by inhibiting KLF4.* Molecular Medicine Reports, 2018. **17**(5): p. 7005–7016.
54. Xiang, J., et al., *MiR-25 is up-regulated in non-small cell lung cancer and promotes cell proliferation and motility by targeting FBXW7.* International Journal of Clinical and Experimental Pathology, 2015. **8**(8): p. 9147.
55. Liu, B. and X. Sun, *miR-25 promotes invasion of human non-small cell lung cancer via CDH1.* Bioengineered, 2019. **10**(1): p. 271–281.
56. Ren, T., et al., *Hsa_circ_0043265 suppresses proliferation, metastasis, EMT and promotes apoptosis in non-small cell lung cancer through miR-25-3p/FOXP2 pathway.* OncoTargets and Therapy, 2020. **13**: p. 3867–3880.
57. Bray, F., et al., *Global cancer statistics 2018: GLOBOCAN estimates of incidence and mortality worldwide for 36 cancers in 185 countries.* CA: A Cancer Journal for Clinicians, 2018. **68**(6): p. 394–424.
58. Tarupi, W., et al., *Stagnation in decreasing gastric cancer incidence and mortality in Quito: Time trend analysis, 1985–2013.* Journal of Cancer Epidemiology, 2019. **2019**.
59. Venerito, M., et al., *Prevention and management of gastric cancer.* 2020. **25**: p. e12740.
60. Lordick, F., et al., *Unmet needs and challenges in gastric cancer: The way forward.* Cancer Treatment Reviews, 2014. **40**(6): p. 692–700.
61. Corso, G., et al., *Somatic mutations and deletions of the E-cadherin gene predict poor survival of patients with gastric cancer.* Journal of Clinical Oncology, 2013. **31**(7): 868–875.

62. Miao, Z.-F., et al., *Effect of neoadjuvant chemotherapy in patients with gastric cancer: A PRISMA-compliant systematic review and meta-analysis.* BMC Cancer, 2018. **18**(1): p. 1–10.
63. Yu, Y., et al., *Circ_0021087 acts as a miR-184 sponge and represses gastric cancer progression by adsorbing miR-184 and elevating FOSB expression.* European Journal of Clinical Investment, 2021. **51**(11): p. e13605.
64. Tang, K.W., et al., *Circ_0049447 acts as a tumor suppressor in gastric cancer through reducing proliferation, migration, invasion, and epithelial-mesenchymal transition.* Chinese Medical Journal (English), 2021. **134**(11): p. 1345–1355.
65. Yin, G.H., et al., *Hsa_circ_101882 promotes migration and invasion of gastric cancer cells by regulating EMT.* Journal of Clinical Laboratory Analysis, 2019. **33**(9): p. e23002.
66. Zhang, R., et al., *Silencing of circRNA circ_0001666 represses EMT in pancreatic cancer through upregulating miR-1251 and downregulating SOX4.* Frontiers in Molecular Biosciences, 2021. **8**: p. 684866.
67. Gao, X., et al., *HMGA 2 regulates lung cancer proliferation and metastasis.* Thoracic Cancer, 2017. **8**(5): p. 501–510.
68. Sun, Y., et al., *miR-503-3p induces apoptosis of lung cancer cells by regulating p21 and CDK4 expression.* Cancer Biomarkers, 2017. **20**(4): p. 597–608.
69. Sun, J., et al., *HMGA2 promotes vasculogenic mimicry and tumor aggressiveness by upregulating Twist1 in gastric carcinoma.* Scientific Reports, 2017. 7(1): p. 1–13.
70. Wu, J., et al., *Transcriptional activation of FN1 and IL11 by HMGA2 promotes the malignant behavior of colorectal cancer.* Carcinogenesis, 2016. **37**(5): p. 511–521.
71. Dai, F.-Q., et al., *miR-150-5p inhibits non-small-cell lung cancer metastasis and recurrence by targeting HMGA2 and β-catenin signaling.* Molecular Therapy. Nucleic Acids, 2019. **16**: p. 675–685.
72. Li, W., et al., *HMGA2 regulates epithelial-mesenchymal transition and the acquisition of tumor stem cell properties through TWIST1 in gastric cancer.* Oncology Reports, 2017. **37**(1): p. 185–192.
73. Cai, X., et al., *Circ_0000267 promotes gastric cancer progression via sponging MiR-503-5p and regulating HMGA2 expression.* Molecular Genetics & Genomic Medicine, 2020. **8**(2): p. e1093.

74. Tang, J., et al., *Knockdown of Circ_0081143 mitigates hypoxia-induced migration, invasion, and EMT in gastric cancer cells through the miR-497-5p/EGFR axis.* Cancer Biotherapy and Radiopharmaceuticals, 2021. **36**(4): p. 333–346.
75. Visse, R. and H. Nagase, *Matrix metalloproteinases and tissue inhibitors of metalloproteinases: structure, function, and biochemistry.* Circulation Research, 2003. **92**(8): p. 827–839.
76. Murphy, G. and H. Nagase, *Progress in matrix metalloproteinase research.* Molecular Aspects of Medicine, 2008. **29**(5): p. 290–308.
77. Gomis-Rüth, F.X., *Catalytic domain architecture of metzincin metalloproteases.* The Journal of Biological Chemistry, 2009. **284**(23): p. 15353–15357.
78. Li, L., H. Li, *Role of microRNA-mediated MMP regulation in the treatment and diagnosis of malignant tumors.* Cancer Biology and Therapy, 2013. **14**(9): p. 796–805.
79. Curran, S. and G.I. Murray, *Matrix metalloproteinases: Molecular aspects of their roles in tumour invasion and metastasis.* European Association for Cancer Research, 2000. **36**(13): p. 1621–1630.
80. Egeblad, M., *New functions for the matrix metalloproteinases in cancer progression.* Nature Reviews. Cancer, 2001. **2**: p. 163–176.
81. López-Otín, C. and L.M. Matrisian, *Emerging roles of proteases in tumour suppression.* Nature Reviews. Cancer, 2007. 7(10): p. 800–808.
82. Yasmin, I.A., et al., *Netrin-like domain of sFRP4, a Wnt antagonist inhibits stemness, metastatic and invasive properties by specifically blocking MMP-2 in cancer stem cells from human glioma cell line U87MG.* Experimental Cell Research, 2021. **409**(2): p. 112912.
83. Cousin, R., et al., *A marine λ-oligocarrageenan inhibits migratory and invasive ability of MDA-MB-231 human breast cancer cells through actions on heparanase metabolism and MMP-14/MMP-2 axis.* Marine Drugs, 2021. **19**(10).
84. Chen, P.N., et al., *Oral submucous fibrosis stimulates invasion and epithelial-mesenchymal transition in oral squamous cell carcinoma by activating MMP-2 and IGF-IR.* Journal of Cellular and Molecular Medicine, 2021. **25**(20): p. 9814–9825.
85. Chen, H.L., et al., *Heteronemin suppresses lymphangiogenesis through ARF-1 and MMP-9/VE-cadherin/vimentin.* Biomedicines, 2021. **9**(9).

86. Huang, C.Y., et al., *Fluoroquinolones suppress TGF-β and PMA-induced MMP-9 production in cancer cells: Implications in repurposing quinolone antibiotics for cancer treatment.* International Journal of Molecular Sciences, 2021. **22**(21).
87. Chen, C.J., et al., *Bisdemethoxycurcumin suppresses human brain glioblastoma multiforme GBM 8401 cell migration and invasion via affecting NF-κB and MMP-2 and MMP-9 signaling pathway in vitro.* Environmental Toxicology, 2022.
88. Li, Z., et al., *Circ_0016347 promotes osteosarcoma progression by regulating miR-1225-3p/KCNH1 axis.* Cancer Biotherapy and Radiopharmaceuticals, 2021.
89. Liu, F., et al., *Circ_0006948 drives the malignant development of bladder cancer via activating the epithelial-mesenchymal transition.* JBUON, 2021. **26**(4): p. 1491–1497.
90. Zheng, Y., et al., *Circ_KATNAL1 regulates prostate cancer cell growth and invasiveness through the miR-145-3p/WISP1 pathway.* Biochemistry and Cell Biology, 2020. **98**(3): p. 396–404.
91. Li, Y., S. Lin, and N. An, *Hsa_circ_0009910: Oncogenic circular RNA targets microRNA-145 in ovarian cancer cells.* Cell Cycle, 2020. **19**(15): p. 1857–1868.
92. Gong, J., et al., *Circular RNA hsa_circ_0005397 promotes hepatocellular carcinoma progression by regulating the miR-326/PDK2 axis.* The Journal of Gene Medicine, 2021. **23**(6): p. e3332.
93. Shi, P., et al., *Hsa_circ_0084927 regulates cervical cancer advancement via regulation of the miR-634/TPD52 axis.* Cancer Management and Research, 2020. **12**: p. 9435–9448.
94. Folkman, J., *Tumor angiogenesis: Therapeutic implications.* The New England Journal of Medicine, 1971. **285**(21): p. 1182–1186.
95. Liu, J., et al., *The role of long non-coding RNAs in angiogenesis and anti-angiogenic therapy resistance in cancer.* Molecular Therapy — Nucleic Acids, 2022. **28**: p. 397–407.
96. Liu, X., et al., *HBXIP accelerates glycolysis and promotes cancer angiogenesis via AKT/mTOR pathway in bladder cancer.* Experimental and Molecular Pathology, 2021. **121**: p. 104665.
97. Shiau, J.P., et al., *FAK regulates VEGFR2 expression and promotes angiogenesis in triple-negative breast cancer.* Biomedicines, 2021. **9**(12).

98. Sasahira, T., et al., *SERPINE2 is an oral cancer-promoting factor that induces angiogenesis and lymphangiogenesis.* International Journal of Clinical Oncology, 2021. **26**(10): p. 1831–1839.
99. Zhou, L. and X. Xie, *RNA-binding protein CELF2 inhibits breast cancer cell invasion and angiogenesis by downregulating NFATc1.* Experimental and Therapeutic Medicine, 2021. **22**(2): p. 898.
100. Zou, J., et al., *LINC00261 elevation inhibits angiogenesis and cell cycle progression of pancreatic cancer cells by upregulating SCP2 via targeting FOXP3.* Journal of Cellular and Molecular Medicine, 2021. **25**(20): p. 9826–9836.
101. Yin, H., et al., *Cancer-associated fibroblasts-derived exosomes upregulate microRNA-135b-5p to promote colorectal cancer cell growth and angiogenesis by inhibiting thioredoxin-interacting protein.* Cell Signalling, 2021. **84**: p. 110029.
102. Zang, M., et al., *Crocetin suppresses angiogenesis and metastasis through inhibiting sonic hedgehog signaling pathway in gastric cancer.* Biochemical and Biophysical Research Communication, 2021. **576**: p. 86–92.
103. Huang, X.Y., et al., *Exosomal circRNA-100338 promotes hepatocellular carcinoma metastasis via enhancing invasiveness and angiogenesis.* Journal of Experimental & Clinical Cancer Research, 2020. **39**(1): p. 20.
104. Yang, C., et al., *Circ_0006988 promotes the proliferation, metastasis and angiogenesis of non-small cell lung cancer cells by modulating miR-491-5p/MAP3K3 axis.* Cell Cycle, 2021. **20**(13): p. 1334–1346.
105. Siegel, R.L., K.D. Miller, and A. Jemal, *Cancer statistics, 2019.* CA: A Cancer Journal for Clinicians, 2019. **69**(1): p. 7–34.
106. Gallardo, E., et al., *SEOM clinical guideline thyroid cancer (2019).* Clinical & Translational Oncology, 2020. **22**(2): p. 223–235.
107. Gur, E.O., et al., *Multifocality related factors in papillary thyroid carcinoma.* Asian Journal of Surgery, 2019. **42**(1): p. 297–302.
108. Tumino, D., F. Frasca, and K. Newbold, *Updates on the management of advanced, metastatic, and radioiodine refractory differentiated thyroid cancer.* Frontiers in Endocrinology, 2017. **8**: p. 312.
109. Pazaitou-Panayiotou, K., et al., *Cerebellar metastasis as first metastasis from papillary thyroid carcinoma.* Endocrine Journal, 2005. **52**(6): p. 653–657.

110. Kunavisarut, T., *Diagnostic biomarkers of differentiated thyroid cancer.* Endocrine, 2013. **44**(3): p. 616–622.
111. Ma, Y., D. Yang, and P. Guo, *Circ_0000144 acts as a miR-1178-3p decoy to promote cell malignancy and angiogenesis by increasing YWHAH expression in papillary thyroid cancer.* Journal of Otolaryngology — Head & Neck Surgery, 2022. **51**(1): p. 28.
112. Ou, Y., et al., *Circ-AFAP1 promote clear cell renal cell carcinoma growth and angiogenesis by the Circ-AFAP1/miR-374b-3p/VEGFA signaling axis.* Cell Death Discovery, 2022. **8**(1): p. 68.
113. Zheng, X., et al., *Circ_0056618 promoted cell proliferation, migration and angiogenesis through sponging with miR-206 and upregulating CXCR4 and VEGF-A in colorectal cancer.* European Review for Medical and Pharmacological Sciences, 2020. **24**(8): p. 4190–4202.
114. Kashfi, K., J. Kannikal, and N. Nath, *Macrophage reprogramming and cancer therapeutics: Role of iNOS-derived NO.* Cells, 2021. **10**(11).
115. Zhou, Z., et al., *Noncoding RNA-mediated macrophage and cancer cell crosstalk in hepatocellular carcinoma.* Molecular Therapy — Oncolytics, 2022. **25**: p. 98–120.
116. Wang, S., et al., *Landscape and perspectives of macrophage-targeted cancer therapy in clinical trials.* Molecular Therapy — Oncolytics, 2022. **24**: p. 799–813.
117. Entezari, M., et al., *Non-coding RNAs and macrophage interaction in tumor progression.* Critical Reviews in Oncology/Hematology, 2022. **173**: p. 103680.
118. Ma, J., et al., *M2 macrophage facilitated angiogenesis in cutaneous squamous cell carcinoma via circ_TNFRSF21/miR-3619-5p/ROCK axis.* The Kaohsiung Journal of Medical Sciences, 2022.
119. Zhang, X., et al., *hsa_circRNA_001587 upregulates SLC4A4 expression to inhibit migration, invasion, and angiogenesis of pancreatic cancer cells via binding to microRNA-223.* American Journal of Physiology-Gastrointestinal and Liver Physiology, 2020. **319**(6): p. G703–G717.
120. Pei, L., et al., *Circular RNA circSDHC (hsa_circ_0015004) regulates tumor growth and angiogenesis via regulating centrosomal protein 55 expression in renal cell carcinoma.* Histology & Histopathology, 2022: p. 18467.

121. Shen, L., et al., *CircRNA VPRBP inhibits tumorigenicity of cervical cancer via miR-93-5p/FRMD6 axis.* Reproductive Sciences, 2022.
122. Zhou, Y., et al., *circ_0006089 promotes gastric cancer growth, metastasis, glycolysis, and angiogenesis by regulating miR-361-3p/TGFB1.* Cancer Science, 2022. **113**(6): p. 2044–2055.
123. Chi, X., et al., *Circ_0003221 downregulation restrains cervical cancer cell growth, metastasis and angiogenesis by governing the miR-139-3p/S100A14 pathway.* Reproductive Sciences, 2022. **29**(6): p. 1822–1835.
124. Gao, T., et al., *Dysfunction of miR-802 in tumors.* Journal of Clinical Laboratory Analysis, 2021. **35**(11): p. e23989.
125. Zou, Y., et al., *MiR-873-5p: A potential molecular marker for cancer diagnosis and prognosis.* Frontiers in Oncology, 2021. **11**: p. 743701.
126. Mirzaei, S., et al., *The long and short non-coding RNAs modulating EZH2 signaling in cancer.* Journal of Hematology & Oncology, 2022. **15**(1): p. 18.
127. Paskeh, M.D.A., et al., *Emerging role of exosomes in cancer progression and tumor microenvironment remodeling.* Journal of Hematology & Oncology, 2022. **15**(1): p. 83.
128. Mirzaei, S., et al., *Regulation of nuclear factor-KappaB (NF-κB) signaling pathway by non-coding RNAs in cancer: Inhibiting or promoting carcinogenesis?* Cancer Letters, 2021. **509**: p. 63–80.
129. Zhang, Y., et al., *CircRNA_0043691 sponges miR-873-3p to promote metastasis of gastric cancer.* Mammalin Genome, 2021. **32**(6): p. 476–487.
130. Wang, G. and H. Yang, *CircRNA DUSP16 knockdown suppresses colorectal cancer progression by regulating the miR-432-5p/E2F6 axis.* Cancer Management and Research, 2021. **13**: p. 6599–6609.
131. Zheng, G.-L., et al., *Elevated LOXL2 expression by LINC01347/miR-328-5p axis contributes to 5-FU chemotherapy resistance of colorectal cancer.* American Journal of Cancer Research, 2021. **11**(4): p. 1572.
132. Zhiani, M., et al., *Apoptosis induction by siRNA targeting integrin-β1 and regorafenib/DDAB-mPEG-PCL hybrid nanoparticles in regorafenib-resistant colon cancer cells.* American Journal of Cancer Research, 2021. **11**(4): p. 1170.

133. Chen, P.-H., et al., *Uracil-tegafur vs fluorouracil as postoperative adjuvant chemotherapy in Stage II and III colon cancer: A nationwide cohort study and meta-analysis.* Medicine (Baltimore), 2021. **100**(18).
134. Silveira, M.J., et al., *Immunomodulatory nanomedicine for colorectal cancer treatment: A landscape to be explored?* Biomaterials Science, 2021. **9**(9): p. 3228–3243.
135. Zhu, T., et al., *Low miR-16 expression induces regulatory CD4+ NKG2D+ T cells involved in colorectal cancer progression.* American Journal of Cancer Research, 2021. **11**(4): p. 1540.
136. Xu, Y., et al., *CircRNA_002178 as a ceRNA promotes the development of colorectal cancer by regulating miR-542-3p/CREB1.* American Journal of Translational Research, 2021. **13**(9): p. 10038–10055.
137. Ashrafizadeh, M., et al., *Nanotechnological approaches in prostate cancer therapy: Integration of engineering and biology.* Nano Today, 2022. **45**: p. 101532.
138. Chang, A.J., et al., *High-risk prostate cancer — classification and therapy.* Nature Reviews. Clinical Oncology, 2014. **11**(6): p. 308–323.
139. Grozescu, T. and F. Popa, *Prostate cancer between prognosis and adequate/proper therapy.* Journal of Medicine and Life, 2017. **10**(1): p. 5.
140. Komura, K., et al., *Current treatment strategies for advanced prostate cancer.* International Journal of Urology, 2018. **25**(3): p. 220–231.
141. Wang, G., et al., *CircRNA pappalysin 1 facilitates prostate cancer development through miR-515-5p/FKBP1A axis.* Andrologia, 2021. **53**(11): p. e14227.
142. Ashrafizadeh, M., et al., *(Nano) platforms in bladder cancer therapy: Challenges and opportunities.* Bioengineering & Translational Medicine. p. e10353.
143. Li, G., et al., *CircRNA hsa_circ_0014130 function as a miR-132-3p sponge for playing oncogenic roles in bladder cancer via upregulating KCNJ12 expression.* Cell Biology and Toxicology, 2021.
144. Yu, X.Y., C.Q. Ma, and Y.H. Sheng, *circRNA CRIM1 regulates the migration and invasion of bladder cancer by targeting miR182/Foxo3a axis.* Clinical and Translational Oncology, 2022. **24**(6): p. 1195–1203.
145. Njei, B., et al., *Emerging trends in hepatocellular carcinoma incidence and mortality.* Hepatology, 2015. **61**(1): p. 191–199.

146. Akinyemiju, T., et al., *The burden of primary liver cancer and underlying etiologies from 1990 to 2015 at the global, regional, and national level: Results from the global burden of disease study 2015.* JAMA Oncology, 2017. **3**(12): p. 1683–1691.
147. Qian, X., et al., *Hepatocellular carcinoma surveillance and treatment: A way to reduce cancer-related mortality in cirrhotic patients.* Journal of Clinical and Translational Hepatology, 2019. **7**(1): p. 1.
148. Berkel, C. and E. Cacan, *DYNLL1 is hypomethylated and upregulated in a tumor stage-and grade-dependent manner and associated with increased mortality in hepatocellular carcinoma.* Experimental and Molecular Pathology, 2020. **117**: p. 104567.
149. Wang, M., et al., *Circular RNA expression profiles and the pro-tumorigenic function of circRNA_10156 in hepatitis B virus-related liver cancer.* International Journal of Medical Sciences, 2020. **17**(10): p. 1351.
150. Banaudha, K.K. and M. Verma, *Epigenetic biomarkers in liver cancer.* Methods in Molecular Biology, 2015: p. 65–76.
151. Jin, Y., Y. Zhang, and X. Luo, *circRNA_PTPRA functions as a sponge of miR-582-3p to regulate hepatocellular carcinoma cell proliferation, migration, invasion and apoptosis.* Experimental and Therapeutic Medicine, 2021. **22**(5): p. 1276.
152. Lu, Y., J. Zhang, and Y. Wu, *Interference with circRNA DOCK1 inhibits hepatocellular carcinoma cell proliferation, invasion and migration by regulating the miR-654-5p/SMAD2 axis.* Molecular Medicine Reports, 2021. **24**(2).
153. Zhou, H. and Y. Chen, *CircRNA has_circ_0001806 promotes hepatocellular carcinoma progression via the miR-193a-5p/MMP16 pathway.* Brazilian Journal of Medical and Biological Research, 2021. **54**(12): p. e11459.
154. Zhang, F., T. Su, and M. Xiao, *RUNX3-regulated circRNA METTL3 inhibits colorectal cancer proliferation and metastasis via miR-107/PER3 axis.* Cell Death & Disease, 2022. **13**(6): p. 550.
155. Zhang, C., et al., *Circular RNA hsa_circ_0043280 inhibits cervical cancer tumor growth and metastasis via miR-203a-3p/PAQR3 axis.* Cell Death & Disease, 2021. **12**(10): p. 888.

156. Tan, Q., et al., *Circular RNA circ_0000517 facilitates the growth and metastasis of non-small cell lung cancer by sponging miR-326/miR-330-5p.* Cell Journal, 2021. **23**(5): p. 552–561.
157. Zhong, J.X., et al., *Circular RNA circ-ERBB2 promotes HER2-positive breast cancer progression and metastasis via sponging miR-136-5p and miR-198.* Journal of Translational Medicine, 2021. **19**(1): p. 455.
158. Chen, S., et al., *Circ_0016760 accelerates non-small-cell lung cancer progression through miR-646/AKT3 signaling in vivo and in vitro.* Thoracic Cancer, 2021. **12**(23): p. 3223–3235.
159. Mao, S., et al., *Hsa_circ_0004296 inhibits metastasis of prostate cancer by interacting with EIF4A3 to prevent nuclear export of ETS1 mRNA.* Journal of Experimental & Clinical Cancer Research, 2021. **40**(1): p. 336.
160. Li, Y., et al., *circ-EIF6 encodes EIF6-224aa to promote TNBC progression via stabilizing MYH9 and activating the Wnt/beta-catenin pathway.* Molecular Therapy, 2022. **30**(1): p. 415–430.
161. Luo, N., et al., *Hsa_circ_0000497 and hsa_circ_0000918 contributed to peritoneal metastasis of ovarian cancer via ascites.* Journal of Translational Medicine, 2022. **20**(1): p. 201.
162. Yu, T., et al., *Circular RNA circ-TNPO3 suppresses metastasis of GC by acting as a protein decoy for IGF2BP3 to regulate the expression of MYC and SNAIL.* Molecular Therapy — Nucleic Acids, 2021. **26**: p. 649–664.
163. Jiang, S.F. and R.R. Li, *hsa_circ_0067514 suppresses gastric cancer progression and glycolysis via miR-654-3p/LATS2 axis.* Neoplasma, 2022.
164. Abuduwaili, K., et al., *circ_0008797 attenuates non-small cell lung cancer proliferation, metastasis, and aerobic glycolysis by sponging miR-301a-3p/SOCS2.* Environmental Toxicology, 2022. **37**(7): p. 1697–1710.
165. Zhu, Y., et al., *Circular RNA circ_0010235 sponges miR-338-3p to play oncogenic role in proliferation, migration and invasion of non-small-cell lung cancer cells through modulating KIF2A.* Annals of Medicine, 2021. **53**(1): p. 693–706.
166. Liu, R., et al., *Circ_0082182 promotes oncogenesis and metastasis of colorectal cancer in vitro and in vivo by sponging miR-411 and miR-1205 to activate the Wnt/β-catenin pathway.* World Journal of Surgical Oncology, 2021. **19**(1): p. 51.

167. Wang, Q., et al., *Circ_0019435 exerts its functions in the cellular process of cervical cancer via epigenetically silencing DKK1 and PTEN.* Reproductive Sciences, 2021. **28**(10): p. 2989–2999.
168. Pan, Z., et al., *Hsa_circ_0006948 enhances cancer progression and epithelial-mesenchymal transition through the miR-490-3p/HMGA2 axis in esophageal squamous cell carcinoma.* Aging (Albany NY), 2019. **11**(24): p. 11937–11954.
169. Li, C., et al., *Circ_0058106 promotes proliferation, metastasis and EMT process by regulating Wnt2b/β-catenin/c-Myc pathway through miR-185-3p in hypopharyngeal squamous cell carcinoma.* Cell Death & Disease, 2021. **12**(11): p. 1063.
170. Li, Q.H., et al., *circ-CSPP1 promotes proliferation, invasion and migration of ovarian cancer cells by acting as a miR-1236-3p sponge.* Biomedicine & Pharmacotherapy, 2019. **114**: p. 108832.
171. Wang, H., et al., *CircRNA circ_0000554 promotes ovarian cancer invasion and proliferation by regulating miR-567.* Environmental Science and Pollution Research International, 2022. **29**(13): p. 19072–19080.

https://doi.org/10.1142/9789811267390_0011

Chapter 11

Circular RNAs (CircRNAs) in cancer therapy response: Biological aspects

Sima Orouei[1], Mehrdad Hashemi[2,3], Parham Rahmanian[4], Mohammad Hossein Gholami[5]*, Min Hee Yang[6] and Kwang Seok Ahn[6]

[1]*Department of Biology, Science and Research Branch, Islamic Azad University, Tehran, Iran*
[2]*Department of Genetics, Faculty of Advanced Science and Technology, Tehran Medical Sciences, Islamic Azad University, Tehran, Iran*
[3]*Farhikhtegan Medical Convergence Sciences Research Center, Farhikhtegan Hospital Tehran Medical Sciences, Islamic Azad University, Tehran, Iran*
[4]*Faculty of Veterinary Medicine, Islamic Azad University, Science and Research Branch, Tehran, Iran*
[5]*Faculty of Veterinary Medicine, Kazerun Branch, Islamic Azad University, Kazerun, Iran*
[6]*Department of Science in Korean Medicine, Kyung Hee University, Seoul, Republic of Korea*

*Corresponding author: Mohammad Hossein Gholami, Faculty of Veterinary Medicine, Kazerun Branch, Islamic Azad University, Kazerun, Iran, Email: hoseingholami2020@yahoo.com

Abstract

Biological functions of genes have been investigated in terms of regulating growth and metastasis of cancer cells. Although targeting genetic and epigenetic factors is a promising approach in oncology and tumor suppression, understanding the role of these factors in therapy response of cancer cells is also of interest, since increasing evidence reveals the development of drug resistance and radioresistance. Chemotherapy agents follow the process of cell cycle arrest and apoptosis induction in decreasing tumor progression, and radiotherapy mainly stimulates mitotic catastrophe and DNA damage in cancer therapy. With respect to the activation of factors responsible for DNA damage repair and increasing tumor proliferation, cancer cells have shown the ability to develop therapy resistance. Circular RNAs (circRNAs) are RNA transcripts that do not encode protein and possess regulatory functions in cells. The biological function of circRNAs in terms of regulating proliferation, migration, differentiation, and apoptosis has been understood, and dysregulation of these factors can lead to cancer initiation and development. Due to the role of circRNAs in affecting tumor growth and metastasis and their ability in regulating signaling networks in different cancers, this chapter is allocated to highlight the function of these epigenetic factors in regulating drug resistance and radioresistance in cancers.

1. Introduction

During the last decades, our understanding of molecular events and mechanisms regulating cancer proliferation, metastasis, immune escape, and tumor viability has significantly improved [1]. The project Cancer Genome Atlas is a large-scale program that has greatly helped in the identification of mutations in cancers, and they can be categorized into "driver" and "passenger" mutations [2–4]. Furthermore, the development of functional genomic tools including small interfering RNA (siRNA), CRISPR/Cas system, and short hairpin RNA has resulted in understanding the role of genes and molecular pathways in cancers [5–7]. With the help of these tools, projects, and significant researches, concepts such as tumor microenvironment, cancer stem cells, epithelial–mesenchymal transition, and immune evasion have been introduced [8–11]. These concepts are beneficial when they can come with the help of conventional therapies. Although chemotherapy and radiotherapy are the most common approaches in cancer suppression, they are not completely effective due to the emergence of resistance and therefore, novel therapeutics can greatly help them in tumor therapy. However, this combination and hope have not been achieved yet due to problems, cost, and time in developing novel therapeutics that can affect functional and vital proteins in cancers, since most of these proteins are hard to target and the development of their inhibitors is a troublesome work. Therefore, many cancer targets and pathways cannot be affected by drugs. Therefore, much interest has been directed toward nucleic acid therapy as the main bridge for cancer suppression. The concept of non-coding RNAs led to significant and milestone progress in disease therapy, especially cancer. This is because a huge number of molecular pathways participate in cancer development, and it is impossible for the scientists to target all of them. Therefore, the best strategy is to target master regulators in cancer and since non-coding RNAs are the upstream regulator of many molecular pathways, researches have been directed toward targeting them in cancer therapy [12–16].

2. Cancer therapy resistance

Two major arms in the treatment of cancer are chemotherapy and radiotherapy. Chemotherapy is a gold standard treatment for every cancer and on diagnosis of cancer, physicians first recommend the process of chemotherapy not only for cancer cell elimination but also for improving the prognosis and overall survival of patients. Along with chemotherapy, radiotherapy is also suggested in cancer therapy. Although both chemotherapy and radiotherapy have side effects. For instance, during radiotherapy, it is possible to induce damage in normal cells, but since its benefits are higher than disadvantages, they can be ignored. For chemotherapy, anti-cancer agents may negatively affect major organs of the body. However, the process of chemotherapy and radiotherapy has been more complicated with the emergence of a phenomenon known as resistance that shocked the physicians working on the treatment of cancer patients. Frequent and long-term applications of chemotherapy and radiotherapy have led to the development of therapy resistance that threatens the life of many cancer patients around the world [17–23]. Therefore, it is highly suggested to understand mechanisms involved in therapy resistance in cancer in developing some solutions and overcoming this troublesome problem.

Due to the significant efforts of researchers around the world, some light has been shed on the factors that can mediate therapy resistance in cancer. Acyl-CoA synthetase-4 stimulates radio-resistance and enhances the invasion of breast tumor cells by overexpressing FOXM1 [24]. KRAS has shown oncogenic function, and it can mediate radio-resistance in tumor cells by preventing a mitotic catastrophe and avoiding cell cycle arrest at G2/M phase. Furthermore, KRAS mutation enhances DNA damage repair and promotes the expression level of 53BP1 [25]. Metformin is able to increase radio-sensitivity of pancreatic tumor cells via Numb upregulation [26]. As an upstream mediator, peroxiredoxin IV increases the proliferation rate of tumor cells and induces radio-resistance via the activation of Akt/GSK3 to decrease reactive oxygen species generation and prevent DNA damage [27]. Exosomal transfer of miR-1323 results in radio-resistance in cervical cancer via induction of Wnt/β-catenin signaling that significantly promotes tumor progression [28]. In lung tumor cells, Golgi phosphoprotein 3 is involved in radio-resistance by increasing the stability of EGFR [29]. Therefore, interaction among molecular pathways leads to radio-resistance in cancers [30]. The same phenomenon is also observed in chemo-resistance. Proliferation and metastasis of gastric tumor cells are suppressed by long non-coding RNA (lncRNA) KLF3-AS1, which increases drug sensitivity via miR-223 sponging [31]. In ovarian tumor cells, changes in mitochondrial dynamics result in the development of drug resistance. Downregulation of DRP1 using siRNA results in reversing mitochondrial dynamics, decreasing migration ability of tumor cells, and reducing ATP levels for preventing chemo-resistance in ovarian cancer [32]. Stimulation

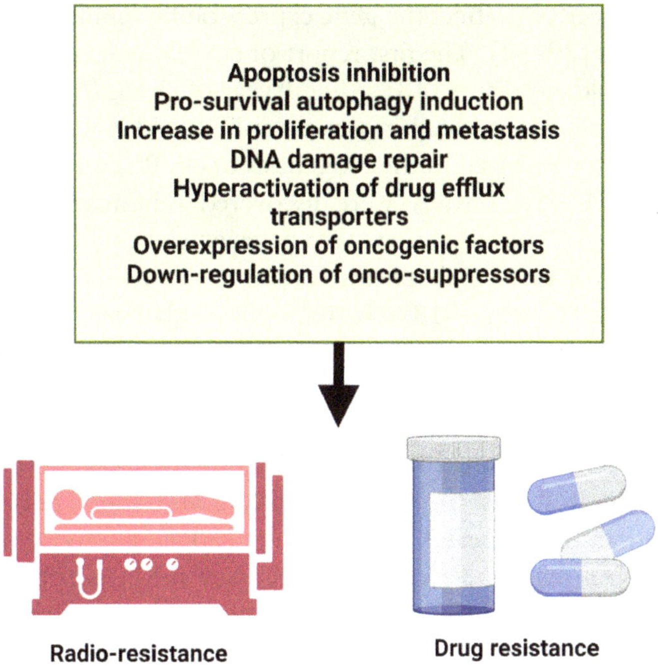

Figure 1. The factors involved in therapy resistance in cancers.

of Akt signaling by LGR6 significantly enhances the survival rate and invasion of glioblastoma cells and induces temozolomide resistance [33]. Based on the studies, changes in proliferation, migration, and metabolism of tumor cells can mediate their resistance to chemotherapy [34–37]. Figure 1 depicts some of the major mechanisms responsible for drug resistance and radio-resistance in cancers.

3. An introduction to the role of circRNAs in oncology

The gene-regulatory RNA transcripts that do not encode proteins are called circular RNAs (circRNAs) and their high stability emanates from their covalently closed loop structure [38]. The expression of circRNAs is tissue specific and even cell specific, and they have obtained much attention in the field of biology due to their vital functions. circRNAs affect the gene expression by regulating miRNAs and proteins [39–42]. The first report of circRNAs was performed in 1976 as viroids in plants [43]. After 1 year of circRNA discovery, an alternative splicing mechanism was described, and it was not considered as a factor involved in the biogenesis of circRNA until the 1990s [44, 45]. In 1991, circRNAs were discovered in humans as scrambled exons and for a long time, they were believed to be pathogenic materials or products of mis-splicing events [43, 45–48]. This belief changed in 2012 and 2013, when a high number of circRNAs were detected in eukaryotic cells using next-gene sequencing technologies and bioinformatic algorithms [39–42]. Therefore, circRNAs result from special selective splicing, and they demonstrate high expression in eukaryotic organisms [49]. In addition to covalently closed loop structure of circRNAs, they lack 5′-end caps and 3′-end tails, making them distinct from linear RNA molecules [50, 51].

circRNAs mainly derive from precursor mRNAs (pre-mRNAs) and their production mechanism is different from the splicing process used for the generation of linear RNA molecules [52]. Back-splicing is a non-canonical form of alternative splicing that is involved in the formation of circRNAs [50, 51]. Although back-splicing has a lower yield compared to linear splicing, circRNAs have higher stability and expression compared to linear RNA molecules due to their covalently closed loop structure making them resistant to exonuclease-mediated degradation [41]. circRNAs are classified into three major groups, including exonic circRNAs, exon–intron circRNAs, and intronic circRNAs [51, 53–55]. Most of the circRNAs are exonic circRNAs that result from exon back-splicing in which 5′ splice donor attacks the downstream 3′ splice acceptor, resulting in the generation of a circRNA with a covalently closed loop structure [56]. In exon–intron circRNAs, they have both exons and introns in their structure and they are produced when introns located in the 5′ donor and the 3′ acceptor on the pre-mRNA) are kept [56].

circRNAs are key players in cancer, and they are capable of regulating cancer hallmarks including proliferation, cell cycle progression, and invasion by affecting various signaling networks [57–61].

hsa-circ-0060937 promotes the expression level of HMGB3 via miR-195-5p inhibition in enhancing lung cancer malignancy [62]. circ-0001821 shows overexpression in multiple myeloma, and it enhances cancer cell growth and mediates undesirable prognosis [63]. hsa-circ-0001806 is involved in glycolysis induction and increasing progression of hepatocellular carcinoma via miR-125b sponging and upregulating HK2 expression [64]. In colorectal cancer patients, hsa-circ-0001944 shows overexpression and mediates poor prognosis [65]. For increasing gastric cancer progression, circ-0027599 sponges miR-21-5p in upregulating RUNX1 expression [66]. hsa-circ-0040809 prevents apoptosis in colorectal cancer by miR-515-5p sponging and overexpression of methyltransferase DNMT1 [67]. hsa-circ-0136666 increases programmed death-ligand 1 (PD-L1) expression via miR-497 inhibition in triggering immune evasion in colorectal cancer [68]. The most well-known downstream target of circRNAs is miRNAs such as miR-876-3p, miR-485-5p, miR-135-5p, miR-455-3p, and miR-590-5p that mediate the regulatory impact of circRNAs on cancer hallmarks [69–73]. In this chapter, the effect of circRNAs in the therapy response of cancer cells is discussed.

4. circRNAs in cancer drug resistance

With respect to the potential role of circRNAs in affecting therapy response, a high number of studies have focused on underlying mechanisms that are regulated by circRNAs in modulating drug resistance. Overexpression of hsa-circ-0046264 is observed in lung cancer, and it shows a positive correlation with tumor stage, size, and lymph node metastasis. High expression level of hsa-circ-0046264 decreases the overall survival of patients and by increasing tumor progression, it is responsible for triggering drug resistance in A549 cells [74]. The interactions among epigenetic factors are of importance in regulating tumor progression. Both circRNAs and miRNAs belong to the non-coding RNA family and are the member of epigenetic factors. Notably, circRNAs mainly regulate tumor progression via miRNA sponging. circ-0026359 overexpression decreases the overall survival of gastric cancer patients and stimulates cisplatin resistance. miR-1200 decreases POLD4 expression and functions as tumor suppressor in increasing the cisplatin sensitivity of gastric tumor cells. circ-0026359 promotes POLD4 expression via miR-1200 sponging to increase gastric cancer progression and induce cisplatin resistance [75]. Overexpression of CDK6 stimulates cisplatin resistance in gastric cancer. hsa-circ-0081143 enhances CDK6 expression via miR-646 inhibition to mediate cisplatin resistance in gastric cancer [76]. In addition to gastric cancer, laryngeal cancer cells can mediate resistance to cisplatin chemotherapy. miR-873 is an onco-suppressor factor that reduces MRP1 expression in increasing cisplatin sensitivity. Upregulation of circ-0004507 is observed in laryngeal cancer and promotes MRP1 expression via miR-873 sponging in triggering cisplatin resistance [77].

Lung cancer is one of the leading causes of death worldwide, and in 2018, it ranked first in terms of cancer-related death rates [78–82]. About 80% of lung cancer cases are non-small cell lung cancer (NSCLC), and 5-year survival rate of patients will be 10%–15% [83, 84]. Chemotherapy is considered as the first-line treatment when there is no immune checkpoint therapy or molecular targeted therapy [85]. Paclitaxel is a chemotherapy agent that impairs dynamics of microtubules and prevents destabilization of microtubules [86]. For advanced NSCLC, paclitaxel chemotherapy is commonly used and it enhances microtubule polymerization and apoptosis [87, 88]. However, different mechanisms have led to the development of paclitaxel resistance in cancer [89]. Upregulation of hsa-circ-0002874 results in paclitaxel resistance in NSCLC. circ-0002874 decreases the expression level of miR-1273f to upregulate MDM2 in mediating paclitaxel resistance in NSCLC [90]. Paclitaxel resistance is also observed in ovarian cancer. CircCELSR1 undergoes overexpression in ovarian cancer and mediates paclitaxel resistance. CircCELSR1 sponges miR-1252 to promote FOXR2 expression in triggering paclitaxel resistance in ovarian cancer [91].

Cervical cancer is the fourth leading cause of death in women, and vaccination and testing have been used for its screening and prevention [79, 92]. In spite of using surgery, chemotherapy, and radiotherapy, cervical cancer cells demonstrate metastasis and death. Although paclitaxel has been used in cervical cancer treatment with treatment benefits [93], circRNAs can lead to the development of drug resistance. circ-ZFR results in paclitaxel resistance in cervical cancer and sponges miR-944 to upregulate interleukin 10 in chemoresistance [94]. The increase in progression of tumor cells can result in paclitaxel resistance. ZEB1 protein is responsible for increasing metastasis of cancer cells and its silencing by CRISPR/Cas9 system decreases the progression of lung cancer cells [95]. Downregulation of ZEB1 reduces metastasis of ovarian cancer and promotes paclitaxel sensitivity [96]. Overexpression of ZEB1 by lncRNA NEAT1 stimulates paclitaxel resistance in ovarian cancer [97]. Upregulation of circ-PVT1 is observed in gastric cancer and enhances the progression of tumor cells. circ-PVT1 promotes the expression level of ZEB1 via miR-124-3p sponging in triggering paclitaxel resistance in gastric cancer [98].

One of the leading causes of death among women is breast cancer [79]. In spite of the use of therapeutic modalities for breast cancer, prognosis of patients is poor [99]. Chemotherapy is a gold standard for breast cancer, but drug resistance has resulted in chemotherapy failure and death of breast cancer patients [100, 101]. Overexpression of circ-RNF111 occurs in breast cancer and silencing circ-RNF111 impairs metastasis, colony formation, and glycolysis in breast tumor cells. circ-RNF111 promotes E2F3 expression via miR-140-5p sponging in increasing tumor progression and mediating paclitaxel resistance in breast cancer [102].

5-Flourouracil (5-FU) is a common chemotherapy agent for colorectal cancer. However, frequent application of 5-FU promotes tumor progression. 5-FU exposure of colorectal cancer cells results in the stimulation of Wnt/β-catenin signaling and an increase in stemness [103]. RNF38 and HNGA2 are among the factors that induce Wnt signaling in triggering 5-FU resistance [104, 105]. Curcumin inhibits EMT and Wnt pathway in enhancing 5-FU sensitivity of colonic tumor cells [106]. Notably, circ-PRKDC decreases miR-375 expression to upregulate FOXM1 expression, resulting in the induction of Wnt/β-catenin signaling and inducing 5-FU resistance [107]. Low expression level of circ-0032833 promotes sensitivity of colorectal tumor cells to 5-FU and oxaliplatin chemotherapy. On silencing circ-0032833, an increase occurs in the expression level of miR-125-5p that downregulates MSI1 expression, reversing 5-FU and oxaliplatin resistance [108]. Based on these studies, circRNAs play a significant role in regulating the response of cancer cells to chemotherapy and knock-down of tumor-promoting circRNAs is important in reversing drug resistance [109–120]. Table 1 and Figure 2 summarize the role of circRNAs in regulating drug resistance in tumors.

5. circRNAs in cancer radio-resistance

The process of radio-resistance in cancer has been complicated by introducing the role of circRNAs. A certain circRNA has not been identified for regulating radio-resistance in cancers, and a high number of them have been shown to play significant role. Furthermore, each circRNA can have both oncogenic and onco-suppressor functions and another complexity is the ability of each circRNA in affecting more than one molecular pathway in regulating radio-resistance in tumors. When circRNAs increase the growth and metastasis of tumor cells, they possess oncogenic functions and can increase the malignant behavior of tumor cells, until they obtain radio-resistance. The process is reversed by onco-suppressor circRNAs that impair proliferation and metastasis of cancer cells for promoting radio-sensitivity. circ-MFN2 shows overexpression in colorectal cancer and enhances proliferation, invasion, and radio-resistance. circ-MFN2 promotes IGF1R expression via miR-574-3p downregulation to increase the malignant behavior of tumor cells in triggering radio-resistance. Silencing circ-MFN2 enhances radio-sensitivity of colorectal cancer cells via downregulating IGF1R expression [150]. Since colorectal cancer is a devastating disease among patients, a combination of surgery and radiotherapy is recommended for its suppression [80, 151].

Table 1. circRNAs and associated molecular pathways in affecting drug resistance.

circRNA	Molecular Pathway	Cancer Type	Drug	Remark(s)	Ref
hsa-circ-0001275	—	Prostate cancer	Enzalutamide	Upregulation of circ-0001275 and its parental gene PLCL2 occurs in cancers and they mediate drug resistance.	[121]
circ-MMP11	miR-153-3p/ANLN	Breast cancer	Lapatinib	circ-MMP11 promotes ANLN expression via miR-153-3p inhibition in increasing tumor progression and triggering chemo-resistance.	[122]
circ-0110805	miR-299-3p/ENDOPDI	Gastric cancer	Cisplatin	circ-0110805 prevents apoptosis and increases growth and invasion of tumor cells. circ-0110805 promotes ENDOPDI via miR-299-3p inhibition in triggering cisplatin resistance.	[123]
circ-0032821	miR-515-5p/SOX9	Gastric cancer	Oxaliplatin	circ-0032821 promotes SOX9 expression via miR-515-5p sponging in mediating drug resistance.	[124]
hsa-circ-0001598	miR-1184/PD-L1	Breast cancer	Trastuzumab	circ-0001598 promotes PD-L1 expression via miR-1184 sponging to induce immune evasion and mediate drug resistance.	[125]
circ-0013587	miR-1227/E-cadherin	Pancreatic cancer	Erlotinib	circ-0013587 promotes E-cadherin levels via miR-1227 inhibition to prevent drug resistance.	[126]
circ-0003998	miR-136-5p/CORO1C	Non-small cell lung cancer	Docetaxel	circ-0003998 sponges miR-136-5p to increase CORO1C expression in triggering docetaxel resistance in lung cancer.	[127]

(*Continued*)

Table 1. (*Continued*)

circRNA	Molecular Pathway	Cancer Type	Drug	Remark(s)	Ref
hsa-circ-0063804	miR-1276/CLU	Ovarian cancer	Cisplatin	circ-0063804 promotes CLU expression via miR-1276 sponging in increasing proliferation of tumor cells and mediating chemo-resistance.	[128]
circ-0007385	miR-519d-3p/HMGB1	Lung cancer	Cisplatin	circ-0007385 promotes malignant behavior of tumor cells and stimulates cisplatin resistance via miR-519d-3p inhibition and subsequent overexpression of HMGB1.	[129]
circ-SETD3	miR-873-5p/APPBP2	Non-small lung cancer	Gefitinib	circ-SETD3 promotes APPBP2 expression by miR-873-5p inhibition to increase tumor progression and to induce drug resistance.	[130]
circ-0076305	miR-296-5p/STAT3	Non-small cell lung cancer	Cisplatin	circ-0076305 stimulates STAT3 signaling via miR-296-5p sponging in mediating drug resistance.	[131]
hsa-circ-0074298	miR-519/SMOC	Pancreatic cancer	Gemcitabine	circ-0074398 increases SMOC expression via miR-519 inhibition in triggering drug resistance.	[132]
circ-0004140	miR-1184/CCL22	Lung cancer	Immune resistance	circ-0004140 increases CCL22 expression via miR-1184 sponging in triggering immune resistance.	[133]
circ-C200rf11	miR-527/YWHAZ	Ovarian cancer	Cisplatin	circ-C200rf11 promotes YWHAZ expression via miR-527 inhibition in inducing M2 polarization of macrophages and mediating drug resistance.	[134]

hsa-circ-0000073	miR-145-5p/miR-151-3p/NRAS	Osteosarcoma	Methotrexate	Enhanced proliferation and invasion of tumor cells and inducing drug resistance by circ-0000073 via miR inhibition and overexpression of NRAS.	[135]
circ-0006528	miR-1236-3p/CHD4	Breast cancer	Adriamycin	circ-0006528 promotes CHD4 expression via miR-1236-3p sponging in increasing tumor progression and inducing drug resistance.	[136]
hsa-circ-0096157	—	Non-small cell lung cancer	Cisplatin	circ-0096157 promotes invasion and proliferation and inhibits apoptosis in triggering drug resistance.	[137]
circ-0002360	miR-6751-3p/ZNF300	Lung cancer	Cisplatin	circ-0002360 promotes ZNF300 expression via miR-6751-3p sponging in apoptosis inhibition and triggering drug resistance.	[138]
hsa-circ-0097922	miR-876-3p/ACTN4	Breast cancer	Tamoxifen	circ-0097922 promotes ACTN4 expression by miR-876-3p sponging in increasing tumor progression and triggering chemo-resistance.	[139]
circ-CPA4	let-7/PD-L1	Non-small cell lung cancer	Cisplatin	circ-CPA4 increases PD-L1 expression via let-7 sponging in increasing tumor malignancy and inducing drug resistance	[140]
hsa-circ-001680	miR-340/BMI1	Colorectal cancer	Irinotecan	circ-001680 increases BMI1 expression via miR-340 inhibition in increasing stemness and triggering chemo-resistance.	[141]
hsa-circ-0025202	miR-197-3p/HIPK3	Breast cancer	Tamoxifen	circ-0025202 enhances HIPK3 expression by miR-197-3p sponging in reversing drug resistance.	[142]

(*Continued*)

Table 1. (*Continued*)

circRNA	Molecular Pathway	Cancer Type	Drug	Remark(s)	Ref
circ-0001721	miR-758/ TCF4	Osteosarcoma	Doxorubicin	circ-0001721 increases TCF4 expression by miR-758 inhibition to induce drug resistance.	[143]
circ-ABCB10	let-7a-5p/ DUSP7	Breast cancer	Paclitaxel	Silencing circ-ABCB10 induces apoptosis and enhances chemo-sensitivity. circ-ABCB10 promotes DUSP7 levels via let-7a-5p inhibition.	[144]
circ-ZFR	miR-195-5p/ KPNA4	Non-small cell lung cancer	Paclitaxel	circ-ZFR increases KPNA4 expression by miR-195-5p inhibition in triggering paclitaxel resistance.	[145]
circ-0001821	miR-526b-5p/ GRK5	Non-small cell lung cancer	Paclitaxel	circ-0001821 increases GRK5 expression by miR-526b-5p sponging to induce chemo-resistance.	[146]
circ-0007031	miR-133b/ ABCC5	Colorectal cancer	5-Flourouracil	circ-0007030 promotes ABCC5 expression by miR-133b in inducing drug resistance.	[147]
hsa-circ-0000520	PI3K/Akt	Gastric cancer	Herceptin	circ-0000520 induces PI3K/Akt signaling in triggering drug resistance.	[148]
circ-0071589	miR-526b-3p/ KLF12	Colorectal cancer	Cisplatin	circ-0071589 increases KLF12 expression by miR-526b-3p sponging in triggering cisplatin resistance.	[149]

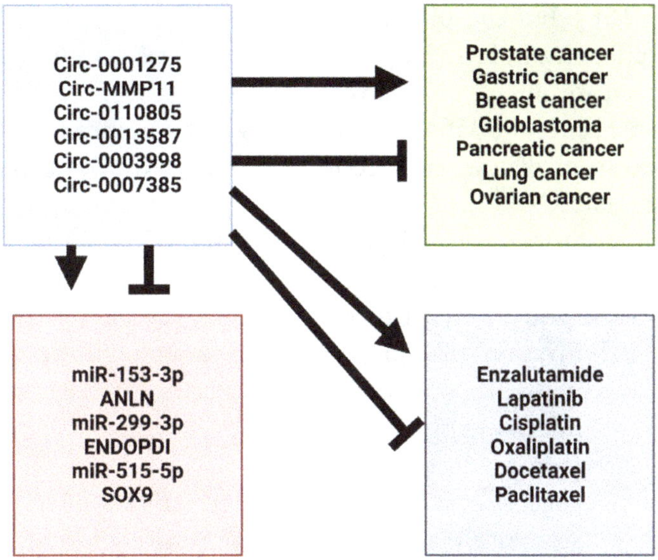

Figure 2. The role of circRNAs in regulating drug resistance in cancers. circRNAs function as key players and by affecting molecular pathways as downstream targets, they regulate drug sensitivity of various cancer; therefore, they can be targeted in cancer therapy.

Unfortunately, irradiation can increase metastasis of colon cancer cells and via c-Jun pathway, and it stimulates EMT in enhancing tumor progression [152, 153]. Silencing circ-0055625 increases radio-sensitivity of colon cancer cells. circ-0055625 promotes MSI1 expression by miR-338-3p sponging to prevent apoptosis and increase proliferation and invasion in triggering radio-resistance in tumor cells [154].

miR-485-5p is a new emerging target in cancer that suppresses progression, EMT, and proliferation of oral cancer cells via downregulating keratin 17 at the mRNA level [155]. Due to tumor suppressor function of miR-485-5p, its downregulation by LINC01224 and NKILA promotes cancer progression [156, 157]. Notably, circRNAs regulate miR-485-5p in regulating tumor progression. CircAPLP2 increases the growth and invasion of colorectal tumor cells by miR-485-5p inhibition and subsequent upregulation of

FOXK1 [158]. hsa-circ-0000554 regulates radio-sensitivity of cancer cells via affecting miR-485-5p. Overexpression of circ-0000554 prevents apoptosis in esophageal cancer cells exposed to irradiation. Noteworthy, circ-0000554 sponges miR-485-5p to increase FERMT1 expression in mediating radio-resistance [159]. Knock-down of such oncogenic circRNAs diminishes the progression of tumor cells and enhances radio-sensitivity. Silencing circ-0009035 impairs the progression of cervical cancer cells and increases their radio-sensitivity. Both in vitro and in vivo experiments have revealed a decrease in growth and invasion of cancer cells on downregulation of circ-0009035. Noteworthy, circ-0009035 increases HOXB7 expression via miR-889-3p sponging in increasing progression and triggering radio-resistance in cervical cancer [160].

Prostate cancer is a leading cause of death among men, and it is a devastating disease of the urological system. Although irradiation and radical proctectomy have been used for prostate cancer treatment, metastasis and chance of relapse threaten the efficacy of irradiation in tumor suppression [161–163]. A single factor is not responsible for the progression of prostate cancer, and it has been shown that non-coding RNAs, activation of pro-survival autophagy, ZEB proteins, and transforming growth factor-β signaling involve in regulating prostate tumor progression [164–166]. Recently, nanostructures have been considered as new therapeutic agents for prostate cancer [167]. circ-ZNF609 is suggested to be involved in radio-resistance in prostate cancer via inducing glycolysis mechanism. miR-501-3p downregulates HK2 expression in inhibiting glycolysis in prostate cancer. However, circ-ZNF609 promotes HK2 expression via miR-501-3p inhibition to induce glycolysis and prevent apoptosis in mediating radio-resistance [168]. Therefore, targeting circRNAs is of importance in regulating radio-resistance in cancers (Figure 3 and Table 2) [169–173].

6. Conclusion and remarks

Based on this chapter, three major problems are currently faced by patients around the world. The first problem is the initiation and

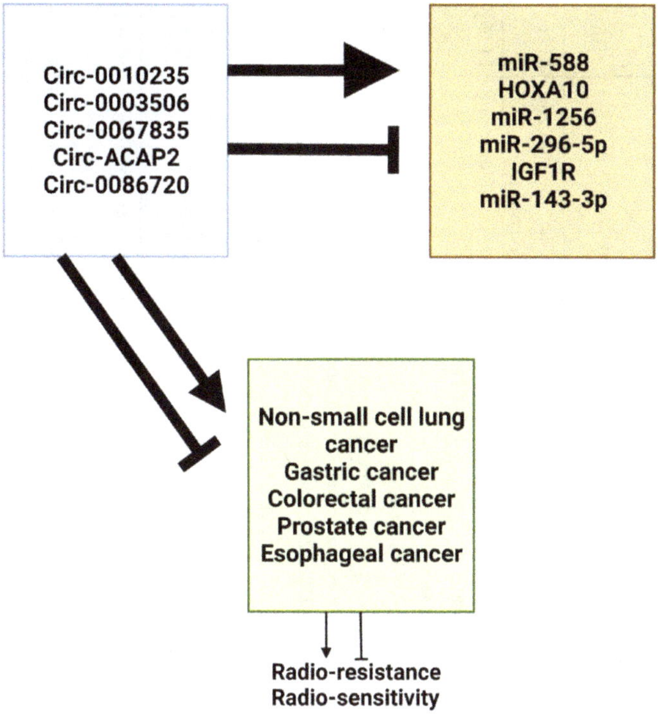

Figure 3. circRNAs and related molecular pathways in regulating radio-resistance in tumors.

development of cancer which is a life-threatening disease, and it negatively affects the life of people and burdens high socioeconomic costs. The second problem is the ability of tumor cells in drug resistance development that endangers the effort of researchers around the world in finding a novel therapeutic for cancer. The third problem is the emergence of radio-resistance. The first problem needs significant changes in the lifestyle of people and an understanding of different kinds of environmental and genetic factors that cause cancer, as a multi-factorial disease. This has been a quite dream for researchers around the world. However, finding a solution for overcoming drug resistance and radio-resistance appears to be more plausible than cancer prevention which was the aim of this chapter. Since circRNAs are

Table 2. The role of circRNAs in regulating radio-resistance in cancers.

circRNA	Molecular Pathway	Cancer Type	Radio-resistance Radio-sensitivity	Remark(s)	Ref
circ-0010235	miR-588/ HOXA10	Non-small cell lung cancer	Radio-resistance	Enhancing tumor progression. circ-0010235 increases HOXA10 expression via miR-588 sponging.	[174]
circ-0003506	miR-1256	Gastric cancer	Radio-resistance	circ-0003506 promotes tumor proliferation and invasion and induces radio-resistance via miR-1256 sponging.	[175]
circ-0067835	miR-296-5p/ IGF1R	Colorectal cancer	Radio-resistance	Overexpression of circ-0067835 on exposure to radiotherapy. circ-0067835 promotes IGF1R expression via miR-296-5p sponging.	[176]
circ-ACAP2	miR-143-3p/ FZD4	Colorectal cancer	Radio-resistance	circ-ACAP2 increases cancer malignancy via miR-143-3p sponging and overexpression of FZD4.	[177]
circ-0086720	miR-375/ SPIN1	Non-small cell lung cancer	Radio-resistance	Increased cancer cell survival and apoptosis inhibition. circ-0086720 increases SPIN1 expression by miR-375 inhibition.	[178]
hsa-circ-0004396	miR-615-5p/ PAK1	Non-small cell lung cancer	Radio-resistance	circ-0004396 increases PAK1 expression by miR-615-5p sponging in triggering therapy resistance.	[179]
circ-0007580	miR-598/ THBS2	Non-small cell lung cancer	Radio-resistance	circ-0007580 induces radio-resistance via miR-598 downregulation and THBS2 upregulation.	[180]
circ-0062020	miR-615-5p/ TRIP13	Prostate cancer	Radio-resistance	circ-0062020 promotes TRIP3 expression via miR-615-5p inhibition. Increasing tumor growth in vivo.	[181]
circ-0007022	miR-338-3p/ neuropilin-1	Esophageal cancer	Radio-resistance	circ-0007022 increases NRP1 expression via miR-338-3p inhibition in increasing tumor progression.	[182]
hsa-circ-0001313	miR-338-3p	Colon cancer	Radio-resistance	Increased cell viability and colony formation. circ-0001313 sponges miR-338-3p in triggering radio-resistance.	[183]

master regulators and modulate different molecular pathways, they are potent influencers of therapy response in cancer. In regulating drug resistance and radio-resistance in cancers, circRNAs mainly affect miRNAs via sponging and decrease their expression to target their downstream factors. Finally, circRNAs are able to regulate molecular pathways, such as STAT3, HMGB1, and PD-L1 to regulate the response of cancer cells to chemotherapy and radiotherapy. For improving the response of cancer patients to chemotherapy and irradiation, the optimal strategy is to silence oncogenic circRNAs in impairing tumor progression. Future studies can focus on translating current findings into the clinic.

Conflict of interest:

The authors declare no conflict of interest.

References

1. MacLeod, A.R. and S.T. Crooke, *RNA therapeutics in oncology: Advances, challenges, and future directions.* Journal of Clinical Pharmacology, 2017. **57**: p. S43–S59.
2. Cancer Genome Atlas Research Network, *Comprehensive genomic characterization defines human glioblastoma genes and core pathways.* Nature, 2008. **455**(7216): p. 1061–1068.
3. Chin, L. and J.W. Gray, *Translating insights from the cancer genome into clinical practice.* Nature, 2008. **452**(7187): p. 553–563.
4. Kim, H., et al., *Integrative genome analysis reveals an oncomir/oncogene cluster regulating glioblastoma survivorship.* Proceedings of the National Academy of Sciences of the United States of America, 2010. **107**(5): p. 2183–2188.
5. Cao, S., et al., *TME-responsive multistage nanoplatform for siRNA delivery and effective cancer therapy.* International Journal of Nanomedicine, 2021. **16**: p. 5909–5921.
6. Cai, W., et al., *Intelligent bio-responsive fluorescent Au-shRNA complexes for regulated autophagy and effective cancer bioimaging and therapeutics.* Biosensors (Basel), 2021. **11**(11).

7. Xu, F., et al., *A combinatorial CRISPR-Cas9 screen identifies Ifenprodil as an adjunct to Sorafenib for liver cancer treatment.* Cancer Research, 2021. **81**(24): p. 6219–6232.
8. Yu, H., D. Pardoll, and R. Jove, *STATs in cancer inflammation and immunity: A leading role for STAT3.* Nature Reviews. Cancer, 2009. **9**(11): p. 798–809.
9. Marshall, L. and R.J. White, *Non-coding RNA production by RNA polymerase III is implicated in cancer.* Nature Reviews. Cancer, 2008. **8**(12): p. 911–914.
10. Ryan, B.M., A.I. Robles, and C.C. Harris, *Genetic variation in microRNA networks: The implications for cancer research.* Nature Reviews. Cancer, 2010. **10**(6): p. 389–402.
11. Weinstein, I.B. and A. Joe, *Oncogene addiction.* Cancer Research, 2008. **68**(9): p. 3077–3080.
12. Liu, Y., et al., *Non-coding RNAs in necroptosis, pyroptosis and ferroptosis in cancer metastasis.* Cell Death & Discovery, 2021. 7(1): p. 210.
13. Peng, Y., *Non-coding RNAs in human cancer.* Seminars in Cancer Biology, 2021. **75**: p. 1–2.
14. Lin, X., et al., *Non-coding RNAs rewire cancer metabolism networks.* Seminars in Cancer Biology, 2021. **75**: p. 116–126.
15. Su, Q., et al., *Exosome-derived long non-coding RNAs as non-invasive biomarkers of bladder cancer.* Frontiers in Oncology, 2021. **11**: p. 719863.
16. Liang, J., L. Zhang, and W. Cheng, *Non-coding RNA-mediated autophagy in cancer: A protumor or antitumor factor?* Biochimica et Biophysica Acta. Reviews on Cancer, 2021. **1876**(2): p. 188642.
17. Ashrafizaveh, S., et al., *Long non-coding RNAs in the doxorubicin resistance of cancer cells.* Cancer Letters, 2021. **508**: p. 104–114.
18. Mirzaei, S., et al., *Nrf2 signaling pathway in cisplatin chemotherapy: Potential involvement in organ protection and chemoresistance.* Pharmacological Research, 2021. **167**: p. 105575.
19. Wu, Q., et al., *YAP drives fate conversion and chemoresistance of small cell lung cancer.* Science Advances, 2021. 7(40): p. eabg1850.
20. Mondal, P. and S.M. Meeran, *microRNAs in cancer chemoresistance: The sword and the shield.* Noncoding RNA Research, 2021. **6**(4): p. 200–210.

21. Pan, Y., et al., *MicroRNAs in pancreatic cancer and chemoresistance.* Pancreas, 2021. **50**(10): p. 1334–1342.
22. Tirinato, L., et al., *Lipid droplets and ferritin heavy chain: A devilish liaison in human cancer cell radioresistance.* Elife, 2021. **10**.
23. Aranza-Martínez, A., et al., *Non-coding RNAs associated with radioresistance in triple-negative breast cancer.* Frontiers in Oncology, 2021. **11**: p. 752270.
24. Kwon, Y.S., et al., *Acyl-CoA synthetase-4 mediates radioresistance of breast cancer cells by regulating FOXM1.* Biochemical Pharmacology, 2021. **192**: p. 114718.
25. Yang, L., et al., *Oncogenic KRAS drives radioresistance through upregulation of NRF2-53BP1-mediated non-homologous end-joining repair.* Nucleic Acids Research, 2021. **49**(19): p. 11067–11082.
26. Zhu, D., et al., *Numb/Notch/PLK1 signaling pathway mediated hyperglycemic memory in pancreatic cancer cell radioresistance and the therapeutic effects of metformin.* Cell Signaling, 2022. **93**: p. 110268.
27. Ding, N., et al., *Peroxiredoxin IV plays a critical role in cancer cell growth and radioresistance through the activation of the Akt/GSK3 signaling pathways.* Journal of Biological Chemistry, 2022. **298**(7): p. 102123.
28. Fang, F., et al., *Exosome-mediated transfer of miR-1323 from cancer-associated fibroblasts confers radioresistance of C33A cells by targeting PABPN1 and activating Wnt/β-catenin signaling pathway in cervical cancer.* Reproductive Sciences, 2022. **29**(6): p. 1809–1821.
29. Chen, G., et al., *Golgi phosphoprotein 3 confers radioresistance via stabilizing EGFR in lung adenocarcinoma.* International Journal of Radiation Oncology, Biology, Physics, 2022. **112**(5): p. 1216–1228.
30. Dong, J., et al., *HMGB1 overexpression promotes a malignant phenotyp. and radioresistance in ESCC.* Journal of Cancer, 2022. **13**(9): p. 2717–2726.
31. Jiang, H., et al., *Long noncoding RNA KLF3-AS1 acts as an endogenous RNA of miR-223 to attenuate gastric cancer progression and chemoresistance.* Frontiers in Oncology, 2021. **11**: p. 704339.
32. Zou, G.P., et al., *Mitochondrial dynamics mediated by DRP1 and MFN2 contributes to cisplatin chemoresistance in human ovarian cancer SKOV3 cells.* Journal of Cancer, 2021. **12**(24): p. 7358–7373.

33. Cheng, Y.Y., et al., *LGR6 promotes glioblastoma malignancy and chemoresistance by activating the Akt signaling pathway.* Experimental and Therapeutic Medicine, 2021. **22**(6): p. 1364.
34. Sharma, R., et al., *BMP4 enhances anoikis resistance and chemoresistance of breast cancer cells through canonical BMP signaling.* Journal of Cell Communication and Signaling, 2022. **16**(2): p. 191–205.
35. Ganguly, K., et al., *Mucin 5AC serves as the nexus for β-catenin/c-Myc interplay to promote glutamine dependency during pancreatic cancer chemoresistance.* Gastroenterology, 2022. **162**(1): p. 253–268.e13.
36. Han, S., et al., *GAS41 mediates proliferation and GEM chemoresistance via H2A.Z.2 and Notch1 in pancreatic cancer.* Cell Oncology (Dordrecht), 2022. **45**(3): p. 429–446.
37. Lang, T., et al., *Disruption of KDM4C-ALDH1A3 feed-forward loop inhibits stemness, tumorigenesis and chemoresistance of gastric cancer stem cells.* Signal Transduction and Targeted Therapy, 2021. **6**(1): p. 336.
38. van Zonneveld, A.J., et al., *Circular RNAs in kidney disease and cancer.* Nature Reviews. Nephrology, 2021. **17**(12): p. 814–826.
39. Salzman, J., et al., *Circular RNAs are the predominant transcrip isoform from hundreds of human genes in diverse cell types.* PLoS One, 2012. 7(2): p. e30733.
40. Memczak, S., et al., *Circular RNAs are a large class of animal RNAs with regulatory potency.* Nature, 2013. **495**(7441): p. 333–338.
41. Jeck, W.R., et al., *Circular RNAs are abundant, conserved, and associated with ALU repeats.* RNA, 2013. **19**(2): p. 141–157.
42. Hansen, T.B., et al., *Natural RNA circles function as efficient microRNA sponges.* Nature, 2013. **495**(7441): p. 384–388.
43. Sanger, H.L., et al., *Viroids are single-stranded covalently closed circular RNA molecules existing as highly base-paired rod-like structures.* Proceedings of the National Academy of Sciences of the United States of America, 1976. **73**(11): p. 3852–3856.
44. Berget, S.M., C. Moore, and P.A. Sharp. *Spliced segments at the 5′ terminus of adenovirus 2 late mRNA.* Proceedings of the National Academy of Sciences of the United States of America, 1977. **74**(8): p. 3171–3175.
45. Nigro, J.M., et al., *Scrambled exons.* Cell, 1991. **64**(3): p. 607–613.

46. Kos, A., et al., *The hepatitis delta (δ) virus possesses a circular RNA.* Nature, 1986. **323**(6088): p. 558–560.
47. Cocquerelle, C., et al., *Mis-splicing yields circular RNA molecules.* FASEB Journal, 1993. 7(1): p. 155–160.
48. Bailleul, B., *During in vivo maturation of eukaryotic nuclear mRNA, splicing yields excised exon circles.* Nucleic Acids Research, 1996. **24**(6): p. 1015–1019.
49. Shen, H., et al., *Circular RNAs: Characteristics, biogenesis, mechanisms and functions in liver cancer.* Journal of Hematology & Oncology, 2021. **14**(1): p. 1–16.
50. Chen, L.-L., *The expanding regulatory mechanisms and cellular functions of circular RNAs.* Nature Reviews. Molecular Cell Biology, 2020. **21**(8): p. 475–490.
51. Kristensen, L.S., et al., *The biogenesis, biology and characterization of circular RNAs.* Nature Reviews. Genetics, 2019. **20**(11): p. 675–691.
52. Ashwal-Fluss, R., et al., *circRNA biogenesis competes with pre-mRNA splicing.* Molecular Cell, 2014. **56**(1): p. 55–66.
53. Rong, Z., et al., *Circular RNA in pancreatic cancer: A novel avenue for the roles of diagnosis and treatment.* Theranostics, 2021. **11**(6): p. 2755–2769.
54. Zhang, Y., et al., *Circular intronic long noncoding RNAs.* Molecular Cell, 2013. **51**(6): p. 792–806.
55. Wang, F., A.J. Nazarali, and S. Ji, *Circular RNAs as potential biomarkers for cancer diagnosis and therapy.* American Journal of Cancer Research, 2016. **6**(6): p. 1167.
56. Guo, Y., et al., *Circular RNAs and their roles in head and neck cancers.* Molecular Cancer, 2019. **18**(1): p. 1–18.
57. Long, F., et al., *Comprehensive landscap. and future perspectives of circular RNAs in colorectal cancer.* Molecular Cancer, 2021. **20**(1): p. 1–22.
58. Wang, S., et al., *Circular RNAs in body fluids as cancer biomarkers: The new frontier of liquid biopsies.* Molecular Cancer, 2021. **20**(1): p. 1–10.
59. Lei, B., et al., *Circular RNA: A novel biomarker and therapeutic target for human cancers.* International Journal of Medical Sciences, 2019. **16**(2): p. 292.

60. Liu, J., W. Yuan, and D. Gong, *Hsa_circ_0000994 inhibits pancreatic cancer progression by clearing immune-related miR-27a and miR-27b.* Jorunal of Oncology, 2022. **2022**: p. 7274794.
61. Liu, D., X. Bi, and Y. Yang, *Circular RNA hsa_circ_0011324 is involved in endometrial cancer progression and the evolution of its mechanism.* Bioengineered, 2022. **13**(3): p. 7485–7499.
62. Xi, J., et al., *Hsa_circ_0060937 accelerates non-small cell lung cancer progression via modulating miR-195-5p/HMGB3 pathway.* Cell Cycle, 2021. **20**(19): p. 2040–2052.
63. Liu, L., F. Zhang, and J. Li, *CircRNA circ_0001821 predicts an unfavorable prognosis and promotes the proliferation of multiple myeloma.* Hematology, 2021. **26**(1): p. 716–723.
64. Chen, X., et al., *Hsa_circ_0001806 promotes glycolysis and cell progression in hepatocellular carcinoma through miR-125b/HK2.* Journal of Clinical Laboratory Analysis, 2021. **35**(12): p. e23991.
65. Duan, H. and J. Qiu, *Association of has_circ_0001944 upregulations with prognosis and cancer progression in patients with colorectal cancer.* Discover Oncology, 2022. **13**(1): p. 23.
66. Han, J., et al., *Circ_0027599 elevates RUNX1 expression via sponging miR-21-5p on gastric cancer progression.* European Journal of Clinical Investigation, 2021. **51**(11): p. e13592.
67. Mao, G., et al., *Hsa_circ_0040809 regulates colorectal cancer development by upregulating methyltransferase DNMT1 via targeting miR-515-5p.* The Journal of Gene Medicine, 2021. **23**(12): p. e3388.
68. Xu, Y.J., et al., *Hsa_circ_0136666 activates Treg-mediated immune escap. of colorectal cancer via miR-497/PD-L1 pathway.* Cell Signaling, 2021. **86**: p. 110095.
69. Wu, G., et al., *Circ-RNF111 aggravates the malignancy of gastric cancer through miR-876-3p-dependent regulation of KLF12.* World Journal of Surgical Oncology, 2021. **19**(1): p. 259.
70. Zhang, Q., et al., *Hsa_circ_0023990 promotes tumor growth and glycolysis in dedifferentiated TC via targeting miR-485-5p/FOXM1 axis.* Endocrinology, 2021. **162**(12).
71. Liu, Q. and H. Dong, *EIF4A3-mediated hsa_circ_0088088 promotes the carcinogenesis of breast cancer by sponging miR-135-5p.* Journal of Biochemical and Molecular Toxicology, 2021. **35**(11): p. e22909.

72. Shi, Y. and C. Liu, *Circular RNA hsa_circ_0043278 inhibits breast cancer progression via the miR-455-3p/EI24 signalling pathway.* BMC Cancer, 2021. **21**(1): p. 1249.
73. Zhao, Y., X. Ma, and W. Shi, *Circ_0069718 promotes the progression of breast cancer by up-regulating NFIB through sequestering miR-590-5p.* Mammalian Genome, 2021. **32**(6): p. 517–529.
74. Liu, Z.H., et al., *Correlations of hsa_circ_0046264 expression with onset, pathological stage and chemotherapy resistance of lung cancer.* European Review for Medical and Pharmacological Sciences, 2020. **24**(18): p. 9511–9521.
75. Zhang, Z., et al., *Circular RNA circ_0026359 enhances cisplatin resistance in gastric cancer via targeting miR-1200/POLD4 pathway.* BioMed Research International, 2020. **2020**: p. 5103272.
76. Xue, M., et al., *hsa_circ_0081143 promotes cisplatin resistance in gastric cancer by targeting miR-646/CDK6 pathway.* Cancer Cell International, 2019. **19**: p. 25.
77. Yi, X., et al., *Circular RNA circ_0004507 contributes to laryngeal cancer progression and cisplatin resistance by sponging miR-873 to upregulate multidrug resistance 1 and multidrug resistance protein 1.* Head & Neck, 2021. **43**(3): p. 928–941.
78. Jemal, A., et al., *Cancer statistics, 2010.* CA: A Cancer Journal for Clinicians, 2010. **60**(5): p. 277–300.
79. Siegel, R.L., K.D. Miller, and A. Jemal, *Cancer statistics, 2019.* CA: A Cancer Journal for Clinicians, 2019. **69**(1): p. 7–34.
80. Bray, F., et al., *Global cancer statistics 2018: GLOBOCAN estimates of incidence and mortality worldwide for 36 cancers in 185 countries.* CA: A Cancer Journal for Clinicians, 2018. **68**(6): p. 394–424.
81. Devesa, S.S., et al., *International lung cancer trends by histologic type: Male: female differences diminishing and adenocarcinoma rates rising.* International Journal of Cancer, 2005. **117**(2): p. 294–299.
82. de Cos, J.S., et al., *Non-small cell lung cancer and silent brain metastasis: Survival and prognostic factors.* Lung Cancer, 2009. **63**(1): p. 140–145.
83. Fellner, S., et al., *Transport of paclitaxel (Taxol) across the blood-brain barrier in vitro and in vivo.* The Journal of Clinical Investigation, 2002. **110**(9): p. 1309–1318.

84. Klimaszewska-Wi niewska, A., et al., *Evaluation of anti-metastatic potential of the combination of fisetin with paclitaxel on A549 non-small cell lung cancer cells.* International Journal of Molecular Sciences, 2018. **19**(3): p. 661.
85. Razi, S.S., et al., *Antitumor activity of paclitaxel is significantly enhanced by a novel proapoptotic agent in non–small cell lung cancer.* The Journal of Surgical Research, 2015. **194**(2): p. 622–630.
86. Ashrafizadeh, M., et al., *Chitosan-based advanced materials for docetaxel and paclitaxel delivery: Recent advances and future directions in cancer theranostics.* The Journal of Surgical Research, 2020. **145**: p. 282–300.
87. Teow, H.M., et al., *Delivery of paclitaxel across cellular barriers using a dendrimer-based nanocarrier.* International Journal of Pharmaceutics, 2013. **441**(1–2): p. 701–711.
88. Reshma, P., et al., *Overcoming drug-resistance in lung cancer cells by paclitaxel loaded galactoxyloglucan nanoparticles.* International Journal of Biological Macromolecules, 2019. **136**: p. 266–274.
89. Ashrafizadeh, M., et al., *New insight towards development of paclitaxel and docetaxel resistance in cancer cells: EMT as a novel molecular mechanism and therapeutic possibilities.* Biomedicine & Pharmacotherapy, 2021. **141**: p. 111824.
90. Xu, J., et al., *Overexpression of hsa_circ_0002874 promotes resistance of non-small cell lung cancer to paclitaxel by modulating miR-1273f/MDM2/p53 pathway.* Aging (Albany NY), 2021. **13**(4): p. 5986–6009.
91. Zhang, S., et al., *circCELSR1 (hsa_circ_0063809) contributes to paclitaxel resistance of ovarian cancer cells by regulating FOXR2 expression via miR-1252.* Molecular Therapy — Nucleic Acids, 2020. **19**: p. 718–730.
92. Lei, J., et al., *Cervical screening and risk of adenosquamous and rare histological types of invasive cervical carcinoma: population based nested case-control study.* BMJ, 2019. **365**.
93. He, L., et al., *Synergistic antitumor effect of combined paclitaxel with FEN1 inhibitor in cervical cancer cells.* DNA Repair (Amsterdam), 2018. **63**: p. 1–9.

94. Long, X., et al., *circ_ZFR is linked to paclitaxel resistance in cervical cancer via miR-944 sponging and IL-10 upregulation.* Analytical Cellular Pathology (Amsterdam), 2022. **2022**: p. 4807287.
95. Mohammadinejad, R., et al., *ZEB1 and ZEB2 gene editing mediated by CRISPR/Cas9 in A549 cell line.* Bratislavské Lekárske Listy, 2020. **121**(1): p. 31–36.
96. Sakata, J., et al., *Inhibition of ZEB1 leads to inversion of metastatic characteristics and restoration of paclitaxel sensitivity of chronic chemoresistant ovarian carcinoma cells.* Oncotarget, 2017. **8**(59): p. 99482–99494.
97. An, J., W. Lv, and Y. Zhang, *LncRNA NEAT1 contributes to paclitaxel resistance of ovarian cancer cells by regulating ZEB1 expression via miR-194.* OncoTargets and Therapy, 2017. **10**: p. 5377–5390.
98. Liu, Y.Y., L.Y. Zhang, and W.Z. Du, *Circular RNA circ-PVT1 contributes to paclitaxel resistance of gastric cancer cells through the regulation of ZEB1 expression by sponging miR-124-3p.* Bioscience Reports, 2019. **39**(12).
99. Sutter, S.A., et al., *Surgical management of breast cancer in Africa: A continent-wide review of intervention practices, barriers to care, and adjuvant therapy.* Journal of Global Oncology, 2017. **3**(2): p. 162–168.
100. Caetano-Pinto, P., et al., *The importance of breast cancer resistance protein to the kidneys excretory function and chemotherapeutic resistance.* Drug Resistance Updates, 2017. **30**: p. 15–27.
101. Broxterman, H.J., K.J. Gotink, and H.M. Verheul, *Understanding the causes of multidrug resistance in cancer: A comparison of doxorubicin and sunitinib.* Drug Resistance Updates, 2009. **12**(4–5): p. 114–126.
102. Zang, H., et al., *Circ-RNF111 contributes to paclitaxel resistance in breast cancer by elevating E2F3 expression via miR-140-5p.* Thoracic Cancer, 2020. **11**(7): p. 1891–1903.
103. Cho, Y.H., et al., *5-FU promotes stemness of colorectal cancer via p53-mediated WNT/β-catenin pathway activation.* Nature Communications, 2020. **11**(1): p. 5321.
104. Xu, X., et al., *HMGA2 enhances 5-fluorouracil chemoresistance in colorectal cancer via the Dvl2/Wnt pathway.* Oncotarget, 2018. **9**(11): p. 9963–9974.

105. Long, Y., Q. Zhao, and Y. Huang, *RNF38 enhances 5-Fluorouracil resistance in colorectal cancer by activating the Wnt pathway.* JBUON, 2021. **26**(4): p. 1246–1251.
106. Lu, Y., et al., *Curcumin may reverse 5-fluorouracil resistance on colonic cancer cells by regulating TET1-NKD-Wnt signal pathway to inhibit the EMT progress.* Biomedicine & Pharmacotherapy, 2020. **129**: p. 110381.
107. Chen, H., et al., *Circ-PRKDC contributes to 5-fluorouracil resistance of colorectal cancer cells by regulating miR-375/FOXM1 axis and Wnt/β-catenin pathway.* OncoTargets and Therapy, 2020. **13**: p. 5939–5953.
108. Li, S. and S. Zheng, *Down-regulation of Circ_0032833 sensitizes colorectal cancer to 5-fluorouracil and oxaliplatin partly depending on the regulation of miR-125-5p and MSI1.* Cancer Management and Research, 2020. **12**: p. 11257–11269.
109. Ou, W., et al., *Circ_0081143 contributes to gastric cancer malignant development and doxorubicin resistance by elevating the expression of YES1 by targeting mziR-129-2-3p.* Gut and Liver, 2022.
110. Niu, R., et al., *Circ_0014235 confers Gefitinib resistance and malignant behaviors in non-small cell lung cancer resistant to Gefitinib by governing the miR-146b-5p/YAP/PD-L1 pathway.* Cell Cycle, 2022. **21**(1): p. 86–100.
111. Li, X., et al., *Hsa_circ_0002483 inhibited the progression and enhanced the Taxol sensitivity of non-small cell lung cancer by targeting miR-182-5p.* Cell Death & Disease, 2019. **10**(12): p. 953.
112. Xu, X., et al., *Exosome-transferred hsa_circ_0014235 promotes DDP chemoresistance and deteriorates the development of non-small cell lung cancer by mediating the miR-520a-5p/CDK4 pathway.* Cancer Cell International, 2020. **20**(1): p. 552.
113. Zhou, Y., et al., *Circular RNA hsa_circ_0004015 regulates the proliferation, invasion, and TKI drug resistance of non-small cell lung cancer by miR-1183/PDPK1 signaling pathway.* Biochemical and Biophysical Research Communications, 2019. **508**(2): p. 527–535.
114. Yuan, S., et al., *Hsa_Circ_0001860 promotes Smad7 to enhance MPA resistance in endometrial cancer via miR-520h.* Frontiers in Cell and Developmental Biology, 2021. **9**: p. 738189.

115. Sun, Y., et al., *Hsa_circ_0020095 promotes oncogenesis and cisplatin resistance in colon cancer by sponging miR-487a-3p and modulating SOX9.* Frontiers in Cell and Developmental Biology, 2020. **8**: p. 604869.
116. Wei, S., L. Qi, and L. Wang, *Overexpression of circ_CELSR1 facilitates paclitaxel resistance of ovarian cancer by regulating miR-149-5p/SIK2 axis.* Anti-cancer Drugs, 2021. **32**(5): p. 496–507.
117. Feng, N., et al., *Circ_PIP5K1A regulates cisplatin resistance and malignant progression in non-small cell lung cancer cells and xenograft murine model via depending on miR-493-5p/ROCK1 axis.* Respiratory Research, 2021. **22**(1): p. 248.
118. Li, X., et al., *A novel circular RNA, hsa_circ_0030998 suppresses lung cancer tumorigenesis and Taxol resistance by sponging miR-558.* Molecular Oncology, 2021. **15**(8): p. 2235–2248.
119. Liu, G., et al., *Circ_0006528 contributes to paclitaxel resistance of breast cancer cells by regulating miR-1299/CDK8 axis.* OncoTargets and Therapy, 2020. **13**: p. 9497–9511.
120. Gao, H., et al., *Depletion of hsa_circ_0000144 suppresses oxaliplatin resistance of gastric cancer cells by regulating miR-502-5p/ADAM9 axis.* OncoTargets and Therapy, 2021. **14**: p. 2773–2787.
121. Lim, M.C.J., et al., *hsa_circ_0001275 is one of a number of circRNAs dysregulated in enzalutamide resistant prostate cancer and confers enzalutamide resistance in vitro.* Cancers (Basel), 2021. **13**(24).
122. Wu, X., et al., *Circular RNA circ-MMP11 contributes to lapatinib resistance of breast cancer cells by regulating the miR-153-3p/ANLN axis.* Frontiers in Oncology, 2021. **11**: p. 639961.
123. Yang, X., Q. Zhang, and B. Guan, *Circ_0110805 knockdown enhances cisplatin sensitivity and inhibits gastric cancer progression by miR-299-3p/ENDOPDI axis.* OncoTargets and Therapy, 2020. **13**: p. 11445–11457.
124. Zhong, Y., et al., *Circular RNA circ_0032821 contributes to oxaliplatin (OXA) resistance of gastric cancer cells by regulating SOX9 via miR-515-5p.* Biotechnology Letters, 2021. **43**(2): p. 339–351.
125. Huang, L., J. Ma, and M. Cui, *Circular RNA hsa_circ_0001598 promotes programmed death-ligand-1-mediated immune escape and*

trastuzumab resistance via sponging miR-1184 in breast cancer cells. Immunology Research, 2021. **69**(6): p. 558–567.

126. Xu, H., et al., *Overexpression of circular RNA circ_0013587 reverses erlotinib resistance in pancreatic cancer cells through regulating the miR-1227/E-cadherin pathway.* Frontiers in Oncology, 2021. **11**: p. 754146.
127. Zhang, W., C. Song, and X. Ren, *Circ_0003998 regulates the progression and docetaxel sensitivity of DTX-resistant non-small cell lung cancer cells by the miR-136-5p/CORO1C axis.* Technology in Cancer Research & Treatment, 2021. **20**: p. 1533033821990040.
128. You, J., et al., *Hsa_circ_0063804 enhances ovarian cancer cells proliferation and resistance to cisplatin by targeting miR-1276/CLU axis.* Aging (Albany NY), 2022. **14**(11): p. 4699–4713.
129. Ye, Y., et al., *circ_0007385 served as competing endogenous RNA for miR-519d-3p to suppress malignant behaviors and cisplatin resistance of non-small cell lung cancer cells.* Thoracic Cancer, 2020. **11**(8): p. 2196–2208.
130. Sheng, J., et al., *Circ_SETD3 regulates gefitinib sensitivity and tumor progression by miR-873-5p-dependent regulation of APPBP2 in non-small cell lung cancer.* Journal of Chemotherapy, 2021: p. 1–13.
131. Dong, Y., et al., *Circ_0076305 regulates cisplatin resistance of non-small cell lung cancer via positively modulating STAT3 by sponging miR-296-5p.* Life Sciences, 2019. **239**: p. 116984.
132. Hong, C., et al., *Hsa_circ_0074298 promotes pancreatic cancer progression and resistance to gemcitabine by sponging miR-519 to target SMOC.* Journal of Cancer, 2022. **13**(1): p. 34–50.
133. Liu, Y., et al., *circ_0004140 promotes LUAD tumor progression and immune resistance through circ_0004140/miR-1184/CCL22 axis.* Cell Death & Discovery, 2022. **8**(1): p. 181.
134. Yin, J., et al., *circ_C20orf11 enhances DDP resistance by inhibiting miR-527/YWHAZ through the promotion of extracellular vesicle-mediated macrophage M2 polarization in ovarian cancer.* Cancer Biology & Therapy, 2021. **22**(7–9): p. 440–454.
135. Li, X., et al., *Circular RNA hsa_circ_0000073 contributes to osteosarcoma cell proliferation, migration, invasion and methotrexate resistance by sponging miR-145-5p and miR-151-3p and upregulating NRAS.* Aging (Albany NY), 2020. **12**(14): p. 14157–14173.

136. Hao, J., et al., *Knockdown of circ_0006528 suppresses cell proliferation, migration, invasion, and adriamycin chemoresistance via regulating the miR-1236-3p/CHD4 axis in breast cancer.* Journal of Surgical Research, 2021. **260**: p. 104–115.
137. Lu, H., et al., *Circular RNA hsa_circ_0096157 contributes to cisplatin resistance by proliferation, cell cycle progression, and suppressing apoptosis of non-small-cell lung carcinoma cells.* Molecular and Cellullar Biochemistry, 2020. **475**(1–2): p. 63–77.
138. Ding, L., L. Li, and Z. Tang, *Cisplatin resistance and malignant behaviors of lung cancer cells are promoted by circ_0002360 via targeting miR-6751-3p to regulate the expression of ZNF300.* Thoracic Cancer, 2022. **13**(7): p. 986–996.
139. Liang, X., et al., *Hsa_circ_0097922 promotes tamoxifen resistance and cell malignant behavior of breast cancer cells by regulating ACTN4 expression via miR-876-3p.* Clinical and Experimental Pharmacology and Physiology, 2022.
140. Hong, W., et al., *Circular RNA circ-CPA4/ let-7 miRNA/PD-L1 axis regulates cell growth, stemness, drug resistance and immune evasion in non-small cell lung cancer (NSCLC).* Journal of Experimental & Clinical Cancer Research, 2020. **39**(1): p. 149.
141. Jian, X., et al., *Hsa_circ_001680 affects the proliferation and migration of CRC and mediates its chemoresistance by regulating BMI1 through miR-340.* Molecular Cancer, 2020. **19**(1): p. 20.
142. Li, H., Q. Li, and S. He, *Hsa_circ_0025202 suppresses cell tumorigenesis and tamoxifen resistance via miR-197-3p/HIPK3 axis in breast cancer.* World Journal of Surgical Oncology, 2021. **19**(1): p. 39.
143. Guan, H., et al., *Circ_0001721 enhances doxorubicin resistance and promotes tumorigenesis in osteosarcoma through miR-758/TCF4 axis.* Cancer Cell International, 2021. **21**(1): p. 336.
144. Yang, W., et al., *Circ-ABCB10 contributes to paclitaxel resistance in breast cancer through Let-7a-5p/DUSP7 axis.* Cancer Management and Research, 2020. **12**: p. 2327–2337.
145. Li, J., R. Fan, and H. Xiao, *Circ_ZFR contributes to the paclitaxel resistance and progression of non-small cell lung cancer by upregulating KPNA4 through sponging miR-195-5p.* Cancer Cell International, 2021. **21**(1): p. 15.

146. Liu, Y., et al., *Circ_0001821 knockdown suppresses growth, metastasis, and TAX resistance of non-small-cell lung cancer cells by regulating the miR-526b-5p/GRK5 axis.* Pharmacology Research & Perspectives, 2021. **9**(4): p. e00812.
147. He, X., et al., *Circ_0007031 enhances tumor progression and promotes 5-fluorouracil resistance in colorectal cancer through regulating miR-133b/ABCC5 axis.* Cancer Biomarkers, 2020. **29**(4): p. 531–542.
148. Lv, X., et al., *hsa_circ_0000520 influences herceptin resistance in gastric cancer cells through PI3K-Akt signaling pathway.* Journal of Clinical Laboratory Analysis, 2020. **34**(10): p. e23449.
149. Zhang, W., et al., *Downregulation of Circ_0071589 suppresses cisplatin resistance in colorectal cancer by regulating the MiR-526b-3p/KLF12 axis.* Cancer Management and Research, 2021. **13**: p. 2717–2731.
150. Liu, D., et al., *Circ-MFN2 positively regulates the proliferation, metastasis, and radioresistance of colorectal cancer by regulating the miR-574-3p/IGF1R signaling axis.* Frontiers in Genetics, 2021. **12**: p. 671337.
151. Påhlman, L., *Indications for neoadjuvant long-term radiotherapy.* Recent Results in Cancer Research, 2005: p. 212–220.
152. De Bacco, F., et al., *Induction of MET by ionizing radiation and its role in radioresistance and invasive growth of cancer.* Journal of the National Cancer Institute, 2011. **103**(8): p. 645–661.
153. Zhang, J., et al., *Suppression of LINC00460 mediated the sensitization of HCT116 cells to ionizing radiation by inhibiting epithelial–mesenchymal transition.* Toxicology Research, 2020. **9**(2): p. 107–116.
154. Gao, C., et al., *Circ_0055625 knockdown inhibits tumorigenesis and improves radiosensitivity by regulating miR-338-3p/MSI1 axis in colon cancer.* World Journal of Surgical Oncology, 2021. **19**(1): p. 131.
155. Jang, T.H., et al., *MicroRNA-485-5p targets keratin 17 to regulate oral cancer stemness and chemoresistance via the integrin/FAK/Src/ERK/β-catenin pathway.* Journal of Biomedical Sciences, 2022. **29**(1): p. 42.
156. Wang, Y., et al., *LncRNA NKILA promotes epithelial-mesenchymal transition of liver cancer cells by targeting miR-485-5p.* Journal of Oncology, 2021. **2021**: p. 1281031.

157. Gu, J., et al., *LINC01224 promotes colorectal cancer progression through targeting miR-485-5p/MYO6 axis.* World Journal of Surgical Oncology, 2021. **19**(1): p. 281.
158. Liu, J., et al., *Knockdown of circAPLP2 inhibits progression of colorectal cancer by regulating miR-485-5p/FOXK1 axis.* Cancer Biotherapy and Radiopharmaceuticals, 2021. **36**(9): p. 737–752.
159. Wang, J., et al., *Circular RNA hsa_circ_0000554 promotes progression and elevates radioresistance through the miR-485-5p/fermitin family members 1 axis in esophageal cancer.* Anti-cancer Drugs, 2021. **32**(4): p. 405–416.
160. Zhao, X., et al., *Silencing of hsa_circ_0009035 suppresses cervical cancer progression and enhances radiosensitivity through microRNA 889-3p-dependent regulation of HOXB7.* Molecular and Cellular Biology, 2021. **41**(6): p. e0063120.
161. Mohler, J.L., et al., *Prostate cancer, version 1.2016.* Journal of the National Comprehensive Cancer Network, 2016. **14**(1): p. 19–30.
162. Hamdy, F.C., et al., *10-year outcomes after monitoring, surgery, or radiotherapy for localized prostate cancer.* The New England Journal of Medicine, 2016. **375**: p. 1415–1424.
163. Chang, A.J., et al., *High-risk prostate cancer — classification and therapy.* Nature Reviews. Clinical Oncology, 2014. **11**(6): p. 308–323.
164. Mirzaei, S., et al., *Transforming growth factor-beta (TGF-β) in prostate cancer: A dual function mediator?* International Journal of Biological Macromolecules, 2022. **206**: p. 435–452.
165. Ashrafizadeh, M., et al., *Targeting autophagy in prostate cancer: Preclinical and clinical evidence for therapeutic response.* Journal of Experimental & Clinical Cancer Research, 2022. **41**(1): p. 1–37.
166. Mirzaei, S., et al., *Molecular landscape of LncRNAs in prostate cancer: A focus on pathways and therapeutic targets for intervention.* Journal of Experimental & Clinical Cancer Research, 2022. **41**(1): p. 1–26.
167. Ashrafizadeh, M., et al., *Nanotechnological approaches in prostate cancer therapy: Integration of engineering and biology.* Nano Today, 2022. **45**: p. 101532.
168. Du, S., et al., *Circ-ZNF609 accelerates the radioresistance of prostate cancer cells by promoting the glycolytic metabolism through miR-501-3p/*

HK2 axis. Cancer Management and Research, 2020. **12**: p. 7487-7499.

169. Li, H.G., et al., *The mechanism of circ_0023990/miR-873-5p/ANXA2 axis regulating radiosensitivity and development of thyroid carcinoma.* Zhonghua Yi Xue Za Zhi, 2021. **101**(40): p. 3329–3337.
170. Yang, X., et al., *Hsa_circ_0079530/AQP4 axis is related to non-small cell lung cancer development and radiosensitivity.* Annals of Thoracic and Cardiovascular Surgery, 2022. **28**(5): 307–319.
171. Kong, D., et al., *Circ_0008500 knockdown improves radiosensitivity and inhibits tumorigenesis in breast cancer through the miR-758-3p/PFN2 axis.* Journal of Mammary Gland Biology and Neoplasia, 2022. **27**(1): p. 37–52.
172. Chen, L., H. Zhou, and Z. Guan, *CircRNA_000543 knockdown sensitizes nasopharyngeal carcinoma to irradiation by targeting miR-9/platelet-derived growth factor receptor B axis.* Biochemical and Biophysical Research Communications, 2019. **512**(4): p. 786–792.
173. Shuai, M., et al., *Upregulation of circRNA_0000285 serves as a prognostic biomarker for nasopharyngeal carcinoma and is involved in radiosensitivity.* Oncology Letters, 2018. **16**(5): p. 6495–6501.
174. Zhu, H., et al., *Circ_0010235 regulates HOXA10 expression to promote malignant phenotypes and radioresistance in non-small cell lung cancer cells via decoying miR-588.* Balkan Medical Journal, 2022. **39**(4): p. 255–266.
175. Zhou, K., et al., *Knockdown of Circ_0003506 impedes radioresistance, cell growth, migration and invasion in gastric cancer.* Digestive Diseases and Sciences, 2022.
176. Wang, P., et al., *Circ_0067835 knockdown enhances the radiosensitivity of colorectal cancer by miR-296-5p/IGF1R axis.* OncoTargets and Therapy, 2021. **14**: p. 491–502.
177. Zhang, G., et al., *Circ-ACAP2 facilitates the progression of colorectal cancer through mediating miR-143-3p/FZD4 axis.* European Journal of Clinical Investment, 2021. **51**(12): p. e13607.
178. Jin, Y., et al., *Circ_0086720 knockdown strengthens the radiosensitivity of non-small cell lung cancer via mediating the miR-375/SPIN1 axis.* Neoplasma, 2021. **68**(1): p. 96–107.

179. Li, D., et al., *Circular RNA hsa_circ_0004396 acts as a sponge of miR-615-5p to promote non-small cell lung cancer progression and radioresistance through the upregulation of P21-activated kinase 1.* Journal of Clinical Laboratory Analysis, 2022. **36**(6): p. e24463.
180. Yang, Z., et al., *Circ_0007580 knockdown strengthens the radiosensitivity of non-small cell lung cancer via the miR-598-dependent regulation of THBS2.* Thoracic Cancer, 2022. **13**(5): p. 678–689.
181. Li, H., et al., *Circ_0062020 knockdown strengthens the radiosensitivity of prostate cancer cells.* Cancer Management and Research, 2020. **12**: p. 11701–11712.
182. Zhang, J., et al., *A Circ-0007022/miR-338-3p/neuropilin-1 axis reduces the radiosensitivity of esophageal squamous cell carcinoma by activating epithelial-to-mesenchymal transition and PI3K/AKT pathway.* Frontiers in Genetics, 2022. **13**: p. 854097.
183. Wang, L., et al., *Inhibition of hsa_circ_0001313 (circCCDC66) induction enhances the radio-sensitivity of colon cancer cells via tumor suppressor miR-338-3p. Effects of cicr_0001313 on colon cancer radio-sensitivity.* Pathology — Research and Practice, 2019. **215**(4): p. 689–696.

https://doi.org/10.1142/9789811267390_0012

Chapter 12

Exosomal circular RNAs (circRNAs) in cancer progression and diagnosis

Rasoul Raesi[1,2], Sam Saghari[3], Farzaneh Bassiri[4,5], Motahhar Motahhary[6], Shokooh Salimimoghadam[7], Abdurrahman Coskun[8] and Ali Zarrabi[9]*

[1]*Department of Health Services Management, Mashhad University of Medical Sciences, Mashhad, Iran*
[2]*Department of Medical-Surgical Nursing, Mashhad University of Medical Sciences, Mashhad, Iran*
[3]*Department of Health Services Management, Tehran Medical Sciences, Islamic Azad University, Tehran Iran*
[4]*Department of Biology, Fars Science and Research Branch, Islamic Azad University, Fars, Iran*
[5]*Department of Biology, Shiraz Branch, Islamic Azad University, Shiraz, Iran*
[6]*General Medicine, Mashhad University of Medical Sciences, Mashhad, Iran*
[7]*Department of Biochemistry and Molecular Biology, Faculty of Veterinary Medicine, Shahid Chamran University of Ahvaz, Ahvaz, Iran*
[8]*School of Medicine, Department of Medical Biochemistry, Acibadem Mehmet ali Aydinlar University, Istanbul, Turkey*
[9]*Department of Biomedical Engineering, Faculty of Engineering and Natural Sciences, Istinye University, Istanbul, Turkey*

*Corresponding author: Ali Zarrabi, Department of Biomedical Engineering, Faculty of Engineering and Natural Sciences, Istinye University, Istanbul, Turkey, Email: ali.zarrabi@istinye.edu.tr

Abstract

One of the diseases affecting and threatening the survival of human life is cancer. Cancer originates from a variety of factors and underlying mechanisms including environmental factors, exposure to toxic chemicals, lifestyle, inactivity, alteration in gene expression, and epigenetic changes. Circular RNAs (circRNAs) are endogenous RNA molecules with covalently closed loop structure and demonstrate high stability due to the resistance to RNase enzymes. They have more expression compared to linear RNA molecules and are potential biomarkers in cancer. Exosomes are small extracellular vesicles that can be secreted by different cells such as tumor cells, normal cells, macrophages, and cancer-associated fibroblasts that contain proteins, lipid and RNA molecules, and even DNA fragments. Dysregulation of circRNAs has been implicated in disease pathogenesis, especially cancer development and initiation. This chapter demonstrates the role of exosomal circRNAs in affecting the growth and invasion of tumor cells, and they can also be used as diagnostic and prognostic factors in cancer.

1. Introduction

Globally, cancer is the leading cause of death [1] after cardiovascular diseases [2, 3]. Based on the reports of WHO, 19.3 million people were diagnosed with cancer in 2020 which led to 10 million deaths [4]. Based on the new reports, one in five people around the world suffers from cancer and the age of onset is reducing. Furthermore, symptoms are still unknown and atypical, and most of the patients are diagnosed at advanced stages that lead to unfavorable prognosis [4]. Currently, both conventional and modern therapies including chemotherapy, radiotherapy, surgery, immunotherapy, and targeted therapy are utilized for the treatment of cancer patients. Besides, the chance of resistance to chemotherapy and radiotherapy has complicated the process of cancer treatment [5, 6].

Circular RNAs (circRNAs) are new emerging targets in cancer therapy, and these endogenous RNA molecules originate from non-canonical back-splicing process [7–10]. The downstream splice-donor site in circRNA can be covalently bound to upstream splice-acceptor site in circRNAs. The first identification of circRNA is related to an RNA virus in 1976, and using electron microscopy in 1991, circRNAs were diagnosed in eukaryotic cells [11–13]. For a long time, circRNAs were considered as products of aberrant splice events [14]. Using next-generation sequencing data, a high number of circRNAs has been identified in eukaryotic cells [15–19].

Most of the circRNAs are expressed from protein coding genes and contain one or more than one exon [20]. The products of basic kinds of alternative splicing of all linear RNA molecules can be found in circRNAs and notably, a number of circRNAs consist of exons that cannot be observed in linear transcripts [21]. circRNAs mainly position in cytoplasm, and they lack polyadenylation and capping [13, 17, 22, 23]. However, there is also a type of circRNAs known as exon–intron circRNAs that internal intron retention can lead to the generation of circRNAs with sequences of both introns and exons [24]. Furthermore, there is another kind of circRNA called circular intronic circRNAs that results from the debranching of intronic lariats during canonical splicing [25]. Exon–intron circRNAs and circular intronic circRNAs are found in the nucleus where they can enhance the transcription of their parental genes [24]. Figure 1 demonstrates circRNA biogenesis in cells.

circRNAs have received much attention in the field of oncology in recent years. CircDLG1 shows overexpression in gastric cancer and by downregulating miR-141-3p expression, it promotes CXCL12 expression in increasing cancer progression and triggering programmed death-ligand 1 (PD-L1) resistance [26]. CircRNF13 promotes the expression level of SUMO2 in elevating growth and invasion of nasopharyngeal carcinoma cells [27]. In liver cancer–initiating cells, circIPO11 stimulates hedgehog signaling in enhancing self-renewal capacity [28]. circPTEN1 inhibits transforming growth factor β (TGF-β)/Smad signaling and decreases the invasion of colorectal tumor cells [29]. circRNA ANAPC7 sponges miR-373 to inhibit cancer proliferation and muscle wasting in vitro and in vivo to mediate Akt dephosphorylation in pancreatic cancer [30]. circRNA

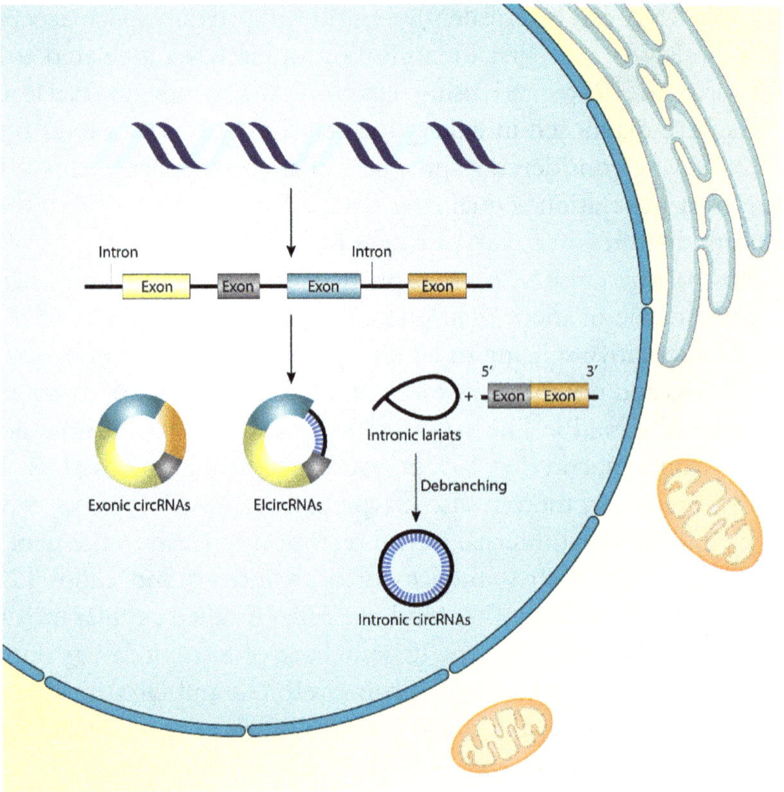

Figure 1. An overview of circRNA biogenesis in cells. Based on this figure, circRNAs can be derived from different locations in the genome between exons and introns, and therefore there are various kinds of these RNA transcripts in cells.

ATCN4 recruits YBX1 to increase the expression level of FZD7 to enhance the progression of intrahepatic cholangiosarcoma cells [31]. Circcia_MAF promotes the expression and transcription activation of MAFF in increasing self-renewal capacity of liver tumor–initiating cells [32]. Based on these studies, circRNAs modulate cancer hallmarks including growth and invasion [33–38], and this chapter focuses on the role of exosomal circRNAs in regulating tumor progression.

2. Exosomes as extracellular vesicles: Basics and biogenesis

Several types of cells such as normal cells, cancer cells, macrophages, and cancer-associated fibroblasts (CAFs) are capable of secreting small extracellular vesicles (EVs) known as exosomes [39, 40]. These subtypes of EVs have a size in the range of 40–160 nm, and cancer cells have demonstrated high capacity in the production and secretion of exosomes [41–43]. The examination of boy fluids has shown that exosomes can be found in blood, lymph, urine, cerebrospinal fluid, bile, saliva, and milk [44–49]. The membranous and cytoplasmic substances derived from parental cells can be carried by exosomes, and these small EVs can contain proteins, lipids, RNA molecules, metabolite, and DNA fragments [50–53]. There are surface receptors on cells that are vital for the capture of exosomes by target cells, and they can be used for transferring genetic materials and reprogramming cellular functions [51].

The biogenesis of exosomes depends on endocytic pathways: first, invaginations of cytoplasmic membrane generate an early secretory endosome and then sprouts are produced inward to form intraluminal vesicles (ILVs) processed within endosome which is known as multivesicular body (MVB) biogenesis. In the next step, acidification is vital for late endosome maturation, and finally, on fusion of ILVs with the cell membrane, secretion of exosomes occurs [53–55]. The biogenesis of exosomes is tightly regulated by proteins called endosomal sorting complex required for transports (ESCRTs), and it is a large family containing 20 proteins. It contains four complexes including ESCRT-0, I, II, and III that have associations with proteins, such as ALIX, VTA1, VPS4, and TSG101 [56, 57]. Each of the aforementioned complexes plays a significant role in the process of exosome biogenesis. For instance, ESCRT-0 is recruited by ubiquitinated cargo and it is necessary for MVB biogenesis to endosomal membrane. ESCRT-I and -II are involved in membrane deformation into buds, and ESCRT-III is vital for the separation of vesicles from the cytoplasmic membrane [58, 59]. In addition, there are mechanisms responsible for exosome biogenesis that are independent of ESCRT and include sphingomyelinase 2-dependent pathway, heterogeneous

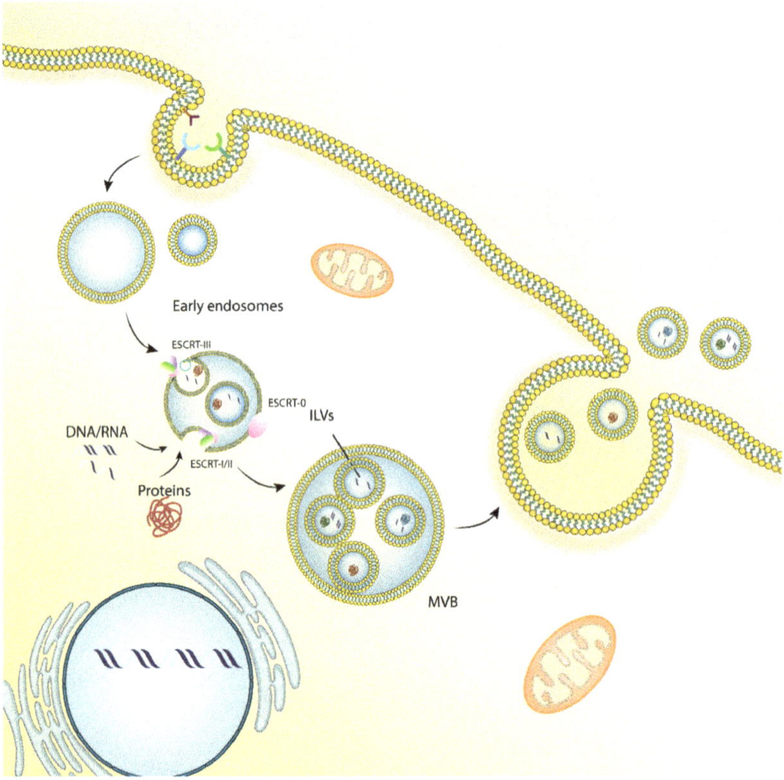

Figure 2. Exosome biogenesis in cells that can occur in an ESCRT-dependent and -independent manner and after the formation of MVBs, exosomes are secreted from the cell.

nuclear ribonucleoprotein-dependent pathway, and microRNA (miRNA) post-transcriptional 3′-end modification, among others [60]. Figure 2 schematically represents exosome biogenesis. Based on the important functions of exosomes for cell-to-cell communication, isolation methods have been developed for them. Ultracentrifugation, ultrafiltration, size exclusion chromatography, precipitation, immuno-affinity-based capture, and microfluidics can be used for the isolation of exosomes from body fluids, examining their contents and using them as biomarkers for disease diagnosis [61–67].

3. Exosomes: Basics in cancer

Exosomes have been mainly attributed to cancer progression [68]. For example, exosomes can stimulate angiogenesis, immune evasion, and tumor microenvironment (TME) remodeling in enhancing the progression of lung tumor cells [69]. Cancer cells secrete exosomes that stimulate hedgehog signaling in increasing the progression of hepatocellular carcinoma and mediating tumor recurrence [70]. The release of exosomes from liver tumor cells is RAB27A dependent and by enhancing Nanog expression, these exosomes mediate regorafenib resistance in hepatocellular carcinoma [71]. In addition to cancer cells, CAFs secrete exosomes containing long non-coding RNA (lncRNA) OIP5-AS1 that increase PD-L1 expression via miR-142-5p sponging in mediating lung tumor malignancy and progression [72]. Although the secretion of exosomes is a vital process in affecting tumor progression, internalization of these small EVs in cancer cells is also important. There is a ligand on exosomes called ADAM17 that can bind to integrin $\alpha5\beta1$ on colorectal cancer cells for internalization [73].

One of the most important challenges in the field of cancer therapy is drug resistance which can be acquired or intrinsic chemo-resistance [74]. In acquired chemo-resistance, a certain population of tumor cells demonstrates resistance to chemotherapy after exposure to anti-cancer agents for long term and frequently. However, in intrinsic chemo-resistance, there is no need for previous exposure to chemotherapy agents and due to the stimulation of oncogenic molecular pathways, hyperactivation of drug efflux transporters, and over-expression of anti-apoptotic proteins, cancer cells can obtain resistance to chemotherapy and sometimes, this further progresses into multi-drug resistance (MDR) [75–79]. CAFs have the ability of secreting exosomes containing gremlin-1 that induces Wnt/β-catenin and BMP molecular pathways in EMT induction, enhancing tumor progression and mediating sorafenib resistance [80]. The exosomes derived from mesenchymal stem cells are able to stimulate AMPK signaling in preventing apoptosis, increasing invasion, and EMT induction for malignant behavior and transformation of lung tumor cells [81].

Enrichment of CD151 in exosomes can result in an increase in metastasis of breast tumor cells [82]. Furthermore, exosomes derived from cancer cells can have lncRNA MALAT1 for miR-1-3p sponging and VASP protein upregulation in increasing breast cancer invasion and drug resistance development [83]. During hypoxia, colorectal tumor cells secrete exosomes containing miR-210-3p, which is vital for the process of carcinogenesis [84]. With respect to the important function of exosomes, there have been efforts to their engineering and providing new insight into cancer treatment. For instance, miR-6785-5p has been loaded in exosomes derived from mesenchymal stem cells and by downregulation of INHBA, they can suppress angiogenesis and invasion of gastric tumor cells [85]. In addition, exosomes can be considered as biomarkers for cancer patients [86]. Enrichment of PLAG10 in exosomes is associated with aggressive behavior of lung tumor cells [87]. The following sections focus on the role of exosomal circRNAs in regulating tumor progression.

4. Exosomal circRNAs in cancer proliferation

Exosomal circRNAs are potent regulators of cancer proliferation. For example, the progression of gastric tumor cells is boosted by exosomal circSHKBP1, owing to its tumor-promoting function. Exosomal circSHKBP1 sponges miR-582-3p to enhance the expression level of HUR in promoting VEGF mRNA stability and preventing ubiquitination of HSP90 via avoiding its interaction with STUB1. Both in vitro and in vivo studies demonstrate that exosomal circSHKBP1 increases gastric cancer progression [88]. CAFs are one of the main components of tumor stroma, and they are the key players in the TME [89]. TME is not only involved in providing tumor proliferation and invasion but also in cell-to-cell interaction [90, 91]. CAFs can secrete energy-rich metabolites that are beneficial in increasing the metabolism of cancer cells and providing mitochondrial respiration [92]. In addition to the role of CAFs in mediating the switching of tumor cells, CAFs can provide drug resistance in cancer via the secretion of exosomes [93–95]. Exosomes derived from CAFs can contain circ-0088300 and by sponging miR-1305, they induce

JAK/STAT signaling for increasing the proliferation rate of gastric tumor cells [96].

miR-409-3p is one of the well-known downstream targets of circRNAs in cancers. CircFAT1 enhances the progression of cervical cancer via miR-409-3p sponging and subsequent overexpression of CDK8 [97]. CircCNOT2 induces an EMT mechanism in breast cancer via miR-409-3p inhibition in increasing breast cancer progression [98]. Furthermore, circ-0001658 promotes Twist1 expression via miR-409-3p inhibition in triggering gefitinib resistance in lung cancer [99]. Notably, miR-409-3p can also be affected by exosomal circRNAs in cancer. Exosomal circNEK9 promotes MAP7 expression via miR-409-3p inhibition to increase the growth rate of gastric tumor cells in vivo [100]. On the other hand, exosomal circ-0001190 participates in suppressing the growth and survival of gastric cancer cells. For this purpose, exosomal circ-0001190 promotes SOSTDC1 expression via miR-586 inhibition to interfere with gastric cancer progression [101]. One of the most well-known mechanisms in gastric cancer is autophagy, and its activation/inhibition is a promising approach since autophagy can have both tumor suppressor and tumor-promoting functions [102–106]. Exosomal circRELL1 has been implicated in impairing the progression and proliferation of gastric tumor cells. In this way, circRELL1 promotes EPHB3 expression by miR-637 inhibition to induce autophagy in gastric cancer inhibition [107].

Lung cancer is one of the devastating diseases that is categorized into small-cell lung cancer (SCLC) and non-small cell lung cancer (NSCLC). Most of the cases of lung cancer are composed of NSCLC, and aggressive behavior, high proliferation and migration rates, and ability in developing therapy resistance are some of the features of this heterogeneous disease. Non-coding RNAs such as miRNAs and lncRNAs have been considered as factors involved in the progression of lung cancer and some of the new therapies based on plant-derived natural products have been introduced for its treatment [76, 108–112]. Exosomal circRNAs play a significant role in regulating the progression of lung tumor cells. Stimulation of aerobic glycolysis increases proliferation of NSCLC cells, a process that undergoes inhibition by miR-101-3p. A new experiment has shown that exosomal circ-MEMO1 promotes KRAS expression via miR-101-3p inhibition to induce glycolysis and to promote lung cancer growth [113]. Pyruvate kinase M2 isoform (PKM2) is a critical enzyme for the process of glycolysis in lung cancer. Exosomal circSHKBP1 sponges miR-1294 to promote the expression level of PKM2 in inducing glycolysis and enhancing the proliferation of lung cancer cells [114]. Lung tumor cells have the capacity of secreting exosomes containing circ-0048856, and by reducing miR-1287-5p expression, they increase the proliferation of lung cancer cells and prevent apoptosis [115]. Based on these studies, exosomal circRNAs play a significant role in increasing the progression of tumor cells, and targeting exosomal circRNAs is important in suppressing cancer proliferation [116–118].

5. Exosomal circRNAs in cancer metastasis

Another important challenge in cancer therapy is the migration and invasion of tumor cells to different parts of the body. In colorectal cancer, hypoxia can lead to the secretion of exosomes. circ-133 is enriched in plasma exosomes of colorectal cancer patients and is able to promote tumor progression. The hypoxic cells secrete exosomal circ-133 that is transferred to normoxic cells to enhance the metastasis of colorectal cancer [119]. Tumor-associated macrophages (TAMs) are another component of TME that are involved in regulating survival, proliferation, and metastasis of cancer cells [120, 121]. Infiltration of TAMs in TME is associated with drug resistance and provides poor prognosis in different cancers including lung cancer, breast cancer, and gastric cancer [122–124]. The number of infiltrating TAMs can be considered as an independent factor for prognosis in NSCLC [125, 126]. TAMs have immunosuppressive activity, and they can increase tumor metastasis via the secretion of growth factors, enzymes, and TGF-β [126]. Cancer-derived exosomal circFARSA induces PTEN degradation by ubiquitination to induce PI3K/Akt signaling for mediating M2 polarization of macrophages and enhancing lung cancer progression [127]. Similar to regulating proliferation,

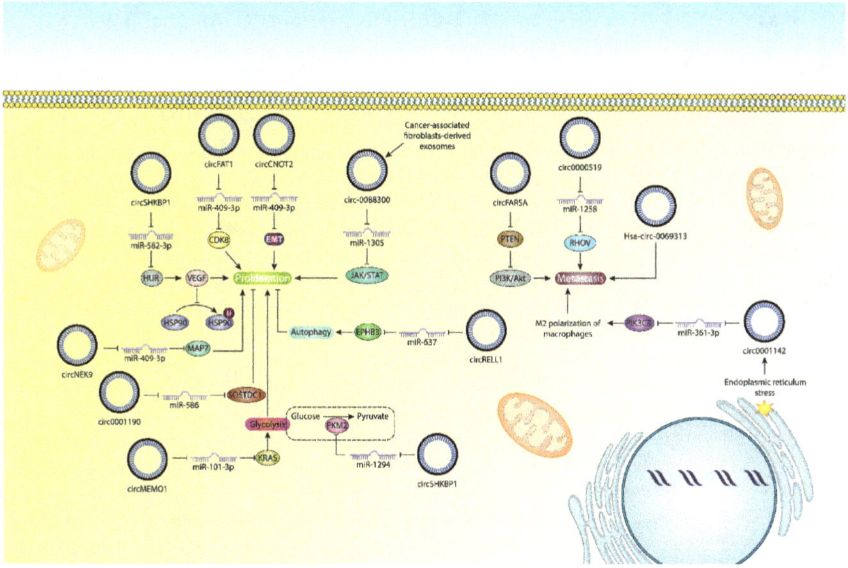

Figure 3. Exosomal circRNAs in regulating proliferation and invasion of tumor cells. Apoptosis, autophagy, glycolysis, polarization of macrophages, and endoplasmic reticulum stress are among the mechanisms and pathways affected by exosomal circRNAs in regulating tumor progression.

exosomal circRNAs mainly affect miRNAs in influencing tumor metastasis. It has been reported that exosomal circ-0000519 promotes RHOV expression via miR-1258 sponging to increase metastasis. Silencing exosomal circ-0000519 decreases metastasis of lung cancer cells [128]. Overexpression of exosomal hsa-circ-0069313 promotes aggressive behavior and mediates lymph node metastasis in NSCLC [129]. The presence of endoplasmic reticulum stress can increase the progression of breast tumor cells. It has been shown that endoplasmic reticulum stress induces the secretion of exosomes from breast tumor cells which in turn, they have circ-0001142 for sponging miR-361-3p, increasing the expression level of PIK3CB, and inducing M2 polarization of macrophages, resulting in breast cancer metastasis [130]. Therefore, exosomal circRNAs are critical regulators of cancer metastasis via affecting various signaling networks [131, 132].

6. Exosomal circRNAs and related molecular pathways

The function of exosomal circRNAs in regulating cancer progression is now obvious based on the previous sections. Based on the experiments, circRNAs affect different molecular pathways in regulating tumor progression. Exosomal circUHRF1 is derived from tumor cells, and it affects the immune system in hepatocellular carcinoma. Exosomal circUHRF1 prevents the secretion of interferon-γ and tumor necrosis factor-α from natural killer cells to induce immune exhaustion and stimulates the resistance to anti-PD1 treatment [133]. On release of exosomal circRNA-0001445, it is absorbed by glioma cells and by sponging miR-127-5p, it promotes SNX5 expression in enhancing tumor progression [134].

LRP6 is a Wnt co-receptor, and its mutation has been observed in various diseases including Alzheimer's disease, osteoporosis, and cancer [135, 136]. LRP6 promotes the progression of hepatocellular carcinoma by activation of Wnt/β-catenin signaling [137]. Exosomal circFBLIM1 is able to induce glycolysis in enhancing hepatocellular carcinoma progression. Overexpression of circFBLIM1 occurs in serum exosomes of hepatocellular carcinoma patients and by sponging miR-338, it promotes LRP6 to induce glycolysis [138]. Sometimes, more than one molecular pathway is affected by circRNAs in enhancing tumor progression. Exosomal circRNA-PED8A is implicated in promoting the progression of pancreatic cancer cells and by sponging miR-338, it simulates MET or Akt signaling [139].

One of the populations at the tumor site is cancer stem cells (CSCs) that express a number of markers including CD44, CD133, ALDH1, and CD90. Overexpression of CD44, SOX2, OCT4, and Nanog provides a high survival rate of CSCs [140]. CSCs are involved in promoting the progression of cancer, and one of the ways is secreting exosomes for transferring information [141–145]. CSCs can secrete exosomal circCARM1 that sponges miR-1252-5p for upregulating PFKFB2 for inducing glycolysis and enhancing breast cancer progression [146]. Furthermore, circRNAs can affect macrophages in regulating cancer progression. Exosomal hsa-circ-0017252 suppresses the progression of gastric cancer. Exosomal hsa-circ-0017252 decreases the expression level of miR-17-5p to suppress M2 polarization of macrophages in impairing gastric cancer progression [147].

One of the oncogenic factors in cancer is STIL, and its overexpression promotes colorectal cancer stemness via the induction of Wnt and Shh pathways [148]. STIL has been also implicated in increasing prostate cancer progression [149], and its silencing inhibits PI3K/Akt signaling in reducing gastric cancer malignancy [150]. Exosomal circ-0000069 is involved in increasing pancreatic cancer progression via STIL overexpression. Silencing exosomal circ-0000069 reduces STIL expression and impairs pancreatic cancer malignancy [151]. The important part of exosomal circRNAs is their ability in regulating cancer stemness. Hypoxic CAFs secrete exosomal circHIF1A that sponges miR-580-5p in enhancing CD44 expression and promoting the stemness of breast cancer [152]. Therefore, different kinds of molecular pathways are regulated by circRNAs in regulating cancer progression.

7. Exosomal circRNAs and drug resistance

The most challenging problem in cancer treatment is the emergence of chemo-resistance. Different factors contribute to the process of drug sensitivity/resistance in cancer. Overexpression of RUNX1 is observed in colorectal cancer and by inducing hedgehog signaling, it induces 5-flourouracil resistance [153]. Due to the endoplasmic reticulum stress, a decrease occurs in the expression level of PHLPP that increases phosphorylation of eIF2α in triggering drug resistance in colon cancer [154]. GPX4, lamin-A, and Hsp90 are other factors involved in triggering drug resistance in cancer [155, 156]. Interestingly, most of the experiments have focused on the role of epigenetic factors in cancer drug resistance. Although significant and increasing evidence highlight the role of miRNAs and lncRNAs in regulating drug resistance [157–160], exosomal circRNAs are new emerging targets that are discussed in this section.

Exosomal circRNA-FBXW7 has shown a role of chemo-sensitivity in colon cancer. Although oxaliplatin is commonly used in the treatment of colon cancer, its resistance has led to chemotherapy failure.

Low expression of exosomal circ-FBXW7 is observed in oxaliplatin-resistant colon cancer cells. Exosomal circ-FBXW7 sponges miR-18b-5p to induce apoptosis in colon cancer cells and enhance their sensitivity to oxaliplatin chemotherapy [161]. The role of exosomal circRNAs in regulating growth and glycolysis in tumor cells has resulted in their impact on chemo-resistance in cancer. Overexpression of exosomal circ-0008928 and its downstream target HK2 is observed in lung cancer, while the expression level of miR-488 decreases. It has been reported that exosomal circ-0008928 promotes HK2 expression via miR-488 inhibition to induce glycolysis and proliferation of lung tumor cells, leading to cisplatin resistance [162]. In addition to cisplatin resistance, lung tumor cells have the capacity of developing resistance to osimertinib chemotherapy. Upregulation of GLUT, HK2, and LDHA leads to glycolysis induction and an increase in the progression of lung tumor cells. hsa-circ-0002130 sponges miR-498 to promote the expression levels of GLUT1, HK2, and LDHA in triggering glycolysis and mediating osimertinib resistance in lung cancer [163].

One of the most devastating diseases of gynecological cancers is ovarian tumor. Increasing evidence has shown the capacity of ovarian tumor cells in developing resistance to cisplatin chemotherapy. The induction of JAK2/STAT3 signaling by ALKBH5–HOXA10 axis results in cisplatin resistance in ovarian cancer [164]. miR-30a inhibits pro-survival autophagy to stimulate apoptosis in increasing cisplatin sensitivity of ovarian tumor cells [165]. Ghrelin and lanthanum chloride are other factors that can increase cisplatin sensitivity in ovarian cancer [166, 167]. Circulating exosomal circFoxp1 participates in developing cisplatin resistance in ovarian cancer. Silencing circFoxp1 impairs the proliferation of ovarian cancer and increases cisplatin sensitivity. Exosomal circFoxp1 promotes the expression levels of CEBPG and FMNL3 via sponging miR-22 and miR-150-3p in mediating cisplatin resistance in ovarian cancer [168]. The same story occurs in esophageal cancer, and exosomal circRNAs regulate cisplatin resistance in these tumor cells. Exosomal circ-0000337 is involved in cisplatin resistance in esophageal cancer, and it sponges miR-377-3p to stimulate JAK2 signaling in enhancing proliferation and invasion of tumor cells and mediating drug resistance [169]. Overall, these studies demonstrate that process of drug resistance is complicated in tumors and exosomal circRNAs are key players.

8. Exosomal circRNAs and radio-resistance

Radio-resistance has been mainly investigated in recent years in terms of understanding the role of biological factors. Skp2 has been implicated in mediating radio-resistance in colorectal cancer, and it promotes Mcl-1 expression [170]. PRMT5 is an arginine methyltransferase that methylates Mxi1 for destabilizing it and inducing radio-resistance in NSCLC [171]. RIOK1 is involved in inducing degradation of p53 via phosphorylation of G3BP2 to mediate radio-resistance in colorectal cancer [172]. Noteworthy, PI3K/Akt signaling is considered as an escape mechanism and induces radio-resistance in renal cancer [173]. Induction of PDP1/PDH axis leads to mitochondrial dysfunction in colorectal cancer and mediates radio-resistance [174]. Therefore, a variety of biological mechanisms are involved in cancer radio-resistance [175, 176]. Exosomal circRNAs have been defined in radio-resistance in cancer. TAMs are capable of secreting exosomal circ-0001610 to increase cancer progression. Exosomal circ-0001610 promotes cyclin B1 expression via miR-139-5p sponging to enhance the progression of endometrial cancer cells and to stimulate radio-resistance [177].

Colorectal cancer is one of the leading causes of death worldwide, and the overall survival of patients with this cancer is unsatisfactory [178, 179]. Irradiation is considered as a main tool in the treatment of colorectal cancer, but radio-resistance has been a main impediment toward the efficacy of radiotherapy in this disease [180, 181]. Exosomal circ-IFT80 is involved in colorectal tumor carcinogenesis, and it reduces the radio-sensitivity of cancer cells. It has been reported that exosomal circ-IFT80 promotes MSI1 expression via miR-296-5p sponging in increasing colorectal cancer progression and mediating radio-resistance [182]. However, exosomal circ-PTPRA functions as onco-suppressor and promotes radio-sensitivity of colorectal tumor cells. The exosomal transfer of circ-PTPRA leads to the

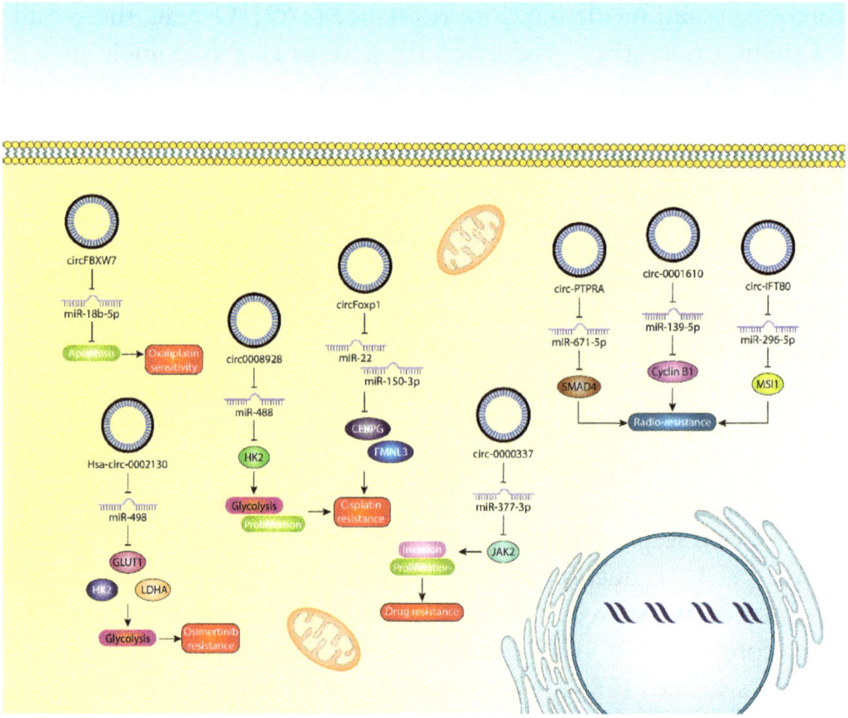

Figure 4. Exosomal circRNAs in regulating drug resistance and radio-resistance in cancers. By inhibition of glycolysis, a significant increase is observed in drug sensitivity of tumor cells, while apoptosis induction by circRNAs is vital for the process of chemo-sensitivity. Furthermore, exosomal circRNAs regulate molecular pathways, such as JAK2, and mainly sponge miRNAs in regulating the drug sensitivity of tumors.

downregulation of miR-671-5p by acting as competing endogenous RNA to promote SMAD4 levels, resulting in radio-sensitivity in colorectal cancer [183]. Therefore, exosomal circRNA modulates the response of cancer cells to radiotherapy, and more experiments should be conducted in terms of revealing the effect of exosomal circRNA on other major pathways and mechanisms such as autophagy in regulating radio-resistance in cancers.

9. Exosomal circRNAs as biomarkers in cancer

One of the interesting points related to exosomes is their presence in body fluids, and in contrast to biopsy which is an invasive approach, they can easily be isolated from the serum of cancer patients and can be analyzed for cancer diagnosis. A recent meta-analysis has shown that exosomal non-coding RNAs can be used as biomarkers in hepatocellular carcinoma and in pooled hazard ratios, downregulated circRNAs were 1.76 [184]. As it was mentioned, biopsy is invasive and is not generally recommended, and recently, a new type of method known as liquid biopsy has been developed that exosomal circRNAs can be used in this case for cancer diagnosis and prognosis [185]. During colorectal cancer progression, the expression level of exosomal circLRAP1 diminishes and it mediates lower survival compared to when it has high expression [186]. In exosomes derived from the plasma of pancreatic cancer patients, hsa-circ-0006220 and hsa-circ-0001666 demonstrate overexpression. These exosomal circRNAs can be considered as diagnostic factors in pancreatic cancer and they mediate lymph node metastasis and increased tumor size [187]. Exosomal circ-0004771 demonstrates overexpression in the serum of colorectal cancer patients, and in postoperative patients, its expression level decreases [188]. Therefore, using exosomal circRNAs is important in cancer diagnosis and prognosis [189–191], and in future experiments, researchers can focus on developing a signature for evaluating the role of exosomal circRNAs. Table 1 provides an overview of exosomal circRNAs in the process of tumorigenesis.

10. Conclusion and remarks

The biogenesis of exosomes has been partially understood, and it has been shown that exosome biogenesis can be performed in an ESCRT-dependent and -independent mechanisms. Therefore, there are still spaces for understanding factors involved in exosome biogenesis. However, it is quite obvious that normal cells, mesenchymal stem cells, cancer cells, macrophages, and fibroblasts can secrete

Table 1. The role of exosomal circRNAs in regulating the progression of tumors.

Exosomal circRNA	Molecular Pathway	Cancer Type	Remark(s)	Ref
circ-0006790	CBX7/S100A11	Pancreatic cancer	Exosomal circ-0006790 recruits CBX7 to induce methylation of S100A11 DNA, resulting in the decrease of tumor progression.	[192]
circ-MID1	miR-506-3p/MID1	Prostate cancer	S100A9 promotes the expression level of exosomal circ-MID1 to sponge miR-506-3p in increasing MID1 expression, resulting in the increase of growth and invasion of tumor cells.	[193]
circ-UBE2D2	miR-200a-3p	Breast cancer	Exosomal circ-UBE2D2 decreases miR-200a-3p expression in increasing tumor progression and mediating tamoxifen resistance.	[194]
circ-PIP5K1A	miR-101/ABCC1	Non-small cell lung cancer	Exosomal circ-PIP5K1A promotes ABCC1 expression via miR-101 inhibition in increasing proliferation and invasion, inhibiting apoptosis, and mediating cisplatin resistance.	[195]
circ-XIAP	miR-1182/TPD52	Prostate cancer	Exosomal circ-XIAP promotes TPD52 expression via miR-1182 sponging to increase cancer progression and to mediate docetaxel resistance.	[196]
circ-0006174	miR-1205/CCND2	Colorectal cancer	Exosomal circ-0006174 stimulates doxorubicin resistance via miR-1205 inhibition and subsequent overexpression of CCND2.	[197]

(Continued)

Table 1. (*Continued*)

circ-102481	miR-30a-5p/ ROR1	Non-small cell lung cancer	Exosomal circ-102481 stimulates EGFR-TKI's resistance via miR-30a-5p sponging and enhances ROR1 expression.	[198]
circPSMA1	miR-637/ Akt1/β-catenin	Triple-negative breast cancer	Exosomal circPSMA1 is involved in carcinogenesis and invasion of tumor cells via miR-637 inhibition, overexpression of Akt1, and induction of β-catenin signaling.	[199]
circEBP41L2	miR-21-5p/ miR-942-5p/ PTEN/Akt	Colorectal cancer	Exosomal circEBP41L2 sponges miR-21-5p and miR-942-5p to induce PTEN signaling, leading to Akt downregulation and a decrease in cancer progression.	[200]
circGDI2	miR-424-5p/ SCAI	Oral cancer	Low expression of exosomal circGDI2 in oral cancer. CircGDI2 promotes SCAI expression via miR-424-5p sponging in impairing tumor progression.	[201]
circRNA-FNDC3B	miR-490-5p/ TXNRD1	Esophageal cancer	circRNA-FNDC3B promotes the expression level of TXNRD1 via miR-490-5p sponging to increase cancer progression.	[202]
circWDR62	miR-370-3p/ MGMT	Glioma	Exosomal circWDR62 promotes MGMT expression via miR-370-3p sponging in enhancing cancer progression and inducing temozolomide resistance.	[203]
circsafb2	miR-620/JAK1/ STAT3	Renal cancer	Exosomal circsafb2 induces JAK1/STAT3 axis via miR-620 sponging to induce M2 polarization of macrophages and to increase cancer progression.	[204]

exosomes comprising different cargoes, such as proteins, lipids, and nucleic acids. With respect to the vital function of exosomes in disease pathogenesis, this chapter was allotted to the understanding role of exosomal circRNAs in regulating tumor progression and as biomarkers. It was shown that the role of exosomes in inhibiting or increasing tumor progression depends on the cargo and if exosomes contain oncogenic circRNAs, they promote the progression of tumor cells and the story is different for onco-suppressor circRNAs. The first hallmark of cancer cells that is affected by exosomal circRNAs is proliferation, so that exosomal circRNAs can affect apoptosis, cell cycle progression, and other cell death mechanisms in affecting the growth rate of tumor cells. One of the mechanisms that have been somewhat overlooked here is ignorance toward the role of exosomal circRNA in regulating glycolysis mechanism in tumors. Another hallmark of cancer is metastasis and exosomal circRNAs are capable of regulating EMT and matrix metalloproteinases in affecting tumor metastasis. Noteworthy, exosomal circRNAs can interact with various molecular pathways in cancer malignancy that STAT3, Wnt/β-catenin, and miRNAs are among them. Besides, exosomal circRNAs are critical regulators of drug resistance and radio-resistance in cancers. Since the diagnosis of cancer patients at early stages is a problem due to the lack of symptoms, they are detected at advanced stages that the prognosis is poor. Exosomal circRNAs can be found in urine, serum, and other body fluids and are used as possible biomarkers in cancer diagnosis.

Conflict of interest:

The authors declare no conflict of interest.

References

1. Gupta, S., et al., *Mailed fecal immunochemical test outreach for colorectal cancer screening: Summary of a Centers for Disease Control and Prevention–sponsored summit.* CA: A Cancer Journal for Clinicians, 2020. **70**(4): p. 283–298.

2. Townsend, N., et al., *Epidemiology of cardiovascular disease in Europe.* Nature Reviews. Cardiology, 2022. **19**(2): p. 133–143.
3. Roth, G.A., et al., *Global, regional, and national age-sex-specific mortality for 282 causes of death in 195 countries and territories, 1980–2017: A systematic analysis for the Global Burden of Disease Study 2017.* Lancet, 2018. **392**(10159): p. 1736–1788.
4. Ju, X., et al., *The emerging role of Circ-SHPRH in cancer.* OncoTargets and Therapy, 2021. **14**: p. 4177–4188.
5. Ashrafizadeh, M., et al., *Doxorubicin-loaded graphene oxide nanocomposites in cancer medicine: Stimuli-responsive carriers, co-delivery and suppressing resistance.* Expert Opinion on Drug Delivery, 2022. **19**(4): p. 355–382.
6. Ashrafizadeh, M., et al., *The interactions and communications in tumor resistance to radiotherapy: Therapy perspectives.* International Immunopharmacology, 2020. **87**: p. 106807.
7. Lei, M., et al., *Translation and functional roles of circular RNAs in human cancer.* Molecular Cancer, 2020. **19**(1): p. 30.
8. Qu, S., et al., *The emerging landscape of circular RNA in life processes.* RNA Biology, 2017. **14**(8): p. 992–999.
9. Jeck, W.R. and N.E. Sharpless, *Detecting and characterizing circular RNAs.* Nature Biotechnology, 2014. **32**(5): p. 453–461.
10. Kristensen, L.S., et al., *The biogenesis, biology and characterization of circular RNAs.* Nature Reviews Genetics, 2019. **20**(11): p. 675–691.
11. Kolakofsky, D.J.C., *Isolation and characterization of Sendai virus DI-RNAs.* Cell, 1976. **8**(4): p. 547–555.
12. Sanger, H.L., et al., *Viroids are single-stranded covalently closed circular RNA molecules existing as highly base-paired rod-like structures.* Proceedings of the National Academy of Sciences of the United States of America, 1976. **73**(11): p. 3852–3856.
13. Hsu, M.-T. and M.J.N. Coca-Prados, *Electron microscopic evidence for the circular form of RNA in the cytoplasm of eukaryotic cells.* Nature, 1979. **280**(5720): p. 339–340.
14. Cocquerelle, C., et al., *Mis-splicing yields circular RNA molecules.* FASEB Journal, 1993. **7**(1): p. 155–160.
15. Wang, P.L., et al., *Circular RNA is expressed across the eukaryotic tree of life.* PLoS One, 2014. **9**(3): p. e90859.

16. Ivanov, A., et al., *Analysis of intron sequences reveals hallmarks of circular RNA biogenesis in animals.* Cell Reports, 2015. **10**(2): p. 170–177.
17. Jeck, W.R., et al., *Circular RNAs are abundant, conserved, and associated with ALU repeats.* RNA, 2013. **19**(2): p. 141–157.
18. Salzman, J., et al., *Cell-type specific features of circular RNA expression.* PLoS Genetics, 2013. **9**(9): p. e1003777.
19. Westholm, J.O., et al., *Genome-wide analysis of drosophila circular RNAs reveals their structural and sequence properties and age-dependent neural accumulation.* Cell Reports, 2014. **9**(5): p. 1966–1980.
20. Guo, J.U., et al., *Expanded identification and characterization of mammalian circular RNAs.* Genome Biology, 2014. **15**(7): p. 1–14.
21. Zhang, X.-O., et al., *Diverse alternative back-splicing and alternative splicing landscape of circular RNAs.* Genome Research, 2016. **26**(9): p. 1277–1287.
22. Memczak, S., et al., *Circular RNAs are a large class of animal RNAs with regulatory potency.* Nature, 2013. **495**(7441): p. 333–338.
23. Salzman, J., et al., *Circular RNAs are the predominant transcript isoform from hundreds of human genes in diverse cell types.* PLoS One, 2012. 7(2): p. e30733.
24. Li, Z., et al., *Exon-intron circular RNAs regulate transcription in the nucleus.* Nature Structural & Molecular Biology, 2015. **22**(3): p. 256–264.
25. Zhang, Y., et al., *Circular intronic long noncoding RNAs.* Melecular Cell, 2013. **51**(6): p. 792–806.
26. Chen, D.L., et al., *The circular RNA circDLG1 promotes gastric cancer progression and anti-PD-1 resistance through the regulation of CXCL12 by sponging miR-141-3p.* Molecular Cancer, 2021. **20**(1): p. 166.
27. Mo, Y., et al., *Circular RNA circRNF13 inhibits proliferation and metastasis of nasopharyngeal carcinoma via SUMO2.* Molecular Cancer, 2021. **20**(1): p. 112.
28. Gu, Y., et al., *Circular RNA circIPO11 drives self-renewal of liver cancer initiating cells via Hedgehog signaling.* Molecular Cancer, 2021. **20**(1): p. 132.

29. Zheng, L., et al., *circPTEN1, a circular RNA generated from PTEN, suppresses cancer progression through inhibition of TGF-β/Smad signaling.* Molecular Cancer, 2022. **21**(1): p. 41.
30. Shi, X., et al., *Circular RNA ANAPC7 inhibits tumor growth and muscle wasting via PHLPP2-AKT-TGF-β signaling axis in pancreatic cancer.* Gastroenterology, 2022. **162**(7): p. 2004–2017.e2.
31. Chen, Q., et al., *Circular RNA ACTN4 promotes intrahepatic cholangiocarcinoma progression by recruiting YBX1 to initiate FZD7 transcription.* Journal of Hepatology, 2022. **76**(1): p. 135–147.
32. Chen, Z., et al., *Circular RNA cia-MAF drives self-renewal and metastasis of liver tumor-initiating cells via transcription factor MAFF.* Journal of Clinical Investigation, 2021. **131**(19).
33. Xie, X., et al., *A circular RNA, circSMARCA5, inhibits prostate cancer proliferative, migrative, and invasive capabilities via the miR-181b-5p/miR-17-3p-TIMP3 axis.* Aging (Albany NY), 2021. **13**(15): p. 19908–19919.
34. Li, X., et al., *Circular RNA circPRMT5 is Upregulated in Breast Cancer and is Required for Cell Proliferation and Migration.* Turkish Journal of Medical Sciences, 2021.
35. Gao, R., et al., *Inhibition of circular RNA_0000285 prevents cell proliferation and induces apoptosis in thyroid cancer by sponging microRNA-654-3p.* Oncology Letters, 2021. **22**(3): p. 673.
36. Qin, C., et al., *Circular RNA 0006349 augments glycolysis and malignance of non-small cell lung cancer cells through the microRNA-98/MKP1 axis.* Frontiers in Cell and Developmental Biology, 2021. **9**: p. 690307.
37. Sun, Y., et al., *Circular RNA circ_ASAP2 regulates drug sensitivity and functional behaviors of cisplatin-resistant gastric cancer cells by the miR-330-3p/NT5E axis.* Anti-cancer Drugs, 2021. **32**(9): p. 950–961.
38. Zhang, W., et al., *Circular RNA hsa_circ_0007507 May Serve as a Biomarker for the Diagnosis and Prognosis of Gastric Cancer.* Frontiers in Oncology, 2021. **11**: p. 699625.
39. Zhu, L., et al., *Isolation and characterization of exosomes for cancer research.* Journal of Hematology & Oncology, 2020. **13**(1): p. 152.

40. Zhang, L. and D. Yu, *Exosomes in cancer development, metastasis, and immunity.* Biochimica et Biophysica Acta — Reviews on Cancer, 2019. **1871**(2): p. 455–468.
41. Ruivo, C.F., et al., *The biology of cancer exosomes: Insights and new perspectives biology of cancer exosomes.* Cancer Research, 2017. 77(23): p. 6480–6488.
42. Golan-Gerstl, R., et al., *Characterization and biological function of milk-derived miRNAs.* Molecular Nutrition and Food Research, 2017. **61**(10): p. 1700009.
43. Dai, J., et al., *Exosomes: Key players in cancer and potential therapeutic strategy.* Signal Transduction and Targeted Therapy, 2020. **5**(1): p. 1–10.
44. Boukouris, S. and S. Mathivanan, *Exosomes in bodily fluids are a highly stable resource of disease biomarkers.* Proteomics. Clinical Applications, 2015. **9**(3–4): p. 358–367.
45. Salido-Guadarrama, I., et al., *MicroRNAs transported by exosomes in body fluids as mediators of intercellular communication in cancer.* OncoTargets and Therapy, 2014. 7: p. 1327.
46. Cappello, F., et al., *Exosome levels in human body fluids: A tumor marker by themselves?* European Journal of Pharmaceutical Sciences, 2017. **96**: p. 93–98.
47. Keller, S., et al., *Body fluid derived exosomes as a novel template for clinical diagnostics.* Journal of Translational Medicine, 2011. **9**(1): p. 1–9.
48. Pan, B.-T., et al., *Electron microscopic evidence for externalization of the transferrin receptor in vesicular form in sheep reticulocytes.* The Journal of Cell Biology, 1985. **101**(3): p. 942–948.
49. Johnstone, R. and C. Biology, *Maturation of reticulocytes: Formation of exosomes as a mechanism for shedding membrane proteins.* Biochemistry and Cell Biology, 1992. **70**(3–4): p. 179–190.
50. Admyre, C., et al., *Exosomes with immune modulatory features are present in human breast milk.* Journal of Immunology, 2007. **179**(3): p. 1969–1978.
51. Kalluri, R. and V.S. LeBleu, *The biology, function, and biomedical applications of exosomes.* Science, 2020. **367**(6478): p. eaau6977.

52. Rani, S., et al., *Isolation of exosomes for subsequent mRNA, MicroRNA, and protein profiling*, in *Gene expression profiling*, 2011. Springer. p. 181–195.
53. Wortzel, I., et al., *Exosome-mediated metastasis: Communication from a distance.* Developmental Cell, 2019. **49**(3): p. 347–360.
54. Dai, J., et al., *Exosomes: Key players in cancer and potential therapeutic strategy.* Signal Transduction and Targeted Therapy, 2020. **5**(1): p. 145.
55. Ibrahim, A. and E. Marbán, *Exosomes: Fundamental biology and roles in cardiovascular physiology.* Annual Review of Physiology, 2016. **78**: p. 67.
56. Colombo, M., et al., *Analysis of ESCRT functions in exosome biogenesis, composition and secretion highlights the heterogeneity of extracellular vesicles.* Journal of Cell Science, 2013. **126**(24): p. 5553–5565.
57. Hessvik, N.P. and A. Llorente, *Current knowledge on exosome biogenesis and release.* Cellular and Molecular Life Sciences, 2018. **75**(2): p. 193–208.
58. Schöneberg, J., et al., *Reverse-topology membrane scission by the ESCRT proteins.* Nature Reviews. Molecular Cell Biology, 2017. **18**(1): p. 5–17.
59. Hurley, J.H. and P.I. Hanson, *Membrane budding and scission by the ESCRT machinery: It's all in the neck.* Nature Reviews. Molecular Cell Biology, 2010. **11**(8): p. 556–566.
60. Tian, X., et al., *Tumor-derived exosomes, myeloid-derived suppressor cells, and tumor microenvironment.* Journal of Hematology & Oncology, 2019. **12**(1): p. 1–18.
61. Paskeh, M.D.A., et al., *Emerging role of exosomes in cancer progression and tumor microenvironment remodeling.* Journal of Hematology & Oncology, 2022. **15**(1): p. 83.
62. Alzhrani, G.N., et al., *Exosomes: Isolation, characterization, and biomedical applications.* Cell Biology International, 2021. **45**(9): p. 1807–1831.
63. Jiang, Z., G. Liu, and J. Li, *Recent progress on the isolation and detection methods of exosomes.* Chemistry, an Asian Journal, 2020. **15**(23): p. 3973–3982.

64. Jafari, D., et al., *Designer exosomes: A new platform for biotechnology therapeutics.* Nature Public Health Emergency Collection, 2020. **34**(5): p. 567–586.
65. Whiteside, T.L., B. Diergaarde, and C.-S. Hong, *Tumor-derived exosomes (Tex) and their role in immuno-oncology.* International Journal of Molecular Sciences, 2021. **22**(12): p. 6234.
66. Burkova, E.E., S.E. Sedykh, and G.A. Nevinsky, *Human placenta exosomes: Biogenesis, isolation, composition, and prospects for use in diagnostics.* International Journal of Molecular Sciences, 2021. **22**(4): p. 2158.
67. Romano, E., P.A. Netti, and E. Torino, *Exosomes in gliomas: Biogenesis, isolation, and preliminary applications in nanomedicine.* Pharmaceuticals, 2020. **13**(10): p. 319.
68. Wang, Y., et al., *Natural killer cell-derived exosomal miR-1249-3p attenuates insulin resistance and inflammation in mouse models of type 2 diabetes.* Signal Transduction and Targeted Therapy, 2021. **6**(1): p. 409.
69. Jiang, C., et al., *Tumor-associated exosomes promote lung cancer metastasis through multiple mechanisms.* Molecular Cancer, 2021. **20**(1): p. 117.
70. Li, L., et al., *Cancer cell-derived exosomes promote HCC tumorigenesis through hedgehog pathway.* Frontiers in Oncology, 2021. **11**: p. 756205.
71. Huang, H., et al., *RAB27A-dependent release of exosomes by liver cancer stem cells induces Nanog expression in their differentiated progenies and confers regorafenib resistance.* Journal of Gastroenterology and Hepatology, 2021. **36**(12): p. 3429–3437.
72. Jiang, Y., et al., *Cancer-associated fibroblasts-derived exosomes promote lung cancer progression by OIP5-AS1/miR-142-5p/PD-L1 axis.* Molecular Immunology, 2021. **140**: p. 47–58.
73. Cardeñes, B., et al., *Cellular Integrin $\alpha5\beta1$ and Exosomal ADAM17 Mediate the Binding and Uptake of Exosomes Produced by Colorectal Carcinoma Cells.* International Journal of Molecular Sciences, 2021. **22**(18).
74. Mirzaei, S., et al., *Caffeic acid and its derivatives as potential modulators of oncogenic molecular pathways: New hope in the fight against cancer.* Pharmacological Research, 2021. **171**: p. 105759.

75. Ashrafizaveh, S., et al., *Long non-coding RNAs in the doxorubicin resistance of cancer cells.* Cancer Letters, 2021. **508**: p. 104–114.
76. Ashrafizadeh, M., et al., *Lung cancer cells and their sensitivity/resistance to cisplatin chemotherapy: Role of microRNAs and upstream mediators.* Cell Signalling, 2021. **78**: p. 109871.
77. Mirzaei, S., et al., *Nrf2 signaling pathway in chemoprotection and doxorubicin resistance: Potential application in drug discovery.* Antioxidants (Basel), 2021. **10**(3): p. 349.
78. Barik, G.K., et al., *Keep your eyes peeled for long noncoding RNAs: Explaining their boundless role in cancer metastasis, drug resistance, and clinical application.* Biochimica et Biophysica Acta — Reviews on Cancer, 2021. **1876**(2): p. 188612.
79. Crudele, F., et al., *The molecular networks of microRNAs and their targets in the drug resistance of colon carcinoma.* Cancers (Basel), 2021. **13**(17).
80. Qin, W., et al., *CAF-derived exosomes transmitted Gremlin-1 promotes cancer progression and decreases the sensitivity of hepatoma cells to sorafenib.* Molecular Carcinogenesis, 2022. **61**(8): p. 764–775.
81. Wang, L., et al., *Mesenchymal stem cells and their derived exosomes promote malignant phenotype of polyploid non-small-cell lung cancer cells through AMPK signaling pathway.* Analytical Cellular Pathology (Amsterdam), 2022. **2022**: p. 8708202.
82. Li, D., et al., *CD151 enrichment in exosomes of luminal androgen receptor breast cancer cell line contributes to cell invasion.* Biochimie, 2021. **189**: p. 65–75.
83. Tao, S., et al., *Exosomes derived from tumor cells initiate breast cancer cell metastasis and chemoresistance through a MALAT1-dependent mechanism.* Journal of Oncology, 2022. **2022**: p. 5483523.
84. Ge, L., et al., *Hypoxic colorectal cancer-secreted exosomes deliver miR-210-3p to normoxic tumor cells to elicit a protumoral effect.* Experimental Biology and Medicine (Maywood), 2021. **246**(17): p. 1895–1906.
85. Chen, Z., et al., *microRNA-6785-5p-loaded human umbilical cord mesenchymal stem cells-derived exosomes suppress angiogenesis and metastasis in gastric cancer via INHBA.* Life Sciences, 2021. **284**: p. 119222.

86. Hofmann, L., et al., *Cargo and functional profile of saliva-derived exosomes reveal biomarkers specific for head and neck cancer.* Frontiers in Medicine (Lausanne), 2022. **9**: p. 904295.
87. Chen, Y., et al., *PLA2G10 incorporated in exosomes could be diagnostic and prognostic biomarker for non-small cell lung cancer.* Clinica Chimica Acta, 2022. **530**: p. 55–65.
88. Xie, M., et al., *Exosomal circSHKBP1 promotes gastric cancer progression via regulating the miR-582-3p/HUR/VEGF axis and suppressing HSP90 degradation.* Molecular Cancer, 2020. **19**(1): p. 112.
89. Zhao, X., Y. He, and H. Chen, *Autophagic tumor stroma: Mechanisms and roles in tumor growth and progression.* International Journal of Cancer, 2013. **132**(1): p. 1–8.
90. Bu, L., et al., *Biological heterogeneity and versatility of cancer-associated fibroblasts in the tumor microenvironment.* Oncogene, 2019. **38**(25): p. 4887–4901.
91. Jang, I. and K.A. Beningo, *Integrins, CAFs and mechanical forces in the progression of cancer.* Cancers (Basel), 2019. **11**(5): p. 721.
92. Shan, T., et al., *Cancer-associated fibroblasts enhance pancreatic cancer cell invasion by remodeling the metabolic conversion mechanism.* Oncology Reports, 2017. **37**(4): p. 1971–1979.
93. Xing, F., et al., *Cancer associated fibroblasts (CAFs) in tumor microenvironment.* Frontiers in Bioscience, 2010. **15**: p. 166.
94. Au Yeung, C.L., et al., *Exosomal transfer of stroma-derived miR21 confers paclitaxel resistance in ovarian cancer cells through targeting APAF1.* Nature Communications, 2016. **7**(1): p. 1–14.
95. Ren, J., et al., *Carcinoma-associated fibroblasts promote the stemness and chemoresistance of colorectal cancer by transferring exosomal lncRNA H19.* Theranostics, 2018. **8**(14): p. 3932.
96. Shi, H., et al., *Exosomal circ_0088300 Derived From Cancer-Associated Fibroblasts Acts as a miR-1305 Sponge and Promotes Gastric Carcinoma Cell Tumorigenesis.* Frontier in Cellular and Developmental Biology, 2021. **9**: p. 676319.
97. Zhou, B., et al., *CircFAT1 facilitates cervical cancer malignant progression by regulating ERK1/2 and p38 MAPK pathway through miR-409-3p/CDK8 axis.* Drug Development Research, 2021. **82**(8): p. 1131–1143.

98. Su, Q., et al., *Circular RNA CNOT2 knockdown regulates twist family BHLH transcription factor via targeting microRNA 409-3p to prevent breast cancer invasion, migration and epithelial-mesenchymal transition.* Bioengineered, 2021. **12**(1): p. 9058–9069.
99. Yu, X., et al., *Circ_0001658 regulates gefitinib resistance of non-small cell lung cancer through miR-409-3p/TWIST1 axis.* Anti-cancer Drugs, 2022. **33**(2): p. 158–166.
100. Yu, L., et al., *Plasma Exosomal CircNEK9 Accelerates the Progression of Gastric Cancer via miR-409-3p/MAP7 Axis.* Digestive Diseases and Sciences, 2021. **66**(12): p. 4274–4289.
101. Liu, C., et al., *Exosomal circ_0001190 Regulates the Progression of Gastric Cancer via miR-586/SOSTDC1 Axis.* Biochemical Genetics, 2022.
102. Yuan, Y., et al., *Narciclasine induces autophagy-mediated apoptosis in gastric cancer cells through the Akt/mTOR signaling pathway.* BMC Pharmacology and Toxicology, 2021. **22**(1): p. 70.
103. Kim, T.W. and H.G. Lee, *Apigenin induces autophagy and cell death by targeting EZH2 under hypoxia conditions in gastric cancer cells.* International Journal of Molecular Sciences, 2021. **22**(24).
104. Wang, M., et al., *High ATF4 expression is associated with poor prognosis, amino acid metabolism, and autophagy in gastric cancer.* Frontiers in Oncology, 2021. **11**: p. 740120.
105. Xu, C., et al., *Costunolide-induced apoptosis via promoting the reactive oxygen species and inhibiting AKT/GSK3β pathway and activating autophagy in gastric cancer.* Frontiers in Cell and Developmental Biology, 2021. **9**: p. 722734.
106. Ma, X., et al., *A 1,10-phenanthroline derivative selectively targeting telomeric G-quadruplex induces cytoprotective autophagy, causing apoptosis of gastric cancer cells.* Life Sciences, 2021. **287**: p. 120095.
107. Sang, H., et al., *Exosomal circRELL1 serves as a miR-637 sponge to modulate gastric cancer progression via regulating autophagy activation.* Cell Death & Disease, 2022. **13**(1): p. 56.
108. Ashrafizadeh, M., et al., *Versatile role of curcumin and its derivatives in lung cancer therapy.* Journal of Cellular Physiology, 2020. **235**(12): p. 9241–9268.

109. Entezari, M., et al., *Long non-coding RNAs and exosomal lncRNAs: Potential functions in lung cancer progression, drug resistance and tumor microenvironment remodeling*. Biomedicine & Pharmacotherapy, 2022. **150**: p. 112963.
110. Cheng, G., et al., *lncRNA PSMA3-AS1 promotes the progression of non-small cell lung cancer through targeting miR-17-5p/PD-L1*. Advances in Clinical and Experimental Medicine, 2021. **30**(10): p. 1043–1050.
111. Chen, S.W., et al., *Cancer cell-derived exosomal circUSP7 induces CD8(+) T cell dysfunction and anti-PD1 resistance by regulating the miR-934/SHP2 axis in NSCLC*. Molecular Cancer, 2021. **20**(1): p. 144.
112. Lu, X., et al., *MiR-27a-3p Promotes Non-Small Cell Lung Cancer Through SLC7A11-Mediated-Ferroptosis*. Frontiers in Oncology, 2021. **11**: p. 759346.
113. Ding, C., et al., *Exosomal Circ-MEMO1 promotes the progression and aerobic glycolysis of non-small cell lung cancer through targeting MiR-101-3p/KRAS axis*. Frontiers in Genetics, 2020. **11**: p. 962.
114. Chen, W., et al., *Exosomal circSHKBP1 participates in non-small cell lung cancer progression through PKM2-mediated glycolysis*. Molecular Therapy — Oncolytics, 2022. **24**: p. 470–485.
115. He, Y., et al., *Exosomal circ_0048856 derived from non-small cell lung cancer contributes to aggressive cancer progression through downregulation of miR-1287-5p*. Pathology — Research and Practice, 2022. **232**: p. 153659.
116. Lin, Q., et al., *Exosomal circular RNA hsa_circ_007293 promotes proliferation, migration, invasion, and epithelial-mesenchymal transition of papillary thyroid carcinoma cells through regulation of the microRNA-653-5p/paired box 6 axis*. Bioengineered, 2021. **12**(2): p. 10136–10149.
117. Huang, G., et al., *Exosomal circKDM4A induces CUL4B to promote prostate cancer cell malignancy in a miR-338-3p-dependent manner*. Biochemical Genetics, 2022.
118. Shang, A., et al., *Exosomal circPACRGL promotes progression of colorectal cancer via the miR-142-3p/miR-506-3p- TGF-β1 axis*. Molecular Cancer, 2020. **19**(1): p. 117.

119. Yang, H., et al., *Hypoxia induced exosomal circRNA promotes metastasis of colorectal cancer via targeting GEF-H1/RhoA axis.* Theranostics, 2020. **10**(18): p. 8211–8226.
120. Wu, T., et al., *Immune contexture defined by single cell technology for prognosis prediction and immunotherapy guidance in cancer.* Cancer Communications, 2019. **39**(1): p. 1–9.
121. Thielmann, C.M., et al., *Iron accumulation in tumor-associated macrophages marks an improved overall survival in patients with lung adenocarcinoma.* Science Reports, 2019. **9**(1): p. 1–9.
122. Malfitano, A.M., et al., *Tumor-associated macrophage status in cancer treatment.* Cancers (Basel), 2020. **12**(7): p. 1987.
123. Choi, J., et al., *The role of tumor-associated macrophage in breast cancer biology.* Histology and Histopathology, 2018.
124. Lopez-Yrigoyen, M., L. Cassetta, and J.W. Pollard, *Macrophage targeting in cancer.* Annals of the New York Academy of Sciences, 2021. **1499**(1): p. 18–41.
125. Sumitomo, R., et al., *M2 tumor-associated macrophages promote tumor progression in non-small-cell lung cancer.* Experimental and Therapeutic Medicine, 2019. **18**(6): p. 4490–4498.
126. Guo, X., et al., *Hypoxia promotes glioma-associated macrophage infiltration via periostin and subsequent M2 polarization by upregulating TGF-beta and M-CSFR.* Oncotarget, 2016. 7(49): p. 80521.
127. Chen, T., et al., *Tumor-derived exosomal circFARSA mediates M2 macrophage polarization via the PTEN/PI3K/AKT pathway to promote non-small cell lung cancer metastasis.* Cancer Treatment and Research Communications, 2021. **28**: p. 100412.
128. Wang, R., et al., *Exosomal hsa_circ_0000519 modulates the NSCLC cell growth and metastasis via miR-1258/RHOV axis.* Open Medicine (Warsaw), 2022. **17**(1): p. 826–840.
129. Chen, Y., et al., *Serum exosomal hsa_circ_0069313 has a potential to diagnose more aggressive non-small cell lung cancer.* Clinical Biochemistry, 2022. **102**: p. 56–64.
130. Lu, C., et al., *Endoplasmic reticulum stress promotes breast cancer cells to release exosomes circ_0001142 and induces M2 polarization of macrophages to regulate tumor progression.* Pharmacological Research, 2022. **177**: p. 106098.

131. Li, J., et al., *Circular RNA IARS (circ-IARS) secreted by pancreatic cancer cells and located within exosomes regulates endothelial monolayer permeability to promote tumor metastasis.* Journal of Experimental & Clinical Cancer Research, 2018. **37**(1): p. 177.
132. Zhao, H., S. Chen, and Q. Fu, *Exosomes from CD133(+) cells carrying circ-ABCC1 mediate cell stemness and metastasis in colorectal cancer.* Journal of Cellular Biochemistry, 2020. **121**(5–6): p. 3286–3297.
133. Zhang, P.F., et al., *Cancer cell-derived exosomal circUHRF1 induces natural killer cell exhaustion and may cause resistance to anti-PD1 therapy in hepatocellular carcinoma.* Molecular Cancer, 2020. **19**(1): p. 110.
134. Han, Y., et al., *Exosomal circRNA 0001445 promotes glioma progression through miRNA-127-5p/SNX5 pathway.* Aging (Albany NY), 2021. **13**(9): p. 13287–13299.
135. Go, G.-w., *Low-density lipoprotein receptor-related protein 6 (LRP6) is a novel nutritional therapeutic target for hyperlipidemia, non-alcoholic fatty liver disease, and atherosclerosis.* Nutrients, 2015. 7(6): p. 4453–4464.
136. Wang, Z., et al., *Harnessing low-density lipoprotein receptor protein 6 (LRP6) genetic variation and Wnt signaling for innovative diagnostics in complex diseases.* The Pharmacogenomics Journal, 2018. **18**(3): p. 351–358.
137. Tung, E.K.-K., et al., *Upregulation of the Wnt co-receptor LRP6 promotes hepatocarcinogenesis and enhances cell invasion.* PLoS One, 2012. 7(5): p. e36565.
138. Lai, Z., et al., *Exosomal circFBLIM1 promotes hepatocellular carcinoma progression and glycolysis by regulating the miR-338/LRP6 axis.* Cancer Biotherapy and Radiopharmaceuticals, 2020.
139. Li, Z., et al., *Tumor-released exosomal circular RNA PDE8A promotes invasive growth via the miR-338/MACC1/MET pathway in pancreatic cancer.* Cancer Letters, 2018. **432**: p. 237–250.
140. Hwang, W.-L., et al., *Tumor stem-like cell-derived exosomal RNAs prime neutrophils for facilitating tumorigenesis of colon cancer.* Journal of Hematology & Oncology, 2019. **12**(1): p. 1–17.
141. Fanale, D., et al., *Circular RNA in exosomes.* Advances in Experimental Medicine and Biology, 2018: p. 109–117.

142. Li, Y., et al., *Circular RNA is enriched and stable in exosomes: A promising biomarker for cancer diagnosis.* Cell Research, 2015. **25**(8): p. 981–984.
143. Kristensen, L., et al., *Circular RNAs in cancer: Opportunities and challenges in the field.* Oncogene, 2018. **37**(5): p. 555–565.
144. Hou, J., et al., *Circular RNAs and exosomes in cancer: a mysterious connection.* Clinical & Translational Oncology, 2018. **20**(9): p. 1109–1116.
145. Wang, Y., et al., *Exosomal circRNAs: Biogenesis, effect and application in human diseases.* Molecular Cancer, 2019. **18**(1): p. 1–10.
146. Liu, Y., et al., *Exosomal circCARM1 from spheroids reprograms cell metabolism by regulating PFKFB2 in breast cancer.* Oncogene, 2022. **41**(14): p. 2012–2025.
147. Song, J., et al., *Exosomal hsa_circ_0017252 attenuates the development of gastric cancer via inhibiting macrophage M2 polarization.* Human Cell, 2022.
148. Pradhan, T., et al., *STIL endows oncogenic and stem-like attributes to colorectal cancer plausibly by Shh and Wnt signaling.* Frontiers in Oncology, 2021. **11**: p. 581671.
149. Wu, X., et al., *The human oncogene SCL/TAL1 interrupting locus (STIL) promotes tumor growth through MAPK/ERK, PI3K/Akt and AMPK pathways in prostate cancer.* Gene, 2019. **686**: p. 220–227.
150. Wang, J., et al., *Knockdown of STIL suppresses the progression of gastric cancer by down-regulating the IGF-1/PI3K/AKT pathway.* Journal of Cellular and Molecular Medicine, 2019. **23**(8): p. 5566–5575.
151. Ye, Z., et al., *Hsa_circ_0000069 Knockdown Inhibits Tumorigenesis and Exosomes with Downregulated hsa_circ_0000069 Suppress Malignant Transformation via Inhibition of STIL in Pancreatic Cancer.* International Journal of Nanomedicine, 2020. **15**: p. 9859–9873.
152. Zhan, Y., et al., *Carcinoma-associated fibroblasts derived exosomes modulate breast cancer cell stemness through exonic circHIF1A by miR-580-5p in hypoxic stress.* Cell Death & Discovery, 2021. 7(1): p. 141.
153. Li, Q., et al., *RUNX1 regulates the proliferation and chemoresistance of colorectal cancer through the Hedgehog signaling pathway.* Journal of Cancer, 2021. **12**(21): p. 6363–6371.

154. Guo, B., et al., *Downregulation of PHLPP induced by endoplasmic reticulum stress promotes eIF2α phosphorylation and chemoresistance in colon cancer.* Cell Death & Disease, 2021. **12**(11): p. 960.
155. Wang, Y., et al., *Lamin-A interacting protein Hsp90 is required for DNA damage repair and chemoresistance of ovarian cancer cells.* Cell Death & Disease, 2021. **12**(8): p. 786.
156. Liu, W., et al., *Glutathione peroxidase 4-dependent glutathione high-consumption drives acquired platinum chemoresistance in lung cancer-derived brain metastasis.* Clinical and Translational Medicine, 2021. **11**(9): p. e517.
157. Chen, Q., et al., *MiR-873-5p targets THUMPD1 to inhibit gastric cancer cell behavior and chemoresistance.* Journal of Gastrointestinal Oncology, 2021. **12**(5): p. 2061–2072.
158. Xing, Z., et al., *LINC00337 induces tumor development and chemoresistance to paclitaxel of breast cancer by recruiting M2 tumor-associated macrophages.* Molecular Immunology, 2021. **138**: p. 1–9.
159. Mao, T.L., et al., *LncRNA MALAT1 facilitates ovarian cancer progression through promoting chemoresistance and invasiveness in the tumor microenvironment.* International Journal of Molecular Sciences, 2021. **22**(19).
160. Tuo, Z., L. Liang, and R. Zhou, *LINC00852 is associated with poor prognosis in non-small cell lung cancer patients and its inhibition suppresses cancer cell proliferation and chemoresistance via the hsa-miR-145-5p/KLF4 axis.* The Journal of Gene Medicine, 2021. **23**(12): p. e3384.
161. Xu, Y., et al., *Exosomal transfer of circular RNA FBXW7 ameliorates the chemoresistance to oxaliplatin in colorectal cancer by sponging miR-18b-5p.* Neoplasma, 2021. **68**(1): p. 108–118.
162. Shi, Q., et al., *Serum exosomes-based biomarker circ_0008928 regulates cisplatin sensitivity, tumor progression, and glycolysis metabolism by miR-488/HK2 axis in cisplatin-resistant nonsmall cell lung carcinoma.* Cancer Biotherapy and Radiopharmaceuticals, 2021.
163. Ma, J., G. Qi, and L. Li, *A novel serum exosomes-based biomarker hsa_circ_0002130 facilitates osimertinib-resistance in non-small cell lung cancer by sponging miR-498.* OncoTargets and Therapy, 2020. **13**: p. 5293–5307.

164. Nie, S., et al., *ALKBH5-HOXA10 loop-mediated JAK2 m6A demethylation and cisplatin resistance in epithelial ovarian cancer.* Journal of Experimental & Clinical Cancer Reseach, 2021. **40**(1): p. 284.
165. Cai, Y., et al., *MicroRNA miR-30a inhibits cisplatin resistance in ovarian cancer cells through autophagy.* Bioengineered, 2021. **12**(2): p. 10713–10722.
166. Leng, Y., et al., *Ghrelin enhances cisplatin sensitivity in HO-8910PM human ovarian cancer cells.* Journal of Ovarian Research, 2021. **14**(1): p. 162.
167. Fang, S., et al., *Lanthanum chloride sensitizes cisplatin resistance of ovarian cancer cells via PI3K/Akt pathway.* Frontiers in Medicine (Lausanne), 2021. **8**: p. 776876.
168. Luo, Y. and R. Gui, *Circulating exosomal circFoxp1 confers cisplatin resistance in epithelial ovarian cancer cells.* Journal of Gynecologic Oncology, 2020. **31**(5): p. e75.
169. Zang, R., et al., *Exosomes mediated transfer of Circ_0000337 contributes to cisplatin (CDDP) resistance of esophageal cancer by regulating JAK2 via miR-377-3p.* Frontiers in Cell and Developmental Biology, 2021. **9**: p. 673237.
170. Yu, X., et al., *Skp2 stabilizes Mcl-1 and confers radioresistance in colorectal cancer.* Cell Death & Disease, 2022. **13**(3): p. 249.
171. Yang, X., et al., *Arginine methyltransferase PRMT5 methylates and destabilizes Mxi1 to confer radioresistance in non-small cell lung cancer.* Cancer Letters, 2022. **532**: p. 215594.
172. Chen, Y., et al., *RIOK1 mediates p53 degradation and radioresistance in colorectal cancer through phosphorylation of G3BP2.* Oncogene, 2022. **41**(25): p. 3433–3444.
173. Wanigasooriya, K., et al., *Patient derived organoids confirm that PI3K/AKT signalling is an escape pathway for radioresistance and a target for therapy in rectal cancer.* Frontiers in Oncology, 2022. **12**: p. 920444.
174. Shi, Y., et al., *Mitochondrial dysfunction induces radioresistance in colorectal cancer by activating [Ca(2+)](m)-PDP1-PDH-histone acetylation retrograde signaling.* Cell Death & Disease, 2021. **12**(9): p. 837.
175. Zhou, Y., et al., *And-1 O-GlcNAcylation regulates homologous recombination repair and radioresistance in colorectal cancer.* Clinical and Translational Medicine, 2022. **12**(4): p. e785.

176. Zhang, J., et al., *SERPINE2/PN-1 regulates the DNA damage response and radioresistance by activating ATM in lung cancer.* Cancer Letters, 2022. **524**: p. 268–283.
177. Gu, X., et al., *Exosomal transfer of tumor-associated macrophage-derived hsa_circ_0001610 reduces radiosensitivity in endometrial cancer.* Cell Death & Disease, 2021. **12**(9): p. 818.
178. Bray, F., et al., *Global cancer statistics 2018: GLOBOCAN estimates of incidence and mortality worldwide for 36 cancers in 185 countries.* CA: A Cancer Journal for Clinicians, 2018. **68**(6): p. 394–424.
179. Siegel, R., et al., *Cancer statistics, 2014.* CA: A Cancer Journal for Clinicians, 2014. **64**(1): p. 9–29.
180. Dell'Acqua, V., et al., *Stereotactic radiation therapy in oligometastatic colorectal cancer: Outcome of 102 patients and 150 lesions.* Clinical and Experimental Metastasis, 2019. **36**(4): p. 331–342.
181. Park, S.-Y., et al., *The JAK2/STAT3/CCND2 Axis promotes colorectal cancer stem cell persistence and radioresistance.* Journal of Experimental & Clinical Cancer Research, 2019. **38**(1): p. 1–18.
182. Li, L., et al., *Exosomal circ_IFT80 enhances tumorigenesis and suppresses radiosensitivity in colorectal cancer by regulating miR-296-5p/MSI1 axis.* Cancer Management and Research, 2021. **13**: p. 1929–1941.
183. Yang, Y., N. Yang, and J. Jiang, *Exosomal circ_PTPRA inhibits tumorigenesis and promotes radiosensitivity in colorectal cancer by enriching the level of SMAD4 via competitively binding to miR-671-5p.* Cytotechnology, 2022. **74**(1): p. 51–64.
184. Nie, G., et al., *Prognostic value of exosomal noncoding RNA in hepatocellular carcinoma: A meta-analysis.* Carcinogenesis, 2022.
185. Baassiri, A., et al., *Exosomal non coding RNA in LIQUID biopsies as a promising biomarker for colorectal cancer.* International Journal of Molecular Sciences, 2020. **21**(4).
186. Zheng, R., et al., *Exosomal circLPAR1 functions in colorectal cancer diagnosis and tumorigenesis through suppressing BRD4 via METTL3-eIF3h interaction.* Molecular Cancer, 2022. **21**(1): p. 49.
187. Hong, L., et al., *Exosomal circular RNA hsa_circ_0006220, and hsa_circ_0001666 as biomarkers in the diagnosis of pancreatic cancer.* Journal of Clinical Laboratory Analysis, 2022. **36**(6): p. e24447.

188. Pan, B., et al., *Identification of serum exosomal hsa-circ-0004771 as a novel diagnostic biomarker of colorectal cancer.* Frontiers in Genetics, 2019. **10**: p. 1096.
189. Xie, Y., et al., *RNA-Seq profiling of serum exosomal circular RNAs reveals Circ-PNN as a potential biomarker for human colorectal cancer.* Frontiers in Oncology, 2020. **10**: p. 982.
190. Kang, Y., et al., *Serum and serum exosomal CircRNAs hsa_circ_0001492, hsa_circ_0001439, and hsa_circ_0000896 as diagnostic biomarkers for lung adenocarcinoma.* Frontiers in Oncology, 2022. **12**: p. 912246.
191. Wang, Y., et al., *The potential of serum exosomal hsa_circ_0028861 as the novel diagnostic biomarker of HBV-derived hepatocellular cancer.* Frontiers in Genetics, 2021. **12**: p. 703205.
192. Gao, G., L. Wang, and C. Li, *Circ_0006790 carried by bone marrow mesenchymal stem cell-derived exosomes regulates S100A11 DNA methylation through binding to CBX7 in pancreatic ductal adenocarcinoma.* American Journal of Cancer Research, 2022. **12**(5): p. 1934–1959.
193. Gao, F., et al., *Exosomes derived from myeloid-derived suppressor cells facilitate castration-resistant prostate cancer progression via S100A9/circMID1/miR-506-3p/MID1.* Journal of Translational Medicine, 2022. **20**(1): p. 346.
194. Hu, K., et al., *Exosomes mediated transfer of Circ_UBE2D2 enhances the resistance of breast cancer to tamoxifen by binding to MiR-200a-3p.* Medical Science Monitor, 2020. **26**: p. e922253.
195. Shao, N., L. Song, and X. Sun, *Exosomal circ_PIP5K1A regulates the progression of non-small cell lung cancer and cisplatin sensitivity by miR-101/ABCC1 axis.* Molecular and Cellular Biochemistry, 2021. **476**(6): p. 2253–2267.
196. Zhang, H., et al., *Exosomal Circ-XIAP promotes docetaxel resistance in prostate cancer by regulating miR-1182/TPD52 Axis.* Drug Design, Development and Therapy, 2021. **15**: p. 1835–1849.
197. Zhang, Y., X. Tan, and Y. Lu, *Exosomal transfer of circ_0006174 contributes to the chemoresistance of doxorubicin in colorectal cancer by depending on the miR-1205/CCND2 axis.* Journal of Physiology and Biochemistry, 2022. **78**(1): p. 39–50.

198. Yang, B., et al., *Tumor-derived exosomal circRNA_102481 contributes to EGFR-TKIs resistance via the miR-30a-5p/ROR1 axis in non-small cell lung cancer.* Aging (Albany NY), 2021. **13**(9): p. 13264–13286.
199. Yang, S.J., et al., *Tumor-derived exosomal circPSMA1 facilitates the tumorigenesis, metastasis, and migration in triple-negative breast cancer (TNBC) through miR-637/Akt1/β-catenin (cyclin D1) axis.* Cell Death & Disease, 2021. **12**(5): p. 420.
200. Jiang, Z., et al., *Exosomal circEPB41L2 serves as a sponge for miR-21-5p and miR-942-5p to suppress colorectal cancer progression by regulating the PTEN/AKT signalling pathway.* European Journal of Clinical Investigation, 2021. **51**(9): p. e13581.
201. Zhang, Y., et al., *Exosomal CircGDI2 suppresses oral squamous cell carcinoma progression through the regulation of MiR-424-5p/SCAI axis.* Cancer Management and Research, 2020. **12**: p. 7501–7514.
202. Tang, B., et al., *Exosomal circRNA FNDC3B promotes the progression of esophageal squamous cell carcinoma by sponging miR-490-5p and regulating thioredoxin reductase 1 expression.* Bioengineered, 2022. **13**(5): p. 13829–13848.
203. Geng, X., et al., *Exosomal circWDR62 promotes temozolomide resistance and malignant progression through regulation of the miR-370-3p/MGMT axis in glioma.* Cell Death & Disease, 2022. **13**(7): p. 596.
204. Huang, X., et al., *Exosomal Circsafb2 reshaping tumor environment to promote renal cell carcinoma progression by mediating M2 macrophage polarization.* Frontiers in Oncology, 2022. **12**: p. 808888.

https://doi.org/10.1142/9789811267390_bmatter

Index

CPSIA information can be obtained
at www.ICGtesting.com
Printed in the USA
JSHW051221050523
41226JS00002B/47

9 789811 267383